TREATING ALCOHOL AND DRUG
PROBLEMS IN PSYCHOTHERAPY PRACTICE

TREATING ALCOHOL AND DRUG PROBLEMS IN PSYCHOTHERAPY PRACTICE

Doing What Works

ARNOLD M. WASHTON
JOAN E. ZWEBEN

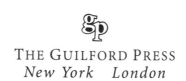

THE GUILFORD PRESS
New York   London

Library of Congress Cataloging-in-Publication Data

Washton, Arnold M.
    Treating alcohol and drug problems in psychotherapy practice : doing what works / Arnold M. Washton, Joan E. Zweben.
        p. cm.
    Includes bibliographical references and index.
    ISBN 1-57230-077-9 (alk. paper)
    1. Substance abuse—Treatment.   2. Alcoholism—Treatment.
3. Psychotherapy.   I. Zweben, Joan E.   II. Title.
    [DNLM: 1. Substance-Related Disorders—therapy.   2. Alcoholism
—therapy.   3. Psychotherapy—methods.   WM 270 W319t 2006]
RC564.W37 2006
616.86′06—dc22

                                                                    2005030403

To my wife, Lori, and my children,
Tala, Danae, and Jacob—the sources
of my inspiration and joy and the
guiding lights of my life
—A. M. W.

In loving memory of my parents,
Benjamin and Ruth Zweben
—J. E. Z.

About the Authors

Arnold M. Washton, PhD, is founder and Executive Director of Recovery Options, a private practice in New York City and Princeton, New Jersey, specializing in the treatment of alcohol and drug problems in professionals and executives. An addiction psychologist and nationally known expert in the field since 1975, he has served on the Substance Abuse Advisory Committee of the U.S. Food and Drug Administration, has been principal investigator of research grants from the National Institute on Drug Abuse, has served as substance abuse advisor to domestic and foreign governments and multinational corporations, and has given expert testimony on addressing drug problems in America before special committees of the U.S. Senate and House of Representatives. Dr. Washton is currently affiliated with Lenox Hill Hospital in New York City, Silver Hill Hospital in New Canaan, Connecticut, and the University Medical Center and Princeton House Behavioral Health in Princeton, New Jersey. In addition to numerous journal articles and book chapters, his professional publications include several books on addiction and its treatment.

Joan E. Zweben, PhD, is founder and Executive Director of the 14th Street Clinic and Medical Group and the East Bay Community Recovery Project, affiliated organizations providing comprehensive treatment in Oakland, California, and Clinical Professor of Psychiatry at the University of California, San Francisco. She is committed to providing flexible, evidence-based treatment to challenging and underserved populations. Dr. Zweben is a clinical psychologist with more than 35 years of experience in treating addiction and training treatment practitioners, including peer counselors, social workers, marriage and family counselors, psychologists, probation officers, nurses, and physicians. She also serves in the Substance Abuse Experts Working Group in the Practice Directorate of the American Psychological Association. Dr. Zweben's activities as an author, teacher, and consultant keep her informed of new developments in the field. She is the author of two previous books and more than 55 articles or book chapters, and editor of 15 monographs on treating addiction.

Acknowledgments

We are indebted to Seymour Weingarten and Jim Nageotte of The Guilford Press for their patience, encouragement, and unfailing confidence in this project. Without their help, it could not have been launched and finished. We are also thankful to our families for the support and understanding they provided throughout this long endeavor. Colleagues and students have contributed through their insightful questions and challenges to our thinking. Above all, we are deeply grateful to the countless men and women who have come to us over the past 30-plus years for help with alcohol and drug problems. They provided the raw material for this volume and are the primary beneficiaries of our clinical work.

Preface

Written specifically for the office-based mental health practitioner, this book is intended to describe what psychotherapists in private practice need to know in order to address alcohol and drug problems competently and routinely in their patients. We describe how therapists can approach and intervene with a range of patients, including those presenting with substance abuse problems and those presenting with other types of mental health problems who also abuse alcohol and drugs.

In very practical and specific terms, we describe how office practitioners can screen, assess, diagnose, engage, motivate, treat, and appropriately refer patients who are using alcohol and other psychoactive substances. This book is intended to serve as a practical "how-to" guide for practitioners from a variety of professional disciplines and schools of thought and for those at all levels of expertise in treating substance use disorders (SUDs), ranging from general psychotherapists with little or no clinical experience in treating alcohol and drug problems to dedicated specialists who, like us, have worked in the addiction treatment field for many years. Our intended readers include psychologists, psychiatrists, social workers, mental health counselors, marriage and family therapists, psychiatric nurses, addiction counselors, and other practitioners who encounter substance-abusing patients in their clinical work. The information in this volume is potentially of value not only to practicing clinicians, but also to students and trainees in advanced courses seeking to enter professional practice. Counselors working in substance abuse treatment settings will find this book useful because it describes an individualized approach to treating alcohol and drug problems that they may not have encountered or had an opportunity to practice in programmatic or agency-based treatment settings.

This book attempts to fill a critical void in the existing literature. Most of what has been written about treating SUDs is geared toward patients with severe addiction problems seen by addiction counselors in agency-based treatment programs. In contrast, this book is geared toward patients presenting with a range of alcohol and drug problems seen by mental health practitioners in office-based psychotherapy practice. These differences are significant in several respects. As compared with those in agency-based treatment programs, office practitioners are in a better position to offer more flexible, individualized care and to engage patients "where they are" when they first appear for treatment. They also are more likely to see patients in the earlier stages of developing or coming to grips with an alcohol or drug problem, including those already in therapy for other mental health problems. Office-based treatment offers an easier entry point for many people who, for a variety of reasons, choose not to seek help at addiction treatment programs. It also offers the option of individual psychotherapy, which is scarcely available in addiction treatment programs owing to a combination of limited resources and the prevailing view in these programs that group therapy is the only effective treatment modality for people with SUDs. Nonetheless, patients often need and want both the personalized attention and the stronger therapeutic relationship that only individual therapy can offer. Individual sessions within drug treatment settings are usually focused on current life challenges and case management issues. Many patients also want the help of a mental health practitioner who has the professional training and skills to address some of the complex psychological issues that are frequently intertwined with alcohol and drug problems. Among such patients are individuals who realize that their personal growth in later stages of recovery requires them to address certain issues (e.g., intimacy, self-esteem, developmental traumas) in ways that Alcoholics Anonymous (AA) or standard addiction treatment programs cannot. The role of mental health training in treating SUDs has become increasingly clear in recent years with recognition of a high rate of comorbidity between SUDs and a broad range of other mental health problems (Kessler et al., 1994, 1997; Kessler, Nelson, & McGonagle, 1996; Kessler, Sonnega, Bromet, Hughes, & Nelson, 1995; Mueser, Noordsy, Drake, & Fox, 2003; U.S. Department of Health and Human Services & Substance Abuse and Mental Health Services Administration, 2002) and that positive treatment outcomes can be expected only when both sets of problems are adequately addressed.

Patients who have the financial resources to access private psychotherapy services are often, but not always, of higher socioeconomic status, more functional, and better educated than those who seek help at public treatment facilities. Although higher pretreatment levels of psychosocial functioning are often associated with better treatment outcomes, an outward appearance of functionality can be deceiving. It can camouflage the true severity of an alcohol or drug problem and reduce the likelihood that it will be diagnosed and treated appropriately. This often happens when an articulate, seemingly high-functioning patient with an undisclosed alcohol or drug problem seeks help from a private therapist for some other type of mental health problem. These patients are remarkable in their ability to look and sound "normal" even when their personal lives are careening out of control. It is well known that when SUDs remain unchecked, they tend to progress over time and are likely to result in increasingly serious consequences that could have been avoided if the progression had been interrupted sooner. To avoid such scenarios, it is essential for all mental health practitioners to have the skills necessary to identify and address SUDs routinely in their patients, regardless of a patient's presenting complaints.

This book is intended to serve as a practical guide, not as a comprehensive textbook or review of the scientific literature. The material covered here extends from a description of the nature and course of SUDs to the particular types of interventions that appear to work best with patients in different stages of the recovery process. At various points in the book, we illustrate specific treatment strategies and bring them to life with case examples. We discuss problems, pitfalls, and key issues encountered most frequently in treating patients with SUDs: how to approach patients about their alcohol and drug use in a nonthreatening way, how to enhance a client's motivation and readiness for change, how to sidestep early resistance and avoid power struggles, when and how to involve family members and significant others, how to assess and treat patients with coexisting psychiatric disorders, how to utilize in-office drug testing as a clinical tool, and a wide variety of other nuts-and-bolts clinical techniques. We also discuss relapse prevention strategies designed to enhance patients' ability to maintain abstinence over the long term, the role of individual psychotherapy in addressing a variety of ongoing and later-stage recovery issues, and the special role of group therapy in treating SUDs.

This book describes an integrated multifaceted approach that is pragmatic, flexible, nondogmatic, and empowering to clinicians from diverse professional backgrounds and theoretical orientations. Among the hallmarks of our integrated approach are (1) giving high priority to developing a therapeutic alliance and maintaining a spirit of collaboration with patients to engage and retain them through different stages of treatment; (2) working from within rather than against the patient's belief system, cognitive style, and conceptual framework; (3) maintaining unfailing respect and positive regard for the patient's autonomy; and (4) maintaining a positive, optimistic stance that instills hope and empowers patients to mobilize their inner resources while overcoming setbacks, disappointments, and mistakes. We describe how to mix, match, and time the delivery of different types of interventions, including motivational, cognitive-behavioral, 12-step recovery, and psychodynamic techniques. We utilize the stages-of-change model (Connors, Donovan, & DiClemente, 2001; DiClemente, 2003; Prochaska, DiClemente, & Norcross, 1992) as a conceptual framework and clinical guide for finding the "best fit" between where the patient is on the continuum of motivation and readiness for change and what the therapist should be doing at each stage to facilitate change.

The population of people with SUDs is heterogeneous, contrary to popular stereotypes about the types of people who develop problems with alcohol and drugs. Substance abusers differ from one another in many important ways, including the severity of their alcohol and drug problems, their chosen goals regarding use (e.g., reduction vs. abstinence), their motivation and readiness to change, their personal strengths and vulnerabilities, their psychological and emotional states, their educational and socioeconomic levels, their personal beliefs and value systems, and their cultural and family histories and frames of reference. Accordingly, different individuals must be approached in different ways, and it is impossible to know in advance what will be acceptable to or work best for a particular patient or work best for him or her. The clinician must have an open mind, a flexible attitude, a willingness to go with the flow or change direction when needed, and an adventurous spirit of trial and error. Regrettably, the addiction treatment field is still permeated with a great deal of ideology, dogma, and rigidity that stifles creativity and limits treatment options. Many clinicians and programs continue to take an unwavering stance that there is only one acceptable pathway to recovery for anyone with an alcohol or drug problem—namely, that abstinence is the only acceptable treatment goal, that 12-step programs such as AA and Narcotics Anonymous (NA) offer the one tried-and-true method for attaining meaningful and lasting recovery, that confrontation of the patient's denial and other intractable defenses is required to motivate him to stop his destructive behaviors, and that recovery is impossible without fully accepting the identity of "addict" or "alcoholic." Although there is some value in each of these notions, we have difficulty with the absolutist thinking and self-righteous extremism that have dominated sectors of the addiction treatment field for so long. The one-size-fits-all approach is likely to be counterproductive with many patients; the broad diversity of people who seek help for alcohol and drug problems points clearly to the need for a more flexible, inclusive, comprehensive approach in order to increase the overall appeal, acceptability, and clinical effectiveness of treatment for SUDs.

It is incorrect to assume that no method of substance abuse treatment really works. Lots of different things work. The key is to figure out what works best for whom at a particular point in time. The literature on SUDs is filled with many excellent ideas, conceptualizations, and treatment techniques. Some have strong empirical validation, and others have never been adequately studied. Clinicians need a menu of different options to choose from so they can tailor the treatment to fit the individual needs of each patient. There is no one best treatment method or approach for everyone with an alcohol or drug problem. The only guide is to do what appears to work best with the types of patients you treat. If you are looking for a cookbook method, this book is not for you. What we offer here are some helpful suggestions, guidelines, and techniques that you can use as you see fit. But they will need to be adapted and modified to fit the patients you encounter. We hope what you read in this book will empower you to more freely exercise your own clinical judgment and unmoor your thinking from the confines of standard approaches, each claiming to be the one and only effective way to deal with people who abuse alcohol and drugs.

OUR CLINICAL ORIENTATION

For most people, SUDs are best understood as emanating from a combination of biological, psychological, personal, and social–cultural factors. In addition to genetic factors that may predispose certain individuals to developing an addiction, a wide spectrum of psychological problems, vulnerabilities, and dynamics, as well as traumatic life events and social or cultural forces, can increase the likelihood that an individual's substance use will become problematic, out of control, and life damaging. We also recognize that substance use plays different roles in different people's lives and that there are unique personal meanings that substance use acquires for various people. By the time alcohol or drug use is causing the types of problems that usually bring people into treatment, the personal factors that encouraged and reinforced the use in the first place are at best obscured. In this regard, clinicians sometimes focus almost exclusively on the negative consequences of a patient's substance use and place too much emphasis on biological and conditioning factors that may have contributed to the development of compulsive use patterns, while paying little attention to the positive benefits and functional role or significance of the substance use in the person's life.

We further recognize that substance use behavior exists along a continuum, ranging from nonpathological or nonproblematic use at one end to chronic relapsing substance dependence characterized by compulsion, loss of control, and severe life-damaging consequences at the other. In between these two extremes is a large undifferentiated area of less severe problems, but problems nonetheless, that fall within the more broadly defined category of substance *abuse* (these categories are discussed in Chapter 2). Although with continued use, progression to more severe forms of the disorder certainly does occur, it is not inevitable in all cases. For many individuals who do progress along this continuum, their substance use moves beyond a point where it is voluntary (or seemingly under volitional control) into a realm where it is involuntary and clearly outside the individual's personal control. This is the syndrome that the *Diagnostic and Statistical Manual of Mental Disorders*, 4th edition (DSM-IV) defines as substance *dependence*, commonly referred to as alcoholism or drug addiction. Many patients we have worked with describe their use as having crossed an "invisible line," on the other side of which they found themselves no longer able to reliably control the amount and frequency of their use, and who continued using even in the face of increasingly severe consequences. It has been hypothesized that the out-of-control nature of addiction is the result of fundamental changes in brain chemistry induced by the chronic drug taking itself. Recent brain research supports the view that after a certain period of alcohol and drug use, varying with each individual, alterations in brain chemistry inevitably occur, and these changes do not reverse completely even with long-term abstinence. It is as if a switch is thrown in the brain that cannot be reset (Leshner, 1997; Volkow et al., 2001). This explanation is consistent with the clinical observation, familiar to all who treat addiction, that when individuals with prior addiction histories relapse after a period of sustained abstinence, their substance use escalates much faster than it did during the original progression from use to dependence, no matter how lengthy the period of abstinence preceding the relapse may have been.

In our clinical work we operate mainly (although neither rigidly nor exclusively) within an abstinence-oriented framework. There is little doubt that total abstinence from alcohol and all other psychoactive substances offers the widest margin of safety for people who develop serious problems with alcohol and drugs, especially when the use is out of control and causing life-damaging consequences. However, we do not view abstinence as the only legitimate treatment goal for all people with alcohol and drug problems. A variety of clinical interventions, described variously in the literature as controlled drinking, moderation management, harm reduction, and behavioral self-control training, have been shown to be effective with many problem drinkers, particularly those whose pattern of alcohol consumption falls most clearly within the categories of harmful or problematic drinking (i.e., alcohol *abuse*) and has never escalated to the level of persisting or chronically relapsing alcohol dependence (Miller & Muñoz, 2005; Sobell & Sobell, 1993; Rotgers, Kern, & Hoeltzel, 2002). Proponents of controlled drinking approaches cite empirical evidence supporting the position that moderate drinking is a reasonable and attainable goal for many individuals with *less severe* drinking problems. And they state that the primary goal of moderation is to help patients establish and maintain a pattern of *responsible* drinking, defined as drinking that provides positive effects (e.g., relaxation, enhanced sociability, etc.) without putting oneself or others at increased risk for suffering negative consequences (Rotgers et al., 2002). Although individuals with severe alcohol problems are clearly not appropriate candidates for controlled drinking approaches, moderation strategies can still be effective as a starting point to engage patients with severe alcohol problems and to help them work incrementally toward achieving abstinence. It is interesting to note that many patients who set out to achieve moderation ultimately choose abstinence after attempts at controlled drinking have failed.

Whereas moderation appears to be a viable option for some drinkers, people dependent on stimulants, opioids, sedatives, and other highly addictive drugs are typically less able to control or moderate their use of these substances reliably. Nonetheless, harm reduction strategies, based on the premise that any clinical interventions aimed at reducing drug-related harm are steps in the right direction, have gained increasing acceptance in recent years (Denning, 2000; Tatarsky, 2002). Although we agree philosophically that reducing drug-related harm makes good sense and is an important contribution to public health, the present book does not emanate from a harm reduction approach, and the interested reader is referred to other publications for details (e.g., Denning, 2000; Denning, Little, & Glickman, 2004; Tatarsky, 2002). Nonetheless, we feel it important to clarify that in our practices we *do* accept and work with patients who are not ready to stop using all psychoactive substances, and we do *not* insist that our patients accept abstinence as their one and only treatment goal or as a prerequisite to receiving our help.

Similarly, we do not discharge or view as treatment failures patients who relapse or change their minds along the way about abstinence as a treatment goal. The guiding principle of "starting where the patient is" has long been a cornerstone of all good psychotherapy, and it is a guiding principle of our integrated approach.

So, what exactly is our clinical orientation? If you had an opportunity to view videotapes of our sessions with different patients, you would see a wide variety of treatment techniques in action. In fact, depending on which tape or portion of a tape you were viewing at a given time, you might draw different conclusions about our clinical orientation. In one tape, you might see us speaking to a patient in AA program language and conclude from that tape that we operate primarily from a traditional abstinence-based disease model. In another session, you might see us using psychoeducational and coping skills training techniques and conclude that our approach is surely cognitive-behavioral. In another session, you might see us exploring a patient's developmental history, addressing transference or trauma issues, or enhancing the patient's awareness of internal conflicts, and surmise from that tape segment that our approach is primarily psychodynamic. In yet another session, you might see us agreeing to help a patient work toward the goal of reducing rather than completely stopping her alcohol or drug use (at least as a first step) and conclude that we operate within a harm reduction or moderation model. The fact is that we do not adhere to any one of these treatment models or approaches. We use them all, and we try our best to be guided in our work as clinicians by three overarching principles:

1. Start where the patient is, not where you want him or her to be.
2. Do what works.
3. Above all, do no harm!

TERMINOLOGY

Throughout this book we use many different terms to describe alcohol and drug problems, including "substance abuse," "substance dependence," "chemical dependence," "addiction," "alcoholism," "alcohol and other drug abuse," "alcohol and other drug problems," "substance-related problems," "psychoactive substance abuse," and "substance use disorders." Given the multiplicity of these terms, some confusion may be inevitable, but it is nonetheless important to point out certain differences between them. The generic term used most frequently by professionals and lay people alike to describe all types of alcohol and drug problems is substance *abuse*. Similarly, we have used this term generically at various points in the book when speaking in broad terms about the spectrum of alcohol and drug problems. For example, we speak about the substance abuse treatment *field*, substance abuse treatment *professionals*, and substance abuse treatment *programs*. It must be noted, however, that within the context of the DSM-IV diagnostic system, the term substance *abuse* is not a generic term but rather connotes a specific category or type of clinical problem involving the use of alcohol and/or drugs. According to DSM-IV, substance *abuse* refers to any repeating maladaptive pattern of substance use that leads to negative consequences. Substance *abuse* is distinguished from substance *dependence,* which is a more severe type of maladaptive use pattern characterized by additional features, such as inability to control amount or frequency of use, preoccupation and obsession about using, and so forth, as explained in more detail in Chapter 3. We adhere to the important diagnostic distinctions between abuse and dependence and are careful to use these terms appropriately in this book wherever it appears necessary to do so. For example, there are many places where we are careful to differentiate *abuse* from *dependence,* especially when discussing screening, assessment, and the appropriateness of specific treatment interventions. Although substance *abuse* is the colloquial term used most commonly to describe alcohol and drug problems, the term now deemed most appropriate for describing the full spectrum of these problems is *substance use disorder,* or SUD, as defined in DSM-IV. The term *substance use disorder* is generic in the sense that it encompasses the categories of abuse and dependence.

Although we and others frequently refer to *alcohol* and *drug* problems, there is increasing recognition that there is little reason to perpetuate the long-standing distinction between these two types of substances. At an earlier time, the distinction was felt to be important when it was seen as maintaining a necessary distinction between use of the legal socially acceptable substance alcohol versus use of illegal street drugs such as heroin and cocaine. As research continues to support the commonalities, rather than the differences, between various psychoactive substances in terms of their effects on brain function and behavior and approaches to treatment, these distinctions no longer seem meaningful. In addition, among clinical populations the combined use of alcohol and other drugs and cross-addiction involving a variety of psychoactive substances (both legal and illicit) has rapidly become the norm. Gone are the days when there were separate treatment programs and separate groups of treatment professionals to deal with alcohol versus drug problems.

Our readers will notice that the terms "addict" and "alcoholic" are all but absent from this book. Despite widespread use in both the professional literature and popular press, these terms continue to have a pejorative connotation that perpetuates negative stereotyping and discriminatory attitudes toward people suffering with alcohol and drug problems. These terms also foster the inaccurate impression that a greater degree of homogeneity exists among people who develop problems with psychoactive substances than clinical observation appears to indicate. When it comes to SUDs, it is too easy to lose sight of essential differences between individuals despite the fact that they may all share the same diagnosis with regard to their substance use behavior.

It should also be noted that the term "substance-using person" (or "patient" or "client") used in this book does not presume a priori that the individual in question has a diagnosable SUD. Regardless of how substance use may be viewed by certain individuals or by society as a whole, there are countless people whose substance use is not pathological and therefore not deserving of formal diagnosis or clinical attention. Although the legal system and government agencies consider any use of illegal drugs whatsoever as abuse, in this book we adhere to the clinical (i.e., not the legal) definitions of these human health care problems. The terms "client" and "patient" are used interchangeably throughout this book. In addition, to maintain gender neutrality, in most instances we alternate between the pronouns "he" and "she."

The term "recovery" appears frequently throughout this book. In the literature on substance abuse treatment and in 12-step programs, recovery refers to the process of personal growth, life enhancement, and diminished vulnerability to relapse that accrues as a person not only remains abstinent from all psychoactive substances but also works actively to make the emotional and lifestyle changes necessary to achieve a reasonable, satisfying lifestyle that does not include alcohol or drug use. An important distinction is drawn between the terms abstinence and recovery. Whereas abstinence is quite simply the absence of alcohol and drug use, recovery refers to an ongoing process of personal transformation that diminishes the likelihood that an individual attempting recovery from an SUD will return to using alcohol and drugs.

LIMITATIONS OF THIS BOOK

It is important for our readers to be aware of an essential qualification and limitation of this book. Although we strongly support the use of evidence-based treatments for SUDs and incorporate many of these strategies into our work, much of the material presented here is based on our own clinical experience and not necessarily on results of scientific research. We have not included comprehensive documentation on topics that do have a strong evidence base, but offer references in the spirit of providing additional reading. Both of us have worked in addiction research and treatment for more than 30 years and have treated thousands of patients with alcohol and drug problems in a variety of clinical settings in both the public and private sectors. Although recent studies support the efficacy of a wide variety of treatment approaches and techniques for SUDs, no one approach has shown itself to be superior to all others (Project MATCH Research Group, 1997). However, what does appear to have an overriding influence on treatment outcome, regardless of the chosen treatment approach or method, is the therapist's attitude, interaction style, and clinical stance toward patients (Miller, 1999; Miller & Rollnick, 2002). Therapists whose style is engaging, respectful, curious, empathetic, nonjudgmental, nonaggressive, optimistic, and encouraging tend to produce better patient retention and outcomes. We emphasize throughout this book the overriding importance of the therapeutic relationship as the primary vehicle for facilitating positive change and the underpinning of all good treatment. The importance of the therapist's attitude and stance toward patients with SUDs cannot be overemphasized, particularly in light of certain psychodynamic issues common to individuals with these problems. Many patients carry a great deal of shame and guilt about their problems even if they are unaware of these feelings and vehemently deny that such problems even exist. These feelings can be elicited and experienced quite intensely if the clinician comes across in any way as nonaccepting or judgmental.

Using the therapeutic relationship to help patients acknowledge that a problem exists and to develop the motivation for change is a challenging but extraordinarily important task. In the integrative treatment model that serves as the framework for what we do, the therapist adjusts and adapts interventions to address the changing tasks that patients face at different stages of treatment and recovery. Various types of clinical techniques and interventions are utilized, as needed, to accomplish agreed-upon treatment goals. Motivation enhancement techniques (an adaptation of Rogerian client-centered therapy) are used to help patients to develop the motivation and readiness to change. Cognitive-behavioral techniques are used to help patients initiate behavior changes, avoid common setbacks, and then maintain these changes. A psychodynamic understanding of the patient and the patient–therapist relationship, coupled with attention to both transference and countertransference phenomena, is helpful at all stages of the treatment process.

Our readers should also know that this book addresses only addictive disorders that involve the use of psychoactive substances. We do not deal separately or specifically with addictive and compulsive behaviors such as those involving food, gambling, work, exercise, spending, or sex (Washton & Boundy, 1989). These behaviors often are intertwined with SUDs (especially drug-related sexual compulsivity) and are discussed here in that context, but not as separate problems per se.

Moreover, in our discussion of SUDs, we do not address nicotine dependence and smoking cessation techniques. Although many, if not most, of the treatment interventions discussed here (particularly cognitive-behavioral techniques for establishing abstinence and preventing relapse) can be adapted and applied to the treatment of nicotine dependence (Fiore et al., 2000) and increasing attention is being focused on the linkage between tobacco smoking and other substance dependencies (Fertig & Allen, 1995), in our view nicotine dependence differs importantly enough from other drug addictions to warrant not addressing it here directly. Perhaps the most important difference is that although the long-term medical consequences of tobacco smoking are quite ominous and potentially fatal, the psychological and behavioral consequences are much less obvious and remain somewhat unclear. Whereas alcohol and other drugs (e.g., cocaine, heroin, etc.) can and often do produce striking changes in mood, affect, and behavior that often disrupt an individual's functioning and mimic a variety of psychiatric disorders, the psychoactive effects and consequences of nicotine, in the overwhelming majority of tobacco smokers, are pale by comparison. (A similar argument can be made for the stimulant drug caffeine, except in individuals who are exquisitely sensitive to this substance). Few, if any, people seek help to alleviate tobacco-related mental health problems, with the possible exception of those embroiled in serious conflicts with significant others who strongly disapprove of the smoking behavior, which may also be a lightning rod for other problems in the relationship.

It is also important for our readers to know that the subject matter of this book is limited primarily to the treatment of functional adults (i.e., employed or otherwise employable adults) who seek the help of an office-based psychotherapist. Our discussions also presume that patients have either insurance benefits to cover the cost of private treatment or the financial resources to pay for it themselves. This book does not address issues specific to treating adolescents, individuals with severe debilitating mental illness, and chronically unemployed persons. Although the presumed treatment setting in this book is a private office-based psychotherapy practice, most if not all of the strategies and techniques we describe here, especially our unfailing emphasis on flexibility and "meeting patients where they are," can be adapted to all types of clinical settings and patient populations.

Contents

PART I

Basic Issues and Perspectives

CHAPTER 1

Introduction

Considering that this book is written specifically for psychotherapists, we begin by discussing why we think all mental health practitioners should be able to address alcohol and drug problems competently and routinely in their patients. We then discuss the unique advantages and limitations of office-based treatment and for which patients it may be best suited. The final section of this chapter addresses logistical considerations in treating patients with substance use disorders (SUDs) in office practice.

Before delving into these issues we feel it is important to address a long-standing problem that has contributed in many ways to our motivations for writing this book. Namely, why practitioners from all of the various mental health disciplines have long overlooked or avoided dealing with the problems of SUDs, and why have so few have developed special expertise or chosen to specialize in this area. Although this situation has been improved somewhat in recent years, lack of adequate clinical attention to such pervasive and potentially destructive disorders, though perplexing at first, can be understood in light of certain barriers that have existed over the course of many decades. These barriers, as discussed later, include gaps in professional education and training on SUDs and their treatment, a stereotyped view of individuals with alcohol and drug problems that discourages therapists from engaging them, and conflicts between certain aspects of traditional psychotherapy and the basic principles of addiction treatment.

The various mental health disciplines that educate and train clinicians need to overcome these barriers because failure to identify, treat, and/or properly refer patients with significant alcohol and drug problems can lead to poor clinical outcomes and may also result in legal liabilities for therapists who misdiagnose or overlook these problems (Zweben & Clark, 1991). Those of us who specialize in treating SUDs frequently see patients who were in therapy for years with well-intentioned psychotherapists who apparently did not assess the nature and extent of a patient's involvement with alcohol and drugs, or knew of the problem but did not recognize the need to intervene until the patient's substance use caused a severe crisis. Regrettably, some therapists find out about a patient's alcohol and drug problems only after the patient ends up in a hospital emergency room for treatment of an overdose or suddenly drops out of therapy to seek specialized help from an addiction treatment program or practitioner.

We recognize, however, that responsibility for poor outcomes with these patients often does not lie with the therapist. Many addicted patients actively withhold information from therapists about their substance use out of fear of rejection or just not being ready to address this issue. Because such patients rarely show detectable signs of intoxication when they appear for therapy sessions, even a seasoned addiction specialist may be unable to accurately identify the problem when the patient is deliberately trying to hide it. We can recall numerous cases in our own clinical experiences when we concluded, based on the available information, that no alcohol or drug problem was present, only to find out at a later time that the patient was arrested, fired from a job, or admitted to an inpatient facility for an untreated addiction. Regrettably, incidents like this sometimes cannot be prevented, despite a clinician's best efforts and intentions.

WHY PSYCHOTHERAPISTS HAVE AVOIDED DEALING WITH SUDs

Education and Training Gaps

The most obvious reason why psychotherapists have avoided dealing with SUDs is that most mental health professionals (we ourselves included) received little if any formal training in the diagnosis and treatment of SUDs during graduate school, internship, or beyond. Despite the extraordinary prevalence of SUDs among people who seek mental health services, astonishingly few training programs in the mental health professions (e.g., psychology, psychiatry, social work, mental health counseling) offer specific course work or clinical supervision in this area and most offer none at all. There is a core knowledge base and skill set for treating SUDs that is glaringly absent from most professional training programs. This deficiency fosters professional disinterest, a sense of clinical impotence, and negative stereotyping of patients with alcohol and drug problems. One consequence is that many therapists assume as a matter of course that patients with SUDs can and should be treated only by specialists or in addiction treatment programs. These therapists are quick to refer patients with alcohol and drug problems, especially those with more severe problems, to other caregivers and/or discharge them from their own practices. This is unfortunate, considering that many substance-abusing patients respond well to intervention by therapists with whom they have established a good therapeutic relationship. The fact is that therapists are often in an excellent position to help patients recognize an alcohol or drug problem and develop the motivation to address it. Even in cases in which the patient's substance abuse problem is more severe than the therapist feels prepared to deal with, cultivating the patient's readiness to accept referral for further assessment and/or specialized treatment, when indicated, is critically important.

The failure of most graduate training programs to address SUDs has led to a continuing dearth of competent practitioners in this area. Although some therapists seek extra training, it may be difficult to assess true proficiency. This situation is beginning to change, however, now that certain professional organizations have developed credentialing mechanisms for practitioners who demonstrate at least basic knowledge and clinical expertise in diagnosing and treating SUDs. For example, the American Psychological Association now offers a certificate of proficiency for psychologists who meet certain criteria including documented hours of clinical experience and clinical supervision in addition to passing a written certification examination. A similar credential is offered by the American Psychiatric Association.

Stereotyped Views of Patients with Alcohol and Drug Problems

Patients who abuse alcohol and drugs have long been stereotyped by mental health professionals as being character disordered and largely unresponsive to psychotherapeutic interventions. Historically, psychotherapists have been influenced by the prevailing view of substance abusers as impulsive, untrustworthy, highly resistant to treatment, and unmotivated to change. Patients with serious alcohol and drug problems are assumed to have borderline, narcissistic, antisocial, and other personality disorders that render them untreatable or as having a poor prognosis at best. Unfortunately, therapists lacking positive experiences with substance-abusing patients have not had an opportunity to see that the distortions in personality and behavior so commonly seen during active addiction often disappear or decrease markedly after the substance use stops. These observations suggest that in many individuals these distortions are often secondary to the alcohol and drug use and not indicative of an underlying personality disorder. Although some substance-abusing patients do indeed exhibit antisocial and other personality disorders that predate their addiction and persist even after they stop using alcohol and drugs, these individuals are the minority, not the majority, of the addicted population. Research has consistently failed to support the notion of a predisposing "addictive personality" common to all people who become addicted to alcohol and drugs. To the contrary, contemporary research shows that chronic use of psychoactive substances *induces* stereotypic distortions in behavior and personality as a result of complex changes in brain activity caused by these substances and the extraordinary behavioral demands of maintaining an active addiction while concealing it from others. Along with cessation of substance use and sufficient time for brain functions to recover from repeated neurological insult by drugs, these aberrations in behavior and personality often resolve quite rapidly. Such observations have led many experts to conclude that addiction is quite literally a substance-induced "brain disease" (Leshner, 1997).

Clinicians familiar with the dynamics of addiction, as compared with those who lack this familiarity, are likely to view the behavior of substance-abusing patients in ways that allow them to respond more effectively. The patient will likely be seen not as character disordered or resistant, but rather as highly ambivalent about relinquishing alcohol and drugs and acting out this internal struggle by giving in to strong urges and cravings to use. The therapist will acknowledge that cravings and urges are common features of the disorder, especially in the early phases of establishing abstinence, and offer helpful suggestions for dealing with such situations. For example, the therapist will offer suggestions about how the patient can avoid "high-risk" situations that stimulate the desire to use and will also teach the patient ways to manage the cravings to prevent them from leading to actual use. The therapist will be less likely to view any lapses to substance use as evidence of resistance, willful noncompliance, or lack of motivation, but rather as a reflection of the ambivalence and lingering attachment to substances that are part of the addictive disorder. The therapist will also acknowledge the inherent difficulties in counteracting what often are physiological and psychological compulsions to use alcohol and drugs even in the face of serious negative consequences. In this way, the more addiction-savvy clinician can join with the patient in acknowledging the struggle involved in achieving abstinence and offer specific behavioral and motivational techniques to enhance the patient's ability to change. This stance fosters development of a strong working alliance that is more empathic and supportive than standard confrontational approaches and more likely to engage and retain patients through the rocky course of early treatment.

Conflicts between Psychodynamic Therapy and Addiction Treatment

Certain aspects of psychodynamic psychotherapy are at odds with some basic principles that inform and guide the treatment of SUDs. For example, many mental health professionals were taught to uncover the underlying or root causes of psychological or behavioral problems as a necessary step in the process of resolving the problems. This can be a setup for failure when dealing with SUDs. As Margolis and Zweben (1998) state, searching for the root causes of an addiction in the early stages of therapy can be likened to a paramedic rushing to the scene of an accident, where victims are lying on the ground bleeding, and taking time out to find out what caused the accident.

Helping an individual to stop using alcohol and drugs requires amazingly little understanding of the factors that may have contributed to development of the problem. Focusing on the presumed underlying causes of alcohol or drug use ignores the fact that substance abuse is a distinct disorder and that there are a multitude of contributing forces that maintain an individual's substance-using behavior having virtually nothing to do with the reasons why he may have started using alcohol and drugs in the first place. It also fosters the dangerous idea that once the underlying causes are adequately resolved, the person's alcohol or drug problem will automatically disappear. In addition, attempting to uncover deep-seated emotionally-laden material too early in treatment often poses a very real danger of stimulating overwhelming affects that are likely to reignite the patient's desire to self-medicate with alcohol and drugs. In the first few weeks and months after stopping substance use, many patients experience labile moods and have great difficulty managing their emotions. They often feel like an emotional "raw nerve," which is quite different from the numbed or anesthetized emotional state in which they existed during their active addiction. Feelings that have been chemically suppressed by alcohol and drugs for many years often surface spontaneously once abstinence is established. A therapist's attempt to elicit these feelings too early in treatment can overwhelm a patient's shaky sense of self and threaten her still fragile commitment to reducing or completely stopping alcohol and drug use. Once the chemical veil of substance use is removed, patients often begin to experience uncomfortable feelings that they have not been accustomed to dealing with for a long time. This is often compounded by intense feelings of shame and guilt that emerge as patients face the reality of negative consequences caused by their prior substance use and the challenging task of dealing with life problems without the buffering effects of alcohol and drugs. A deep sense of loss, grief, and resentment about having to give up alcohol and drugs (feelings often likened to those of losing a "best friend") also contributes to patients' discomfort and instability in the early phases. In light of these considerations, therapists should pay careful attention to the timing of interventions in the early phases and be mindful of the patient's tenuous hold on abstinence.

Discomfort with the Disease Model and 12-Step Program Philosophy

Many therapists, from both psychodynamic and behavioral orientations, have difficulty with the notion that addiction is an incurable disease and with other tenets of 12-step programs. Psychodynamic therapy tends to view addiction as a symptom of unresolved psychological problems rather than as a primary problem requiring targeted intervention. Within this framework, the underlying or "real" problem must be attended to first and sufficiently resolved before the patient will be able to stop using the addictive substances. Similarly, but for entirely different reasons, behaviorally oriented therapists are among the most vociferous opponents of the disease model. They point to the absence of a scientific basis for the disease model and abstinence-only approaches to treatment, viewing addictive substance use not as a permanent incurable disorder, but as a learned behavior perpetuated by a combination of physiological, psychological, and social reinforcers.

These long-standing ideological conflicts have created a rift between the communities of mental health practitioners on the one hand, and mainstream addiction treatment providers and self-help programs on the other. This has led to an unfortunate situation in which therapists sometimes feel threatened by or competitive with AA and traditional treatment. Anti-AA therapists may not only fail to encourage a patient's involvement in AA, but go so far as to devalue the program and actually discourage patients from embracing the 12-step philosophy. Similarly, more than a few people in AA are hostile to the idea of psychotherapy for alcohol- and drug-addicted persons, and especially toward "enabling" therapists who fail to support complete abstinence from all psychoactive substances as essential to recovery. Fueling the antagonism, some AA zealots contend that psychotherapy is harmful to addicted persons and should be categorically avoided by people in recovery.

As discussed in Chapter 4, certain elements of the disease model and 12-step philosophy have enormous therapeutic value and can be utilized for patients' benefit regardless of your theoretical orientation. You need not accept or believe unequivocally in all aspects of the disease model in order to utilize selected aspects of this model to help your patients. To quote an AA slogan, when questioning the value of AA you are advised to "take what you need and leave the rest."

WHY *ALL* THERAPISTS SHOULD KNOW HOW TO TREAT SUDs

There are many compelling reasons why all practicing therapists should acquire the skills required to address SUDs competently and routinely in their patients, as discussed in the following sections.

Prevalence and Consequences of Untreated SUDs

First and foremost among these reasons is that in addition to being highly prevalent in the general population, SUDs are particularly common among people who seek help for other types of mental health problems. Alcohol and drug abuse is so widespread in clinical populations that patients with SUDs are likely to appear in the caseload of every mental health practitioner. Clinicians cannot assume that substance abuse is absent even if there are no clear warning signs. Instead, they must be proactive and assess *all* patients routinely and methodically for SUDs, whether or not substance abuse is a presenting complaint. SUDs are frequently overlooked or misdiagnosed in mental health patients, partly because chronic alcohol and drug use can and often does induce behavioral changes and psychiatric symptoms that mimic almost any type of mental health problem, ranging from anxiety and depressive disorders to personality disorders and psychoses. Moreover, failure to address alcohol and drug problems creates an opportunity for these problems to fester and result in increasingly adverse outcomes. Untreated SUDs not only can diminish or completely nullify the effectiveness of both psychotherapy and pharmacotherapy for other mental health problems, but are associated with extraordinarily high rates of morbidity and mortality. Suicide rates among people with serious alcohol and drug problems are many times greater than the general population rates. Alcohol and drug abuse contributes to deaths and serious injuries resulting from overdose, drowning, homicide, and domestic violence. Substance abuse is associated with a wide variety of other serious health problems, including sexual abuse, exposure to sexually transmitted diseases (e.g., HIV, hepatitis C, genital herpes), drug-induced psychiatric disorders, adverse interactions with medications prescribed for other medical conditions, and with a wide range of serious medical problems directly caused or exacerbated by alcohol and drug use (Institute of Medicine, 1990).

Applicability of Psychotherapy Training and Skills

Miller and Brown (1997) assert unequivocally that well-trained psychologists and other mental health clinicians already possess many of the essential therapeutic skills needed to treat people with alcohol and drug problems and that the challenge for all practitioners is to acquire the relevant core knowledge base about SUDs and to adapt, modify, and refine their clinical skills to work more effectively with these patients. For example, treating patients with alcohol and drug problems requires the therapist to be active, directive, outgoing, open, and supportive, especially in the early stages of treatment where the primary goals are to engage the patient and contain crises. Traditional therapists whose style tends to be passive, quiet, pensive, analytic, and interpretive often find it difficult to step outside this role to meet these patients' needs. This is especially true for therapists who work in a psychodynamic mode, for whom taking a more active and directive stance may be experienced as not doing "real" therapy. Therapists whose orientation is more cognitive-behavioral, however, usually have an easier time adjusting and adapting their skills to work more effectively with addicted patients, particularly in the early stages of treatment where behavior change, not insight, is the primary goal.

There are additional aspects of the training and skills of competent psychotherapists that are highly applicable and potentially of great value in treating SUDs. Therapists' ability to express empathy and forge a positive therapeutic relationship with their patients contributes significantly to retention and positive outcomes in treating SUDs, just as they do in the treatment of other mental health problems. Some authors contend that above and beyond the therapist's theoretical orientation, his or her ability to form a therapeutic alliance with substance-abusing patients is perhaps the most crucial determinant of treatment effectiveness (Gerstley et al., 1989; McLellan, Woody, Luborsky, & Goehl, 1988). Psychotherapists are trained to be good listeners, to convey nonjudgmental acceptance and positive regard for their patients, to work therapeutically with a patient's resistance, not against it, and to remain vigilantly aware of their own countertransference reactions as potential obstacles to the therapeutic work. Studies show consistently that the therapist's attitude and clinical stance toward patients matter a great deal in treating SUDs (Miller, 1983; Miller & Rollnick, 2002). In particular, Rogerian qualities of therapist warmth, friendliness, nonjudgmental acceptance, and empathy are seen as more important predictors of retention and favorable treatment outcomes than the therapist's theoretical orientation, treatment philosophy, or personal addiction history. Psychotherapists are also trained to be highly sensitive and responsive to individual differences. The diversity of the substance-abusing population necessitates clinical flexibility and sophistication to accommodate wide-ranging individual differences. In this regard, psychotherapists are generally well prepared to make important diagnostic distinctions and to individualize treatment according to differing patient needs—essential ingredients for delivering effective treatment.

Other basic psychotherapy techniques that are potentially of great value in treating SUDs include helping patients learn how to identify and appropriately manage internal feeling states, how to anticipate problems and formulate strategies to deal proactively with these problems, how to become more self-observing, and how to recognize and appreciate the influence of unconscious forces on thoughts, feelings, and behaviors. The therapist's tools for accomplishing these tasks are the interviewing and therapy techniques that all well-trained clinicians acquire during graduate and postgraduate training. Included among these are Socratic questioning, reflective listening, reframing, expressing empathy, conveying nonjudgmental acceptance, and offering emotional support.

Opportunities for Early Intervention

Another reason why all psychotherapists should know how to treat SUDs is that office practitioners are in an excellent position to intervene early with patients in the throes of developing more serious problems with alcohol and other drugs. Psychotherapists probably come in contact with more patients who have alcohol and drug problems than any other health care practitioners, with the possible exception of primary care physicians. Furthermore, office practitioners encounter many patients not likely to appear at addiction treatment programs, such as those in the early stages of developing or acknowledging an alcohol or drug problem and those in therapy for other mental health problems who also abuse alcohol and drugs. Psychotherapists are in an ideal position to offer low-threshold, low-intensity interventions that make it easier for reluctant, ambivalent patients to begin to address their alcohol and drug use.

The salient point here is that office practitioners have an important role to play in identifying early warning signs of emerging SUDs and intervening effectively to arrest the problem before it causes severe and possibly irreversible harm. Typically, by the time people arrive at an addiction treatment program, their alcohol and drug problems have already progressed to the point of severe addiction and they have already suffered serious consequences that earlier intervention may have averted. Many people with alcohol and drug problems seek professional consultation and advice from psychotherapists as a first step in trying to decide whether their alcohol and drug use is really a problem and what course of action, if any, to take. Individuals who do not want, need, and/or fit into traditional addiction treatment programs are often good candidates for office-based treatment, including those already in recovery who want individual psychotherapy provided by an office practitioner who is familiar with the obstacles and issues that arise at each stage of the recovery process. All in all, office practitioners are well positioned to provide attractive low-threshold entry points for individuals who are not likely to seek help from traditional treatment programs and those who, for whatever reasons, have not done well in these programs.

Private Practice Opportunities

Clinicians who can deal effectively with SUDs are in an excellent position to expand the range of services they offer in office practice in a marketplace for private mental health services that is increasingly restrictive and competitive. The ongoing trend toward treating SUDs in less restrictive environments (i.e., outpatient rather inpatient settings), heretofore largely spurned by managed care, has created growing opportunities for practitioners who are capable of providing these types of services in their private practices. Some managed care plans routinely refer patients with less severe alcohol and drug problems to qualified therapists instead of routing these patients automatically to specialized addiction treatment programs. This reflects an increasing recognition that office-based practitioners skilled in treating SUDs can provide clinically viable and cost-effective treatment alternatives for patients who do not require intensive inpatient or outpatient treatment. Similarly, there is a growing demand for practitioners who can not only focus on the patient's alcohol and drug problem, but also skillfully address co-occurring mental health problems that may be part of the overall clinical picture. Many patients are often poorly treated by clinicians who may be skilled in dealing with mental health but not SUDs, and by addiction counselors who may be skilled in dealing with substance abuse but not mental health disorders. Relatively few therapists are skilled in dealing with both types of disorders, especially in the complicated clinical situation where both disorders exist simultaneously in the same patient. There are many complex issues that clinicians who treat patients with dual diagnoses must be prepared to deal with, such as psychotropic medication, prioritizing and timing the treatment for one disorder versus the other, and managing the complicated interplay and interaction between the two disorders and their respective clinical courses (as discussed more fully in Chapter 6).

Additional practice opportunities emanate from the fact that substantial numbers of people with alcohol and drug problems are willing and able to self-pay for private office-based treatment. Many of these individuals simply do not want to be treated in a clinic or program and prefer instead to receive the specialized help they need from a private practitioner. Self-pay patients seen in our own practices, for example, include health care professionals, university professors, government officials, business executives, corporate employees, business owners, and others, who are grateful to have the option of being treated as outpatients in a totally private, confidential setting. These individuals could have used their health insurance to obtain help from an agency-based addiction treatment program, but chose instead to seek treatment from a specialist practitioner. In addition to preferring the greater privacy, individualized care, and choice of therapist that only office-based treatment can offer, many people who can afford private treatment do not want to use their health insurance to pay for substance abuse treatment, fearing the very real ramifications of having this information become part of their permanent medical records in a computerized data bank. We have heard many patients complain over the years about being unable to obtain life, disability, or health insurance as a direct result of having previously filed insurance claims for substance abuse treatment.

Professional Gratification

Last, but certainly not least, among the reasons why psychotherapists should address SUDs is that working with patients with these disorders can be extremely gratifying. It is very rewarding to assist patients in their liberating journey from addiction to recovery. Contrary to popular stereotypes that portray substance-abusing patients as extremely difficult to treat, many show rapid, observable, and rather dramatic improvement. This is particularly true for patients with a history of reasonably good functioning prior to the onset of their addiction, although many with premorbid histories of serious dysfunction also show marked improvement. There is no way of knowing just how profoundly chronic substance use is affecting a person's functioning until it is eliminated entirely from the clinical picture. Positive changes often become evident almost immediately in the days and weeks after the substance use stops. Then, as the recovery process unfolds, life-enhancing changes can be seen to reverberate through nearly all aspects of patients' lives, including improvements in physical health and fitness, family and other interpersonal relationships, work productivity and satisfaction, self-esteem, and overall quality of life. Both of us have chosen to work as dedicated specialists in this field, but it is probably more accurate to say that this field chose us. Like most other mental health professionals, neither of us was formally trained in this area during our years of graduate or postgraduate training and we did not go into practice with the intention of becoming specialists in treating addiction. It was the exhilarating experience of participating in the personal transformation of addicted patients and the profound sense of both professional and personal gratification we derived from these clinical experiences that motivated us originally to work with these patients more than three decades ago. It is also what motivates us to continue working with these patients today.

UNIQUE ADVANTAGES
OF OFFICE-BASED TREATMENT

Privacy

In light of the social stigma associated with substance abuse and the very real possibility that serious consequences can result if others find out about it, many individuals with alcohol and drug problems are highly concerned, and rightfully so, about protecting their privacy and confidentiality. Fearing exposure, many of these individuals delay seeking help or avoid seeking help at all unless they can be assured a level of privacy and confidentiality that only a private office-based practice can offer.

Lower Entry Threshold

One of the most valuable features of office-based treatment is its ability to provide a nonthreatening entry point into treatment. It is up to the practitioner, of course, to skillfully seize the moment by making maximum use of an opportunity to intervene proactively. Unlike addiction treatment programs, office-based therapy attracts many individuals in the early stages of developing a problem, as well as those in the early stages of coming to grips with the fact that they have a problem. As stated earlier, it stands to reason that people who do not view their alcohol or drug use as a serious problem are not likely to seek help from a specialized addiction treatment program.

Countless patients in psychotherapy for other problems could be helped to short-circuit an emerging SUD, and thereby spared much pain and suffering, with the help of therapists who have the clinical confidence and skills to intervene appropriately. Many people with alcohol and drug problems seek professional evaluation and guidance from psychotherapists in order to find out whether or not heir alcohol and drug use is really a problem and what type of treatment, if any, may be warranted.

Flexible, Individualized Care

Office-based therapy adds flexibility and choice to the menu of existing treatments for people with alcohol and drug problems. By doing so it enhances the ability to match the treatment more precisely to the specific needs of each individual patient. The office practitioner is not constrained by agency policies and procedures or by institutional control over treatment philosophy and approach. There are no rules dictating which patients are admitted into treatment and how treatment should be done. Perhaps most important, the office practitioner has the freedom and flexibility to "start where the patient is" as an initial engagement strategy instead of requiring immediate compliance with a preplanned treatment program.

Alternative to Traditional Treatment Programs

Psychotherapists who have acquired the requisite knowledge and skills for treating SUDs are in a unique position to offer clinically viable alternatives to mainstream addiction treatment programs for patients who do not want or need what these programs typically offer. Traditional treatment programs sometimes alienate patients in the early stages of addressing an alcohol or drug problem with their devotion to a rigid belief system and dogmatic stance that a 12-step AA-oriented approach, based on the disease model, is the one best method of recovery for everyone who comes through their doors. Clients who do not accept this view and embrace this approach immediately and without challenge are often confronted aggressively as being "in denial." Some patients readily accept the 12-step approach and make good use of it (which we wholly encourage and support), but others are turned off by coercive tactics and fail to engage in treatment that offers them no alternative path. One of the most important functions of office-based treatment is to offer that alternative path. Office practitioners have a unique opportunity, and even a clinical responsibility, to offer treatment that "starts where the patient is" rather than pressure the patient into being where the therapist thinks she should be. The critical importance of working through, joining, or temporarily side-stepping rather than assaulting a patient's resistance is something that every psychotherapist can appreciate.

Supplement or Sequel to Traditional Treatment Programs

Office-based therapy can serve not only as an alternative, but also as a supplement to other forms of treatment a patient may be receiving. For example, many recovering individuals in AA and other self-help programs seek assistance from psychotherapists when they encounter psychological or emotional problems that their AA participation alone cannot adequately address. Similarly, patients involved in addiction treatment programs may benefit from concurrent individual therapy that not only supports, amplifies, and extends the therapeutic work being done in an outpatient recovery group, but provides an additional safety net against premature dropout. Office-based therapy can also be an important component of aftercare treatment for patients who have completed a structured inpatient or outpatient program and want the help of a psychotherapist who knows how to deal with the complicated psychological issues often intertwined with alcohol and drug problems.

WHICH PATIENTS CAN BENEFIT FROM OFFICE-BASED TREATMENT?

Office-based treatment can meet the needs of many different types of patients with alcohol and drug problems. The following list attempts to identify the individuals who may benefit from office-based treatment and those most likely to seek it out. This is by no means intended to be an exhaustive list.

1. Individuals whose problematic use of psychoactive substances falls short of meeting the criteria for serious abuse or dependency.
2. Individuals who want a harm reduction approach offering an option of reducing rather than totally stopping their substance use, at least as a first step in the treatment process.
3. Individuals whose prior experiences with addiction treatment programs have been unhelpful and/or unpleasant, including those who have failed in one or more programs and want to try a different approach.
4. Individuals who cannot work within the traditional disease model and 12-step philosophy of mainstream addiction treatment providers.
5. Individuals who need help with the combination of an SUD and other complex mental health problems that only a trained mental health clinician can adequately address.

6. Individuals who prefer the absolute privacy and individualized attention that only office-based treatment can offer.
7. Individuals who want to choose their own therapist rather than be assigned to a staff counselor at an agency.
8. Individuals in the early stages of facing their alcohol or drug problems who are more likely to respond to an individualized approach using motivational rather than confrontational techniques.
9. Individuals who have already achieved a period of sustained abstinence and want psychotherapy to address addiction-related and other unresolved psychological issues.
10. Individuals who are currently participating in group therapy in an outpatient addiction program and want to supplement this with concurrent individual therapy.
11. Individuals who have already completed an outpatient or inpatient addiction treatment program and want ongoing individual therapy.
12. Individuals who have begun their recovery by participating in AA or other self-help programs and want professional therapy to deal with psychological issues that self-help alone cannot adequately address.

LIMITATIONS OF OFFICE-BASED TREATMENT

Despite its numerous advantages, office-based treatment also has certain limitations, and by no means do we propose it as the answer for all individuals with alcohol and drug problems. Not all people who want office-based therapy are able to access it. Many managed care plans, for example, require that all reimbursable treatment for substance abuse be provided only in state-licensed addiction treatment programs and not by independent practitioners. Even among patients who are employed or have other financial resources, some individuals are simply unable to afford the frequency of visits in the early treatment stages that would be optimal (e.g., three to five sessions per week). Accordingly, where feasible, it is important to be flexible and creative enough to negotiate a treatment plan that adequately addresses patients' clinical needs within the confines of their financial limitations. For example, in addition to reducing or adjusting your fees in selected cases, you can reduce the length of individual sessions (e.g., 30 minutes) and proportionally reduce the fee you charge for these briefer sessions. You can also supplement briefer sessions, where needed, by maintaining close contact with patients by telephone and/or e-mail. Group therapy is a lower-cost alternative (per-session fees for group therapy are often substantially lower than fees for individual therapy), and from a purely clinical perspective group therapy is the treatment of choice for many patients with SUDs. Where appropriate and indicated, you can refer patients to a local addiction treatment program for group therapy (while you continue to provide supportive individual therapy at reduced frequency) or provide group treatment in your own office practice (as discussed in Chapter 12).

PRACTICAL CONSIDERATIONS IN PROVIDING OFFICE-BASED TREATMENT FOR SUDs

Expanding your private practice to include specific treatment services for patients with SUDs is likely to require some changes in office logistics and procedures. For example, you will need to decide at what level you wish to be involved with these patients and what types of clinical services you are prepared to offer them. Such services can range from offering assessment and referral only, to taking major responsibility for the treatment and overall clinical management of patients with serious addictions. You will also need to develop office policies and procedures on how to schedule the first appointment and deal with missed sessions, taking into account that no-show rates with these patients are typically higher than with most others, particularly for the first appointment. Additional issues, such as maintaining a higher level of availability for crisis intervention and implementing clear policies to ensure that you are paid reliably for your services, also require careful consideration.

Scheduling the First Appointment

No-show rates for the initial appointment with patients with serious alcohol and drug problems are notoriously high. Often the appointment is made when the patient is in crisis and seeking immediate relief. If the crisis subsides before the scheduled appointment, there is a good chance that the patient will not show up. Generally, the longer patients must wait before seeing you for the first time, the less likely they are to show up for the appointment. No-shows are very costly for office practitioners. They waste precious time and reduce income. It is highly unlikely that a patient you have never met will pay you for a missed first appointment.

Several strategies can help to reduce no-show rates. One is to see new patients as quickly as possible after the first contact is made. The first visit does not always have to occur on the very same day that the patient initially calls. However, there is much to be said in favor of seizing the moment and "striking while the iron is hot." Whenever possible, you should try to see new patients within 1 or 2 days after they call. If your schedule does not permit this to happen and several days or more must intervene between the initial call and the first visit, you should contact the patient in the interim to both confirm the appointment and restate your willingness to help. Conveying interest and concern often goes a long way toward helping prospective patients overcome their ambivalence about seeking professional help. Another technique for bridging the gap before the first visit is to offer patients the option of filling out your intake questionnaires in advance. You can mail or fax your intake forms to prospective patients and ask them to bring the completed forms with them to the first visit. Similarly, if you have a website for your practice, you can offer new patients the option to download and print the intake forms directly from your website. You may also want to place information on the website about your qualifications and/or experience in treating substance use disorders and the specific types of services you offer.

How should you deal with patients who fail to show up without prior notice for the initial appointment and then call to schedule another appointment? One way is to require prepayment before giving them another appointment. Alternatively, you can offer these patients the option of coming to your office to fill out your intake forms in the waiting room and at that point be given the next available appointment time for an initial consultation. Patients who show up to for the paperwork are more likely to show up for the subsequent appointment.

Appointment Frequency and Missed Sessions

Appointment length and frequency must be adjusted to meet individual patient needs. Patients who are actively using alcohol and drugs, have recently stopped using, and/or have been recently discharged from inpatient care need as much structure and therapeutic contact as you can reasonably provide during the first few weeks. It can be extremely helpful to see these patients two, three, or even four times a week for brief visits of 20–30 minutes each during the beginning phase of treatment, when the tendency to return to using is extraordinarily high. These brief sessions can focus on concrete issues such as time planning, ways to avoid or cope with high-risk situations that could lead to use, and enhancing the patient's motivation to change. As treatment progresses, the frequency of individual sessions can be reduced to once or twice per week, according to patient need, while the length of each session is increased. Patients who are attending group therapy sessions one or more times a week with you and/or other caregivers can be seen individually once every 2 weeks instead of every week, if that seems clinically appropriate and makes treatment more manageable financially for the patient.

Whenever patients miss a scheduled session and fail to call afterward, you should reach out to them as soon as possible. Doing so not only enhances retention and conveys concern, it helps to establish accountability and reinforce the idea that behaving responsibly is an essential part of recovery. Sometimes patients encounter unexpected delays and/or responsibilities at work or home that make it impossible for them to attend a scheduled session. This is understandable and likely to occur at least some of the time, especially with patients who have demanding jobs and family responsibilities. However, if it occurs regularly, you should explore whether the patient may be feeling ambivalent about being in treatment. It is better to address lateness and missed sessions as possible signs of ambivalence and wavering motivation than to confront this behavior as evidence of resistance and noncompliance.

You should be clear with patients from the outset about your policy with respect to charges for missed sessions. Third-party payers long ago outlawed billing for missed sessions. Accordingly, you should avoid this practice and make no exceptions when payments are made by third parties. However, you do have the option to hold self-pay patients personally responsible for missed session fees as long as you inform them of this policy, preferably in writing, upon accepting them into your practice.

Collecting Fees

Making sure that you are compensated for your professional services is not an easy task. Most health care practitioners are not very skilled in practice management, especially when it comes to financial matters. Treating patients with SUDs can pose a variety of obstacles to procuring payment for your services. For example, most third-party payers have different reimbursement criteria for SUDs than for other mental health disorders. The maximum number of reimbursable visits per year is frequently lower for SUDs, as is the reimbursement rate. Moreover, many insurance and managed care plans exclude private practitioners as eligible providers of substance abuse treatment services. Under these plans only treatment services delivered in state-licensed substance abuse treatment programs are authorized for reimbursement. However, exceptions do exist and appear to be growing. An increasing number of third-party payers offer reimbursement to private practitioners who are certified by their respective professional organizations in the treatment of SUDs. Examples include the certificate of proficiency in the treatment of SUDs offered by the College of Professional Psychology of the American Psychological Association and the certificate of added qualification in addiction psychiatry offered by the American Psychiatric Association. Private practitioners certified to treat SUDs are potentially attractive to third-party payers because they offer less expensive and less intensive alternatives to the types of services offered routinely in addiction treatment programs. Office practitioners are in a better position to individualize care and, where appropriate, provide brief therapy and other forms of time-limited intervention for SUDs. This is an important option for patients with mild to moderate severity SUDs who do not require higher levels of care.

The lower reimbursement rates and more stringent eligibility criteria for treatment of SUDs versus mental health disorders can create serious ethical dilemmas for private practitioners. For example, some patients may ask you to omit the SUD diagnosis from their insurance claim forms and indicate a mental health diagnosis instead, the goal being to meet eligibility criteria for reimbursement or a higher reimbursement rate. Moreover, some of these patients will tell you that unless you change the diagnosis they will be unable to afford your fees and be forced to seek help elsewhere. You may be tempted to consider this request, especially for patients who do indeed have coexisting mental health problems, as is often the case with SUDs. Regardless of the patient's plight, you must recognize that falsifying insurance documents and/or clinical records is a serious ethical and legal infraction that may result in very grave consequences for both you and your patients. You should categorically refuse to satisfy any and all of these requests, without exception. You can empathize with the patient's plight while letting him know unequivocally that deliberately changing or omitting a diagnosis in order to qualify for or maximize reimbursement is insurance fraud.

As stated earlier, not all patients need or even want to file for third-party reimbursement for their treatment. Some would rather pay out-of-pocket for private treatment in order to maintain their confidentiality and keep their substance abuse history out of the computerized medical data bank, even if paying for their own treatment causes some financial hardship. Many patients are concerned that this information will come back to haunt them at a later time. When the patient's insurance plan is administered by her employer, potential loss of privacy also is a justifiable concern.

Accepting patients into your practice on a self-pay basis can offer a much-welcomed relief from the difficulties of dealing with managed care and other third-party payers. However, obtaining payment for the services you render to patients who are using alcohol and drugs can be fraught with other types of challenges that you must be prepared to meet. For instance, many patients' finances are already stretched to the limit and some are in serious debt by the time they appear for treatment. Frequently, they have failed to pay bills on time and they have been financially irresponsible in a variety of ways during the course of their active addiction. It is essential that you not add yourself to the list of a patient's disgruntled creditors. Although it is quite natural as a mental health professional to empathize with your patients' plight and feel obliged to help them even if it entails some financial sacrifice of your own, these good intentions can backfire badly in private practice where your livelihood and ability to meet your own financial obligations are at stake. Furthermore, allowing patients to build up large unpaid balances can become a serious obstacle to the therapeutic work. As patients become more indebted to you financially, they also become more hesitant to let you know when they are heading for trouble or are already there. In addition, the more money patients owe you, the more likely they are to drop out of treatment prematurely and without warning. As their financial debt to you rises, so does their inability to tell you face-to-face that they have not stopped using or that the treatment is not doing for them what they had expected. Although patients are usually grateful for your willingness to defer payment, inevitably some will devalue you for having allowed them to "get over" on you. Obviously, this is not a helpful situation for either you or the patient.

FINAL COMMENT

There are many compelling reasons why all psychotherapists should become proficient in addressing SUDs, regardless of patients' presenting complaints. Considering the extraordinarily high rates of comorbidity between SUDs and other mental health problems and the serious consequences that can ensue if both problems are not adequately addressed, all practitioners should know how to assess, treat, and/or properly refer patients with alcohol and drug problems and do so routinely in their practices. Office-based treatment fills some important gaps in the continuum of care and provides treatment options not currently available in the existing treatment system. Treating patients with SUDs in office practice can be a very rewarding experience, but you must be prepared to modify your office policies and procedures, recognizing the special challenges that these patients sometimes present. For example, your ordinary methods of scheduling first appointments and allowing patients to reach you outside normal office hours may require modification for these patients. You will need to be clear and consistent with patients, but perhaps more flexible than usual in certain ways to accommodate individual needs.

CHAPTER 2

Nature, Course, and Diagnosis of Substance Use Disorders

SUDs are complex conditions that must be understood from a variety of perspectives. All practitioners need to understand the nature and course of these disorders in order to decide whether intervention is needed, and if so, what kind. Certainly, many patients present for treatment whose use is occasional and appears to contribute little if at all to their presenting complaints. Nonetheless, you should remain attentive to the possibility that even moderate use can affect a person's mood, mental state, and coping abilities and in ways that can hamper therapeutic progress, or it may represent a transitional phase in the developmental course of more serious substance abuse problems. Thus, it is important to appreciate the factors that can influence the course of these disorders. It is also important to be familiar with the diagnostic criteria and categories that define SUDs.

Addiction specialists view SUDs as conditions that are influenced by complex interaction between biological, psychological, and social factors that are present to differing degrees in each individual. This accounts for the wide variation in patterns in the general as well as the clinical population. Biological factors include, for example, individual differences in a person's response to drugs due to factors such as gender, age, and genetic heritage. Psychological factors include the full spectrum of mental and emotional difficulties, as well as cognitive and behavioral problems that elevate risk or provide resiliency. Social factors include variables such as socioeconomic status, the prevalence of heavy drinking in certain peer groups and subcultures, and religious prohibitions against using psychoactive substances.

Many models and theories have been applied to the study of addiction, and each sheds light on certain dimensions of the problem (Margolis & Zweben, 1998). Different factors come into play in the initiation of substance use and in the progression to serious problems. Expectancies about the positive effects of alcohol and other drugs develop through peer influence, adult examples, and the mass media. These expectations can shape the actual alcohol or drug experience once experimentation begins, during the period when doses are relatively modest. For example, research has demonstrated that study participants given a placebo and placed in a party atmosphere report having just as pleasant a time as those who consumed alcohol (Marlatt, 1985; Yalisove, 2004). If influential peer groups reinforce the desirability of drinking or taking drugs, then occasional use may evolve into regular use. Drinking alcohol or using other drugs thus becomes part of the inclusion requirement—the price of membership. Although adolescents are particularly susceptible to these pressures, adults are by no means immune.

Once alcohol and drug use begins, other factors influence the transition from occasional use to more serious involvement. A large body of literature documents the importance of genetic predisposition to developing problems with alcohol and other drugs (Bierut et al., 1998; Kendler & Prescott, 1998; Pickens, 1997; Pickens et al., 2001; Schuckit, 1989; Schuckit & Smith, 1996; Tsuang et al., 1998; Vanyukov & Tarter, 2000). Genetic and environmental factors have differing levels of influence with each drug, and each drug category (except psychedelics) has influences unique to itself. For example, the genetic factors that influence vulnerability to alcoholism are thought to be somewhat different from those relevant to developing an addiction to cocaine. Genetic factors increase individual vulnerability by shaping individual differences in how psychoactive substances affect an individual's brain and behavior. These may operate through metabolism, sensitivity to particular drug effects, unusually high or low tolerance, and neurological differences. For example, studies have documented that a genetically transmitted high tolerance to alcohol's intoxicating effects, although socially valued, may be predictive in some cases of future alcoholism. Presumably, the ability of some people to remain unaffected by substantial quantities of alcohol sets the stage for future problems because such people lack a warning system to indicate that their drinking is excessive or problematic (Schuckit & Smith, 1996). In some individuals, alcohol is an extremely potent reinforcer, capable of alleviating negative affect states such stress, depression, and anxiety. Progression to serious problems is also influenced by biomedical factors. Women have higher morbidity and mortality with lower levels of alcohol consumption than men, owing to differences in absorption, distribution, and elimination. Although women are less likely than men to drink heavily or even moderately, they are more vulnerable to alcohol-related liver damage, cardiovascular disease, and brain damage. Recent reviews also noted women's relatively greater susceptibility to alcohol's effects on cognitive functions, such as divided attention and memory (National Institute on Alcohol Abuse and Alcoholism, 2000; Zweben, 2002). Therapists should keep in mind that women who drink have a more rapid downhill course, indicating the need for more vigorous early intervention.

THE CONTINUUM OF SUBSTANCE USE

Addiction specialists typically see patients who have developed serious problems with alcohol and drugs, whereas general psychotherapists are more likely to see patients with benign use or mild to moderate problems. Although such patients often do not identify their substance use as an issue, you should nonetheless remain alert to the possibility that it is influencing their moods, their self-esteem, their sense of personal effectiveness, and the like. Relatively small quantities of alcohol and drugs may have pronounced effects in some individuals. Substance use may also interfere with the therapeutic action of various types of psychotropic medications.

Although DSM-IV provides a uniform set of diagnostic criteria for all psychoactive substances (as discussed later in this chapter), it forces all SUDs into only two categories (abuse and dependence) without a methodology for rating the severity of these disorders. This diagnostic schema overlooks the fact that there is not a dichotomy but rather a continuum of substance use and substance-related harm. Some patterns of use fall into the realm of nonpathological or nonproblematic use in the sense that they are associated with no apparent harm or dysfunction. Despite popular cultural beliefs, stereotypes, and biases, many people do seem able to use legal and illegal substances in ways that do not fit neatly into the categories of abuse and dependence. A broader range of substance use categories that include abuse and dependence have been defined as follows:

Experimental use marks the initiation into use and may represent a relatively benign category. People are motivated by curiosity to experience a drug effect and usually try a substance for the first time in a social situation. Their use is limited to a few exposures, they do not develop a regular pattern of use, and no substance-related harm or consequences are evident. It is important to remember that even apparently benign experimentation can and sometimes does result in significant harm. For example, tragic stories continue to emerge yearly from college campuses, in which young people, some of whom normally drank very little or not at all, consume large quantities of alcohol in connection with fraternity events and suffer serious injury or even die. Similarly, infrequent cocaine use can produce cardiac arrhythmia and even sudden death in a partygoer, without prior warning or any evidence of the person's having a pre-existing vulnerability to experiencing such an ominous reaction to the drug. In short, there is no level of substance use that is completely safe and free of risk.

Occasional use is another category that may be relatively benign. This category is sometimes called social or recreational use, but prevention specialists are wary of using any such term that conveys that use at any level is a harmless form of "recreation." Substance use in this category is typically infrequent and irregular, and the quantities consumed are modest. You should inquire carefully and document use over time, because it is common for the patient to report irregular use when in fact a pattern has emerged. It is useful to ask the patient to keep notes describing the circumstances, quantities, and adverse effects for purposes of self-observation. It is important to evaluate the effect on the individual before deciding that a use pattern is benign. For example, marijuana is widely viewed to be a "light" drug, but it has been shown to exacerbate depression in those who are prone to it, as well as producing physical dependency in long-term regular users. Similarly, what passes for "normal" drinking in some social circles is in fact above the level at which physical and social harms have been shown to occur. Problematic drinking can be camouflaged by the user's being part of a peer or social group of heavy drinkers. Even moderate social drinking can depress mood. Enormous variability among individuals means that small amounts of a substance may have surprisingly strong effects, and a period of abstinence may be one of the best ways to identify these effects. Patients with the best of intentions may underreport their use, but even those who report accurately may be impacted more strongly by their alcohol and drug use than they realize.

Regular use is said to be present when a person's use becomes more frequent and patterned. Many people move so slowly from occasional to regular use that they scarcely notice the transition. This may begin with a pattern of drinking heavily every Friday night or using cocaine every weekend. The person becomes habituated, and a regular pattern emerges. In the case of a drug like marijuana, people may develop a pattern of regular use, but if their use does not create any obvious or serious problems, they may feel little cause for concern. People at this stage may not necessarily experience negative consequences, and perhaps the clinician cannot identify obvious negative effects. However, the regularity of use may or may not be a warning sign that some loss of control is beginning to develop. The reinforcing properties of a drug become seductive once a person reliably achieves desirable changes in mood and feeling states by using the drug.

Circumstantial or situational use includes various patterns in which the substance is used to produce specific types of effects deemed desirable to enhance an experience or better cope with certain types of situations. For example, stimulants may be used to study for examinations, meet work deadlines, or enhance sexual arousal. Similarly, alcohol and/or tranquilizers may be used to deal with the anticipatory anxiety of public speaking or being in uncomfortable social situations. This pattern of use can become problematic when the instantly "curative" effects of the substances preclude the person from developing other non-drug coping skills and the types of situations that create the desire for substance use arise more frequently.

Binge use refers to an episodic pattern in which large quantities of alcohol or drugs are consumed intensively in marathon-like fashion during a single episode of use. For example, a drinking binge may involve consumption of enormous quantities of alcohol that continues almost nonstop for an entire weekend. Similarly, some cocaine users disappear on binges for days, until they run out of drugs and/or money or collapse from physical exhaustion. Binges may be punctuated with long periods of abstinence and little or no craving. This can encourage a belief that the use pattern is really not a problem. However, because binge patterns typically involve larger quantities of drugs used per occasion, as compared with maintenance patterns of use, the acute physical impact is generally greater. It is also challenging to address the patient's fluctuating motivation. Immediately following a binge, the person may feel remorseful and overwhelmed by the negative consequences of the intensive use and at that point feel strongly motivated not to repeat the pattern again. However, it is typical for patients to begin to minimize or selectively forget about the drug-related consequences as time passes after the last binge.

Abuse is said to occur when an individual manifests significant substance-related problems repeatedly in important areas of functioning (health, legal, social). For example, a parent may consume enough wine with dinner to become regularly unable to assist a child having difficulties with homework. A college student who has been arrested and is on probation may continue to smoke marijuana despite progressive warnings about the consequences of testing positive in a drug screen. A skier may use whiskey to warm up on the slopes in the late afternoon, despite having previously suffered serious orthopedic injuries due to intoxication. Although many who show signs of abuse do not progress to substance dependence, this does not mean that the therapist should ignore such warning signs. Substance abuse is often related to the patient's presenting problems and, where indicated, an attempt should be made to view it within that context. Most therapists are in an ideal position to do early intervention with substance abusers if they take the stance that it is not necessary to wait for severe problems to emerge before addressing a patient's alcohol and drug use.

Dependence, the most troubling category on the continuum of substance use, is evidenced by a preoccupation with obtaining and using the drug, an inability to control consumption in a dependable manner, impairment in psychosocial functioning, and continued use despite adverse consequences. A diagnosis of dependence does not require evidence of tolerance or withdrawal. For example, a business executive's heavy drinking that begins every evening after work has on numerous occasions caused him to miss important meetings with coworkers and prospective clients the next morning. It has also caused severe conflict with his wife, who is on the verge of leaving him if he does not seek help for his drinking problem. He has promised many times to cut down or stop drinking altogether, but his good intentions do not result in lasting change. He would like to drink less, but cannot imagine life without alcohol. This person clearly meets the criteria for alcohol dependence.

Late Onset of Detectable Signs and Symptoms

Patients who seek private office-based psychotherapy are often (but not always) functional enough that the signs and symptoms of serious alcohol and other drug problems are not readily apparent. Consider the following case:

> James is an astute businessman whose vision and judgment allowed him to build a highly successful company. Charming and gregarious, he was sought after in many business-related social gatherings, where alcohol was plentiful. He was a driven achiever, and had great difficulty unwinding after he finally left his office. His alcohol consumption increased slowly over time until he was consuming substantial amounts daily. He consumed a before-dinner drink, a nightly bottle of wine with dinner, and an aperitif with dessert. High levels of drinking were normal in his business subculture and he never appeared intoxicated, so his drinking behavior passed unnoticed. His frequent brief affairs had disrupted his marriage, and he sought therapy to clarify whether to seek a divorce. A medical checkup for gastric distress revealed elevated liver enzymes and slight gastrointestinal bleeding, both related to alcohol. Upon the advice of his physician, he decided to discontinue drinking and was astonished to find himself struggling to accomplish this. His withdrawal symptoms were sufficient to require medication, and he was chagrined that the type of discipline he applied to his work life was not enough to keep him from drinking. His therapist was able to offer behavioral strategies to establish and consolidate abstinence. This allowed James and his therapist to work on other issues more productively.

Drinkers like James may appear to function well for a long time; then, at some point, the cumulative effect of drinking results in what appears to be a sudden onset of difficulties. At that point, other alcohol-related manifestations, such as irritability, short-temperedness, silent withdrawal, sexual indiscretions, or other interpersonal difficulties, can be examined in a new light. You can reframe the patient's unexpected struggle to stop as a valuable learning experience about how easy it is to underestimate the power of alcohol.

Unpredictable Course: Progression Is Not Inevitable

Addiction specialists typically see patients who have severe problems, and so much of what is written about addiction suggests that progression is inevitable. However, clinical experience, studies of natural recovery, and long-term prospective studies indicate that there are subgroups of people who use alcohol and drugs to varying degrees at different stages of their lives. Excessive or problematic substance use at one point in an individual's life is not necessarily predictive of progression to more serious problems at a later point in her life. Researchers have long understood that it is necessary to understand the natural history of a disorder in order to determine to what extent clinical intervention does or does not affect the developmental course of that disorder. Such work balances a perspective that becomes skewed when generalizations and conclusions are based only on clinical populations, which cannot possibly be truly representative of the entire population of people in society who ever experience problems with alcohol and other drugs. A 50-year prospective study documented a subgroup that continued alcohol abuse for decades without remission or progression to more severe symptoms (Vaillant, 1995). This study followed a college sample and a working-class, core city sample from the Boston area. Findings supported the view that social class is an important mitigating factor in developing more serious problems. The working-class sample had significantly higher rates of death and complete abstinence from alcohol than the group with greater social advantages. The middle-class sample had more than twice as many who continued to abuse alcohol without significant progression. Though your patient may never meet the criteria for a full-blown SUD, this does not mean that the consequences are unimportant for your therapeutic goals. Although the substance abuse pattern may be stable, it may nonetheless undermine your patient's quality of life and ability to make use of resources.

COMPLEX ETIOLOGIES

Considering that the etiology of an SUD in any given person is multidimensional, a variety of risk factors should be considered when formulating a treatment plan. Biological factors include drug properties and genetics.

How prone to abuse is the patient's substance of choice and method of use? Use of highly dependence-producing drugs and/or rapid routes of administration elevate the risk, despite personal and social protective factors. High-dose use of stimulants (i.e., cocaine and methamphetamine) has been shown repeatedly to override most protective factors. On a psychological level, coexisting psychiatric disorders can markedly elevate the risk. The anxiety and mood disorders that propel people into psychotherapy also are associated with high levels of problematic substance use. However, you cannot assume that the presence of an SUD inevitably means "ego deficits" or other psychological problems. Longitudinal studies have demonstrated the hazards of generalizing from contact with individuals in the active stages of their abuse cycles. The psychological and behavioral patterns begin to look similar and obscure the heterogeneity that often is present both before the development of a substance abuse problem and after a period of abstinence.

Social factors are certainly major elements in the etiology of SUDs. Subgroups in which drinking and drug use are socially encouraged contribute significantly to the development of problems in susceptible users, and eventually even individuals with few other risk factors may succumb with sufficient repeated exposure and peer pressure. Poverty factors, with their attendant sense of hopelessness, contribute heavily to people becoming exposed to substances at very young ages, and trapped in these patterns more readily than those with greater options. Recovery resources are certainly fewer. Although the casualty rate is high, many indigent people can and do cease their substance use and go on to live productive lives. The mitigating element of social class may mean that the patient in psychotherapy is less likely to confront the negative consequences of use unless the therapist is astute and willing to make the issue part of the therapy.

RECOVERY WITHOUT TREATMENT

Although clinician intervention is a powerful catalyst for change, it is important to remember that recovery from serious alcohol and drug problems can occur without formal treatment (Biernacki, 1986; Sobell, Ellingstad, & Sobell, 2000). Studies of natural or untreated recovery, though relatively few and methodologically limited, highlight some of the important factors that allow people to overcome problems with alcohol and drugs. Both clinical and nonclinical populations report similar types of consequences that led them to decide to change their substance use behaviors—increasing dysphoria, emotional distress, loss of important relationships, loss of jobs, interference with performance, health problems, financial problems, and legal problems. The most important factor cited as promoting success in "natural recovery" is a supportive social environment that includes family and significant others. Other influences include changes in work and general lifestyle, changes in living arrangements, and involvement in religion. Interestingly, many of the same factors have been identified as contributing to positive outcomes in addiction treatment programs. It has also been observed that many individuals change their patterns of alcohol and drug use as part of a more global "maturing out" process (Peele & Brodsky, 1991) that involves assuming new responsibilities, entering a new stage of development in the life cycle, changing peer groups, and/or developing a new set of values that excludes or competes with substance use.

FAVORABLE PROGNOSIS
WITH APPROPRIATE INTERVENTION

Stigma and stereotypes have conveyed the mistaken assumption that people with serious alcohol and drug problems are fundamentally untreatable. This is far from the case. Those with mild to moderate problems often respond well to brief interventions. Many have been contemplating change, and a brief conversation and recommendation from a therapist or physician is all it takes to initiate a meaningful change process. Others may balk initially, then revise their views and commitments as they continue to engage in a process of self-examination:

> A therapist working with visualizations noted that a patient had unusual difficulty sustaining attention to the imagery and suggested that marijuana use could be a contributing factor. The patient agreed to experiment with discontinuing the marijuana, and after several months he exhibited more normal powers of concentration. He was surprised at the changes he noticed and decided to extend his commitment to abstinence indefinitely.

Results with severely addicted populations also yield reasonably good results if treatment is sufficiently comprehensive to address not only the alcohol and drug use, but also the risk factors undermining stable recovery. Three decades of research document improvement in both middle-class and indigent populations. Treatment of substance abuse has been compared with treatment for diabetes, asthma, and hypertension, three chronic relapsing medical disorders that evoke very different attitudes from treatment providers (McLellan, Lewis, O'Brien, & Kleber, 2000).

Improvement rates are similar across all four disorders and depend heavily on patient compliance with specific treatment recommendations. Low compliance also results from similar factors: poor social support, psychiatric comorbidity, and poverty. If substance abuse is viewed as a chronic, relapsing disorder, then it is unrealistic to expect a single treatment episode to result in lifelong recovery or a "cure" for most people. It is possible that individuals will require additional treatment, as in the case of those with diabetes, who may repeatedly lapse in and out of managing their disease properly. Treatment for an alcohol or drug problem can be intensive, such as inpatient or residential treatment, or can consist of a continuum of outpatient activities fading in intensity as the patient progresses. Recovery maintenance can occur in the self-help system without much costly treatment intervention. In all four disorders, lifestyle changes are among the most important and the key to achieving positive results over the long term.

INTERACTION WITH OTHER
MENTAL HEALTH PROBLEMS

Epidemiological studies have established that co-occurring disorders are the norm, not the exception, among people with SUDs, and thus treatment for SUDs must address these co-occurring problems. General psychotherapists are usually well equipped to address the mental health disorders, but need to learn how to address SUDs in an integrated manner. Substance use can exacerbate or obscure symptoms, lead to earlier onset of serious disorders, and promote premature termination or failure to progress in treatment. For these reasons, the office-based practitioner is well advised to invest the time needed to become proficient in addressing SUDs.

Historically, substance abuse problems were viewed as manifestations of an "underlying" disorder and were presumed to resolve once the "primary" disorder was treated. This view produced a sizeable cohort of treatment failures, as well as patients who were embittered at having lost decades of their lives despite having sought help from professionals. The recovering community developed an intense distrust of professionals. This distrust is gradually dissipating as mental health professionals become more competent in addressing SUDs and people in recovery from addiction receive effective treatment from mental health clinicians for other types of problems. However, one legacy is the idea that the substance abuse must be treated first and other issues put on hold until abstinence is firmly established. This was an appealing idea that proved impractical. It became apparent that many people could not get clean and sober unless their other problems were effectively addressed, and sequential treatment was ineffective for many. Clinicians have been working on principles of integrated treatment, and the research literature documents growing success with complicated populations, including those with severe mental illness. In these models, issues of safety take priority, no matter what the source of danger. Interventions to promote stabilization address substance use issues, other psychiatric issues, medical problems, domestic violence, and any other conditions that may interfere with initiating or sustaining recovery.

SUDs ARE
PRIMARY DISORDERS

A key to treating SUDs successfully is to approach them as independent disorders with a life of their own whether or not they are intertwined with other mental health problems. Although many therapists can cite individual examples of successfully addressing SUDs in psychodynamic therapy, there are no systematic studies confirming the efficacy of nonspecific treatments (e.g., psychodynamic psychotherapy) for substance abuse. Patients present with mood and anxiety disorders and relationship problems believing that their substance use helps them cope with their difficulties. It is always possible to make the case that the patient is engaged in some form of self-medication for character defects or painful feeling states (Khantzian, 1997; Khantzian, Halliday, & McAuliffe, 1990; Krystal, 1988). Usually, there is partial truth in such assertions. The related assumption, that the substance use behavior would change once the "underlying" issues were addressed, allowed patients to remain in therapy for years, if not decades, without the therapist addressing their behavior. In retrospect, it is remarkable how long therapists persisted in this approach despite its inadequacies.

The view of SUDs as independent conditions has allowed for the development of specialized treatment methods that have, in turn, improved the effectiveness of psychotherapy. Substance abuse functions as a "wild card" that promotes early dropout from psychotherapy and undermines therapeutic progress if the patient does remain in treatment. However, SUDs are often intertwined with predisposing, concurrent, and/or resulting mental health problems. As such, they complicate the assessment and treatment of other disorders. Designating an SUD as a primary disorder does not mean you should postpone addressing other issues until the substance use is resolved. In an integrative approach, you must consider how various conditions interact and prioritize treatment tasks appropriately. An extensive literature on co-occurring disorders examines how best to address the challenges of specific combinations of disorders (e.g., Graham, Schultz, Mayo-Smith, & Ries, 2003). In general, clinicians need to focus first on safety, next on behavior change and stabilization, and then on maintenance of gains and/or ways to make progress.

ADDICTION AS A BIOPSYCHOSOCIAL DISORDER

A major challenge for the office-based practitioner is to appreciate the biological, psychological, and social factors involved in the initiation, progression, and maintenance of SUDs. It is certainly expectable for most specialists to conceptualize problems in terms of their own theoretical orientation and clinical expertise, but an integrated model requires a continuing ability to shift perspectives.

A growing literature documents the many ways in which addiction is a complex brain disease. Predisposing characteristics can set the stage for future problems, as in the case of the individual who is endorphin deficient long before using any opioid substances. A predisposed individual is more likely to develop problems because certain drugs are dramatically more rewarding. Continuing drug use changes the brain in ways that may not normalize immediately, if at all, upon cessation of drug use. These changes are thought to contribute to persistent vulnerability to relapse in all stages of recovery even well after drug taking has ceased. In current models, chronic drug use brings a cycle of spiraling dysregulation of the brain's reward systems, progressively increasing, and eventually resulting in loss of control over drug taking and compulsive use. In time, this process changes the reward set point in the brain, resulting in a continuous relapse vulnerability that remains high even though the patient is abstinent (Koob, 2000; Koob & Le Moal, 2001). Research on the brain supports the disease model first proposed by Jellinek (1960) more than 40 years ago.

The disease model forms the basis of nearly all addiction treatment programs in the United States, but, regrettably, this model has been misinterpreted, misused, and misapplied. An essential tenet of the disease model, first developed in relation to a subtype of alcoholism and later applied to drug abuse, is that once a person has crossed the line from controlled to uncontrolled use, he can never return to reliably controlled use. Thus, the remedy (not the cure) for alcoholism is abstinence. Jellinek and subsequent proponents noted that there is no cure for this condition; however, it can be effectively held in remission by refraining from use. A corollary is that abstinence from all intoxicants is required. There are two main reasons for this. The first is the likelihood of drug substitution. For example, it is common for heroin users who have ceased using opioids to escalate their alcohol consumption, often requiring treatment. However, problems with alcohol may escalate slowly, leading the patient to underestimate the connection. The second reason poses more complex clinical challenges. It appears that the use of any intoxicant may stimulate hunger for the primary drug of abuse. Use of the primary drug may occur immediately, or even weeks or months later. For example, both clinical experience and the empirical literature document the frequency of significantly higher relapse rates to stimulant drugs (cocaine and methamphetamine) in individuals who continue to smoke marijuana or drink alcohol. The fact that the return to using stimulant drugs may not occur immediately after using substances makes it more difficult for these individuals to perceive the connection between these events.

A key principle in working with SUDs is that patients are likely to connect immediate consequences much more readily with their substance use, than consequences that unfold over time. Thus, cocaine users will readily acknowledge that if they are in a bar drinking and someone offers them cocaine, their ability to resist temptation and refuse the offer is severely compromised. What appears harder to integrate is that the beer today is a harbinger of the cocaine relapse 3 weeks from now. Even the patient who has repeated this cycle numerous times may continue to defend drinking because "alcohol wasn't a problem before I started using cocaine." Recent work on the neurobiology of craving offers one level of explanation for such phenomena. Once the reward pathways are stimulated by any psychoactive substance, the person is more likely to be drawn back to her primary drug of abuse.

In the biopsychosocial model, behavior is a major focus, especially in early recovery. By avoiding the first drink or drug use, the patient avoids setting in motion the cycle of events that lead to compulsive use. Behavioral interventions assist the patient to change course while choice is still possible and behavior is still voluntary. Various cognitive-behavioral models address motivation, commitment to abstinence, identifying necessary psychological and lifestyle changes, and relapse prevention (Carroll, 1999; Carroll, Libby, Sheehan, & Hyland, 2001; Kadden et al., 1995; Matrix Center 1995, 1997, 1999a, 1999b). These are based in part on the premise that feelings, thoughts, and behaviors interact with the effects of psychoactive drugs on brain chemistry to initiate and maintain compulsive behaviors.

The development of the disease model was a landmark event in the history of treatment, because it provided the framework to move alcoholism out of the realm of a character defect and moral weakness and into the realm of a treatable disorder. The former view justified desperate and abusive practices, further fostering the dangerous assumption that alcohol-dependent persons were untreatable. Once the disease model became more accepted, clinicians were given a way to help these individuals work past their shame and guilt and take personal responsibility for changing their behavior. Although these feelings remained paralyzing for many, the ability to introduce an alternative approach gave therapists a productive place to begin.

The disease of addiction is viewed as sharing certain similarities with other chronic conditions such as heart disease. It has multiple factors contributing to its etiology, including genetic factors in some but not all cases. Using the disease model does not imply that the treatment is solely medical. It is behavior change by the addicted person, not the intervention of treatment professionals, that produces progress. Although the disease model is sometimes misconstrued as giving a rationale for abdicating responsibility for one's alcohol and drug use ("My disease made me do it"), the fact is that the addicted person is deemed fully capable of managing the disease. The remedy is abstinence. In other words, the inability to dependably control his alcohol or drug use existed prior to the first use, and by acknowledging the disease, the person accepts the need to avoid using and beginning the destructive cycle all over again.

Once the disease model became widely accepted, funding followed. The National Institute on Alcohol Abuse and Alcoholism (NIAAA; www. niaaa.gov) was established in the early 1970s and has extensively studied a wide variety of issues. This research has enormously elucidated our understanding of alcoholism and pointed the way to the development of more effective treatment methods.

There is still much misunderstanding of the disease model, even by its proponents, who may interpret it narrowly. Many forget that in Jellinek's seminal work (Jellinek, 1960), progression was inevitable in only some but not all of his five subtypes. Although the disease model states that addiction is to be treated as a primary disorder, this does not mean that other areas of concern are neglected in programs based on this model. In fact, it is important to find out what actually goes on in a treatment program and avoid conclusions based on stereotypes. In an important treatment outcome study that drew participants from highly regarded, accredited substance abuse programs, the patient was more likely to receive psychiatric services in an inpatient program with a traditional orientation to alcohol and other drug dependence treatment than in the inpatient program with a psychiatric orientation (McLellan et al., 1993). Recovering counselors are often stereotyped as being the most rigid, but several studies document that they endorse more varied treatment techniques and a broader range of treatment goals (Humphreys, Noke, & Moos, 1996; Stoffelmayr, Mavis, Sherry, & Chiu, 1999). Careful observation leads us to conclude that inflexibility is not concentrated in any particular therapeutic orientation.

The debate about harm reduction and moderation goals can be a catalyst for depicting programs oriented to the disease model as uniformly harsh and rigid. Though this may occur in programs isolated from the mainstream, most programs based on the disease model have modified their practices in keeping with the treatment outcome literature. One of the most important developments is the emphasis on motivational enhancement strategies as a way of engaging those who are ambivalent about abstinence. Such programs have also developed an understanding of the importance of retention in producing good outcomes and are far less likely to terminate clients who drink or use. They do retain the view that complete abstinence yields the best results, but in recent years at least some outpatient programs have become increasingly willing to work with clients who continue to drink and use in the hope of moving them incrementally toward abstinence. Inpatient or residential facilities do not tolerate active drinking or drug use on-site. This is intended to provide safety for other residents, and does not necessarily preclude transfer to an outpatient component for those who use alcohol or drugs during their residential stay.

DIAGNOSTIC CRITERIA

The diagnostic system used most widely in the United States for mental health problems, the DSM-IV (American Psychiatric Association, 1994), defines two types of SUDs: substance *abuse* and substance *dependence.* These two categories are applied to a wide range of different types of psychoactive substances, including (1) central nervous system depressants (e.g., alcohol, sedatives–hypnotics, and benzodiazepines such as Valium, Xanax, and Ativan); (2) central nervous system stimulants (e.g., cocaine, amphetamine); (3) opioids (e.g., heroin, methadone, morphine, codeine, Demerol, Percoset, Vicodin, OxyContin); (4) cannabinoids (e.g., marijuana, hashish); (5) hallucinogens (e.g., LSD, mescaline); (6) inhalants (e.g., nitrous oxide, butyl nitrate, solvents, glues, aromatic hydrocarbons); and (7) phencyclidine (PCP) and related substances (e.g., ketamine—"Special K").

The DSM-IV definitions of abuse and dependence are based not on quantitative measures of substance use, such as how much or how often a person may use, but rather on the qualitative nature of a person's involvement with psychoactive substances. The definitions hinge primarily on the nature of a person's attachment to alcohol/drugs, the role that substances play in the person's life, and the impact that substance use has on the individual's functioning, as these factors are seen as more clinically relevant to diagnosis and treatment planning than absolute consumption levels. Moreover, these definitions reflect a consensus that pathological use of psychoactive substances is manifested as a *behavioral* syndrome characterized by *behavioral* indicators such as loss of control over use, preoccupation and obsession with use, and continued use despite adverse consequences.

It is important to recognize that a diagnosis of substance dependence can be applied in the absence of signs of physical dependence. In fact, in DSM-IV not only are signs of tolerance or withdrawal not required for a diagnosis of dependence, but in the absence of core behavioral indicators (e.g., loss of control, preoccupation, etc.) these physiological signs alone do not support a diagnosis of dependence. A person who is physically dependent on an adequate dose of prescription painkillers (opioids) but displays no evidence of drug-related obsession, compulsion, or psychosocial dysfunction does not qualify for a diagnosis of substance dependence. For example, many people are physically dependent on prescription painkillers or anxiolytics, but their functioning is improved rather than impaired by the medication and they do not exhibit addictive behaviors. Confusion between physical dependence and addiction (substance dependence) leads to undermedication of pain or anxiety and unnecessary disruption of appropriate treatment for patients who are in fact functioning well.

Although the variable of consumption level is absent from DSM-IV, it can provide useful information as to how easily an individual may be able to quit or cut down and whether medical intervention may be needed to safely manage the withdrawal syndrome associated with certain types of substances (e.g., alcohol. benzodiazepines, and other central nervous system depressants).

The DSM-IV defines substance *abuse* and substance *dependence* as maladaptive patterns of substance use leading to clinically significant impairment or distress over a 12-month period. Substance dependence is manifested by at least three of seven possible indicators. Two of these seven indicators refer to impaired control of substance use: (1) taking the substance in larger amounts or over longer periods of time than originally intended and (2) persistent desire or unsuccessful efforts to control or cut down use. The next three indicators refer to the priority and impact of substance use on the person's behavior and psychosocial functioning: (3) spending a great deal of time acquiring or using the substance or recovering from its effects, (4) reducing or giving up important social, occupational, or recreational activities because of substance use, and (5) continued use despite knowledge that the substance use is associated with persistent or recurrent physical or psychological problems caused or exacerbated by the use. The last two indicators refer to signs of physical dependence: (6) tolerance, defined as the need for increased amounts of the substance to achieve the desired effects or as diminished effects with continued use of the same amount, and (7) emergence of withdrawal symptoms after abruptly reducing or stopping use, or the need to take substitute drugs to prevent or relieve withdrawal symptoms.

A diagnosis of abuse is a less severe than that of dependence and can be applied only to individuals who never previously met the criteria for substance dependence for the same or similar class of substances. Four different criteria define substance abuse, with the patient needing to exhibit only one of the four within a 12-month period to receive a diagnosis of abuse: (1) recurrent substance use resulting in failure to fulfill major role obligations such as those at home, work, or school, (2) recurrent substance use in situations in which it is physically hazardous (e.g., while driving or operating other dangerous machinery), (3) recurrent substance-related legal problems (e.g., arrest for DWI or possession of controlled substances), (4) continued substance use despite persistent or recurrent social or interpersonal problems caused or exacerbated by the use. Both types of substance use disorders (abuse and dependence) are characterized by substance-related dysfunction and continued use despite adverse consequences, but dependence is distinguished by the additional features of impaired control of substance use and preoccupation or compulsion regarding the use. Whereas in substance abuse the person is seen as still having some ability to control or moderate use and is neither obsessed with the substance use nor at a point where it dominates her life, in substance dependence there is clear evidence of an automatic, stereotyped, compulsive pattern of substance use that is occurring without the person's full volitional control and in some cases accompanied by signs of physiological dependence such as tolerance and withdrawal.

It should be noted that where *illegal* drug use is concerned, nonclinical (i.e., moral, cultural, and legal) considerations may complicate the diagnosis of substance *abuse*. It has been argued that because any use of illicit drugs exposes the user to the potential risk of serious legal consequences, it should be considered de facto as *abuse*. Although defining use of all illicit drugs as abuse ignores the fundamental concepts that underlie the DSM-IV definition of substance use disorders, clinicians should refrain from condoning or supporting illicit drug use in their patients but also refrain from being judgmental or recriminating about it.

DSM-IV Specifiers

DSM-IV defines various types of "specifiers" to further delineate a diagnosis of substance abuse or dependence. For example, for persons who have stopped using there are four "remission" specifiers based on time elapsed since the criteria for abuse or dependence were met.

1. *Early full remission.* For at least 1 month but less than 12 months, no criteria for abuse or dependence have been met.

2. *Early partial remission.* For at least 1 month but less than 12 months, one or more criteria for abuse or dependence have been met but the full criteria have not been met.

3. *Sustained full remission.* None of the criteria for abuse or dependence have been met at any time during a period of 12 months.

4. *Sustained partial remission.* Full criteria for dependence have not been met for 12 months or longer; however, one or more criteria for dependence or abuse have been met.

There are also specifiers that denote (1) whether physiological dependence (as evidenced by either tolerance or withdrawal) is part of the clinical picture, (2) whether the patient is receiving substitute medication (e.g., methadone), and (3) whether the patient is residing in a controlled environment (e.g., hospital or rehab) where access to psychoactive substances is precluded.

NIAAA Categories of "Low-Risk" and "At-Risk" Drinking

Recognizing that most people who drink do not develop problems related to their alcohol consumption, the NIAAA defines "low-risk" or nonproblematic drinking as no more than two drinks per day for adult males and no more than one drink per day for adult women, with never more than four drinks per occasion for men and three for women. (A standard "drink" is defined as 12 grams of pure ethyl alcohol, which is equal to one 12-ounce serving of beer or wine cooler, one 5-ounce glass of wine, or 1.5 ounces of liquor or other distilled spirits.) These consumption limits are based on extensive research on the levels above which physical and social harms can be documented (National Institute on Alcohol Abuse and Alcoholism, 2000; Yalisove, 2004). The definition of "low risk" must also take into account individual characteristics such as age, body weight, metabolic rate, psychiatric status, overall health status, and family (genetic) history, all of which can affect a person's sensitivity to alcohol and lead to adverse interactions with a wide variety of medical conditions and prescribed medications. Some people are highly sensitive to alcohol, as evidenced by negative changes in mood, behavior, and personality in response to relatively small doses of alcohol, whereas in other drinkers these same doses have no such effects. Being at "increased risk" for developing alcohol-related problems is defined by the NIAAA by one or more of the following: (1) drinking above the aforementioned low-risk consumption levels, (2) drinking by people whose use of alcohol or other central nervous system depressants has ever met DSM-IV criteria for substance abuse or dependence, (3) drinking by pregnant women, (4) drinking by people with medical conditions adversely affected by alcohol, (5) being under the influence of alcohol in situations that are of high risk, such as driving an automobile or operating other dangerous machinery. The concept of low-risk consumption is highly controversial and usually not applied to use of illicit drugs. As might be expected, no safe levels of illegal drug use have been formally defined by health organizations or government agencies. Although reducing levels of drug use and drug-related harm may be desirable intermediate steps, complete abstinence from illegal drugs is generally recommended as the only acceptable goal.

FINAL COMMENT

We have discussed in this chapter the nature and course of SUDs, emphasizing that these problems are multidetermined primary disorders that have complex etiologies. Often there is neither a linear nor an inevitable progression from initial use to addiction. Although therapists must be careful not to downplay or ignore their patients' use of alcohol and drugs, especially when other types of mental health problems are the primary presenting complaints, they also should not overreact and overdiagnose (pathologize) substance use when it falls short of meeting the criteria for abuse or dependence. DSM-IV provides a uniform set of diagnostic criteria for all substance use disorders, but forcing all disorders into only two categories (abuse and dependence) without a methodology for rating the severity of these disorders overlooks the fact that there is not a dichotomy but rather a continuum of substance use and related problems.

CHAPTER 3

Pharmacology and Overview of Psychoactive Substances

Acquiring a basic understanding and working knowledge of the pharmacology of psychoactive substances is essential for all mental health practitioners. Although there is no need for every clinician to become an expert on the subject, familiarity with the various types of psychoactive drugs, how they are used, and how they affect mental and physiological functioning is essential. Acquiring this familiarity is important for at least several reasons. First, without this knowledge it is extremely difficult, if not impossible, to perform a valid clinical assessment and arrive at an accurate diagnosis. Second, choosing an appropriate course of treatment must take into account certain aspects of the particular substances that the patient is using and the current pattern of use. For example, it is critical that you to be able to determine when medical detoxification is needed to ensure safe and effective withdrawal before encouraging a substance-dependent patient to abruptly discontinue use. Third, being familiar with the various drugs of abuse and how they are used is essential in establishing your credibility with substance-using patients. Often they are highly attuned to signs of a therapist's ignorance about drugs and lack of fluency in discussing the particulars. For them to feel confident in your ability to be of help, they need assurance that you actually know what you are talking about when it comes to drug use. You should know at least as much about the pharmacology of psychoactive drugs as your patients do.

The purpose of this chapter is to familiarize you with the clinically relevant pharmacology of the most commonly used psychoactive drugs. It is not intended to provide in-depth coverage of the subject, which can be obtained elsewhere, including some of the texts that served as primary resources for material in this chapter (Giannini & Slaby, 1989; Graham & Schultz, 1998; Graham, Schultz, Mayo-Smith, & Ries, 2003; Lowinson, Ruiz, Millman, & Langrod, 2005; Miller, 1991; Schuckit, 2000). Additional information on drugs and their effects is available from a wide variety of publications that can be obtained at no cost from the National Clearinghouse for Alcohol and Drug Information (1-800-729-6686 or www.health.org). Absent from this chapter, for example, is information about the intricate chemical structure of drug molecules, the complex physiological effects of drugs on various organ systems, and details of how psychoactive drugs affect neurotransmitter systems in the brain. Instead, what we have attempted to provide here is information about alcohol and other drugs of abuse that is directly relevant to clinical practice. We begin by defining some of the basic pharmacological terms and phenomena used to describe the nature of drug actions in the human body. We then present for each category of psychoactive substances a description of the types of drugs that fall into that category, how they are most commonly used, characteristics of their psychoactive and other pharmacological effects, and adverse consequences associated with their use.

BASIC CONCEPTS

Psychoactive substances are pharmacological agents that chemically alter brain function sufficiently to cause changes in an individual's mood, perception, and/or state of consciousness. The target organ of all psychoactive substance use is the brain. In order for a drug to be psychoactive, it must get into the bloodstream, cross the blood–brain barrier, and alter neurochemical activity in certain target areas of the brain.

Route of Administration

The particular method used to deliver a drug into the bloodstream is known as the route of administration. For any given drug, route of administration determines how quickly the drug gets into the bloodstream and reaches the brain, as well as how quickly and intensely the user experiences the drug-induced euphoria ("high") and other effects. Some routes of administration are more rapid and efficient than others. The most rapid drug delivery methods are intravenous (iv) injection and pulmonary inhalation (smoking). Both yield almost instantaneous onset of drug effects. Typically, the drug-induced euphoria produced by these rapid routes of administration is extremely intense but relatively short-lived. In comparison, drug effects produced by intranasal ("snorting") and oral routes of administration have a slower onset, are less intense, and are of longer duration. In general, for any given drug, more rapid routes of administration are associated with more rapid development of tolerance and addictive patterns of use.

Half-Life

Duration or persistence of drug actions in the body is determined not only by route of administration, but also by the characteristic rate at which a drug is metabolized, commonly known as the drug's "half-life." The half-life is the time it takes for the concentration of a drug in the bloodstream to drop 50% from its initial peak concentration. Drugs such as heroin and cocaine, for example, have very short half-lives as compared with methadone and methamphetamine, which take much longer to be metabolized. In general, the longer the half-life of a drug, the longer its duration of action and the longer it can be detected in body fluids (e.g., blood and urine).

Tolerance, Cross-Tolerance, and Physical Dependence

The phenomena of tolerance, cross-tolerance, and physical dependence are crucial to understanding the development of substance dependence. Most drug effects diminish with repeated use such that the user must take progressively larger doses in order to achieve the same effects. This phenomenon is known as tolerance. Cross-tolerance exists between different drugs within the same category. Thus, an individual tolerant to alcohol will be comparably tolerant to equivalent doses of sedative–hypnotic drugs such as benzodiazepines and barbiturates. Similarly, an individual tolerant to codeine (an opioid) will be tolerant to equivalent doses of other opioids such as heroin and morphine. Physical dependence refers to an altered physiological state produced by repeated use of a drug and is manifested by the emergence of a withdrawal syndrome upon cessation of use or marked reduction in the amount or frequency of use. Continued use of the drug prevents the emergence of the withdrawal syndrome and may become one of the compelling reasons why some individuals continue using certain drugs even after they have become tolerant to the drugs' reinforcing psychoactive effects. The most predictable and stereotyped withdrawal syndromes are associated with opioids (narcotics), alcohol, and sedatives–hypnotics. In contrast, there is no clearly definable withdrawal syndrome associated with stimulant drugs such as cocaine and methamphetamine or with hallucinogens such as LSD.

DRUG CATEGORIES

Psychoactive drugs are categorized according to certain defining features of their pharmacological actions and, to a lesser extent, similarities in chemical structure. The eight main categories are:

1. Alcohol
2. Benzodiazepines and other sedatives–hypnotics
3. Stimulants
4. Opioids (narcotics)
5. Marijuana and other cannabinoids
6. LSD and other hallucinogens
7. "Club" drugs, PCP, and inhalants
8. Nicotine

Alcohol

Alcohol is the most widely used psychoactive drug in the world. In the United States it is estimated that 95 million or 60% of adults (individuals at least 18 years old) drink at some level and 7% of adults drink daily. Approximately 26% of 12- to 17-year-olds are classified as "regular" drinkers. Alcohol-dependent persons die at 2.5 times the rate of nondependent individuals. The suicide rate among alcohol-dependent persons is estimated to be 20 times that of the general population (Institute of Medicine, 1990).

Many types of beverages contain ethyl alcohol ($C_2 H_6 O_2$), including beer, wine, and various types of distilled spirits. The alcohol content of these beverages ranges from 1.6% in "lite" beer to upwards of 40% in distilled spirits such as gin and whiskey. Doubling the percentage of alcohol by volume yields the beverage's "proof" rating. Thus, a beverage that is 40% alcohol is referred to as 80 proof.

Alcohol requires no digestion. It is absorbed directly into the bloodstream from the gastrointestinal tract. Carbonation increases this absorption rate. Thus, champagne intoxicates more quickly than noncarbonated alcoholic beverages. Conversely, the presence of food in the stomach decreases the rate of alcohol absorption and diminishes its psychoactive effects.

The impact of alcohol on an individual's behavior is assessed by measuring blood alcohol concentration (BAC). Breathalyzers measure the concentration of alcohol in expired air, which is directly related to blood concentration. The amount of alcohol present in the blood is reported in terms of the number of grams of alcohol present in 100 milliliters of blood, expressed as a percentage. For example, 100 milligrams per 100 milliliters = 0.10 grams per 100 milliliters or 0.1%. In most states an alcohol concentration of 0.08–0.10% or higher is the legal threshold for a charge of driving while intoxicated (DWI).

Alcohol is a depressant of the entire central nervous system. All brain functions are affected by alcohol, including behavior, cognition, judgment, respiration, psychomotor coordination, and sexuality. Alcohol impairs motor coordination and judgment simultaneously—a dangerous combination. In dose-dependent fashion, alcohol alters brain functions that normally exercise the restraints responsible for maintaining inhibition of social behavior, thus giving freer reign to impulses. Accordingly, alcohol is often said to be a disinhibitor. At low to moderate doses alcohol induces euphoria or relieves dysphoria. Many people use alcohol to relax after a hard day's work or to feel less anxious in social situations. With increasing doses, buoyancy decreases while psychomotor functioning becomes slower and more impaired. Continued drinking will often induce sleep or, in a worst case, coma. Alcohol has the potential to cause a fatal overdose. Individuals who consume large quantities of alcohol in a short period of time may experience respiratory depression and ultimately death. The effects of alcohol on the central nervous system correlate to some degree with BAC. At 0.03% there is little noticeable effect; at 0.05% a person's responses and reactions are slowed to some extent and performance in skilled tasks deteriorates; at 0.10–0.15% most drinkers are noticeably intoxicated as demonstrated by slurred speech and impaired motor coordination. A BAC of 0.30% is often associated with loss of consciousness, and a concentration of 0.40% or more can cause death.

The effects of alcohol on mood, mental state, and behavior depend not only on the amount that is ingested, but also the chronicity of use. For example, alcohol may relieve anxiety in the early stages of an individual's drinking history, but actually induce anxiety in the latter stages of use. Similarly, it may enhance sexuality in the early phases and then impair sexual performance in the latter stages. One of the hallmarks of alcohol dependence is continued drinking even though alcohol is inducing negative rather than positive psychoactive effects. The earlier benefits and pleasures of alcohol-induced mood states are long gone, but the alcohol consumption continues anyway.

Alcohol consumption is typically measured according to how many ounces of each type of alcoholic beverage are consumed (e.g., beer, wine, or distilled spirits). A standard "drink unit" is defined as a beverage containing 13.6 grams of ethyl alcohol. Accordingly, a standard drink unit is equivalent to one 5-ounce glass of wine, one 12-ounce bottle of beer, or one 1.5-ounce glass of distilled spirits. When an person says, "I don't have a problem with alcohol, I only drink beer or wine, I never touch hard liquor," keep in mind that it is the total amount (dose) of alcohol consumed in a given time period and not the particular type of alcoholic beverage a person drinks that determines its effects. The impact of alcohol on an individual's brain function and behavior are determined by the dose of alcohol that actually reaches the brain, irrespective of the particular type of alcoholic beverage that is ingested into the stomach.

The adverse effects of alcohol on various internal organ systems are well documented and are not discussed at length here. Suffice it to say that diseases of the liver, pancreas, heart, and endocrine systems are often associated with chronic excessive drinking. Heavy drinkers also experience surprisingly high mortality from cancers of the mouth, larynx, esophagus, and liver. It is well known that high-dose alcohol consumption can induce loss of memory or a "blackout" for the period of intoxication. Individuals who experience a blackout may have no memory of the drinking episode, including where they were, whom they were with, or what they did during that time period.

Individuals who consume alcohol chronically and repeatedly become progressively tolerant to its effects. As a result, larger and larger amounts of alcohol must be consumed in order to achieve the same effects. Individuals who have developed tolerance to alcohol may have high BACs, in the range of 0.2% or greater, without exhibiting obvious signs of intoxication. Increasing tolerance to alcohol is accompanied by increasing physical dependence, and withdrawal from alcohol can lead to health-threatening or even life-threatening consequences if not managed appropriately. Individuals tolerant to alcohol are cross-tolerant to other central nervous system depressants, including benzodiazepines, barbiturates, and nonbarbiturate sedative–hypnotics. Benzodiazepines (e.g., Valium, Librium, Ativan) are usually the drugs of choice for managing alcohol withdrawal. The alcohol withdrawal syndrome usually appears within 24–48 hours after cessation of drinking. Mild withdrawal symptoms include tremor, insomnia, sweating, weakness, nausea, and vomiting. A severe and potentially life-threatening withdrawal syndrome, known as delirium tremens, can emerge after 48 hours if high-dose alcohol consumption is discontinued too abruptly and no substitute medication (e.g., benzodiazepines) is administered. The symptoms of delirium tremens include extreme agitation and anxiety, profound depression and lethargy, increasing mental confusion, profuse sweating, elevated pulse rate, and a rise in body temperature. Hallucinations and grand mal seizures may also occur in severe cases. Medical management of the alcohol withdrawal syndrome is beyond the scope of this discussion; protocols describing alcohol detoxification procedures are readily available in the medical literature (Graham & Schultz, 1998).

Benzodiazepines and Other Sedatives–Hypnotics

The category of nonalcohol central nervous system depressants, also known as sedatives–hypnotics, includes a wide variety of different types of drugs, all having the ability to depress brain activity in a manner similar to that of alcohol. The best known and most widely used sedatives–hypnotics are the barbiturates and benzodiazepines.

All of these substances are cross-tolerant with alcohol. Accordingly, alcohol withdrawal is frequently managed pharmacologically with equivalent doses of barbiturates (e.g., phenobarbital) or benzodiazepines (e.g., Librium or Valium). The cross-tolerance that exists between alcohol and all other sedative drugs is an essential factor that must be taken into account when evaluating a patient's level of physical dependence, inasmuch as the dependence-producing effects of these substances are synergistic and thus additive. For instance, a person who drinks four cans of beer and takes 20 milligrams of diazepam (Valium) every day will have higher overall levels of alcohol tolerance and physical dependence than a person who drinks the same amount of beer but takes no other sedative drugs whatsoever.

Like alcohol, all sedatives cause dose-dependent changes in mood in conjunction with impairment of psychomotor and cognitive functions. Low doses produce mild sedation accompanied by antianxiety or tranquilizer effects, whereas moderate doses are more likely to produce overt signs of intoxication such as impaired motor performance and slurred speech accompanied by gross changes in mental status and behavior. Large doses can produce unresponsive stupor, respiratory depression, and even death. All sedatives are capable of producing pharmacologic tolerance and physical dependence, with a withdrawal syndrome nearly identical to that of alcohol. Medical management of the sedative withdrawal syndrome is essential because, like withdrawal from alcohol, it can be health- or even life-threatening, especially if chronic high-dose sedative use is discontinued too abruptly without appropriate tapering with the use of substitute medication. A full-blown sedative withdrawal syndrome may include psychotic delirium, repeated seizures, and even cardiovascular collapse.

Barbiturates

The barbiturates, originally introduced into clinical medicine in the early 1900s, were thought initially to be safe and effective agents for treating anxiety and insomnia, but were later found to have a high potential for dependence and to be particularly lethal in terms of overdose, especially when combined with alcohol. Abuse of barbiturates (e.g., Seconal, Tuinal) has declined dramatically since the 1960s when these drugs were more popular and more readily available. There are several other sedative–hypnotic drugs whose effects are nearly identical to those of barbiturates, although, strictly speaking, their chemical structure does not warrant classification as barbiturates. These include glutethimide (Doriden), ethchlorvynol (Placidyl), and methaqualone (Quaalude). Supplies of these drugs have dwindled as their legal manufacture and distribution were outlawed some years ago by the U.S. Food and Drug Administration (FDA).

Benzodiazepines

Benzodiazepines such as Valium (diazepam) are sedative drugs used primarily to treat anxiety and insomnia. By 1977, benzodiazepines were the most widely prescribed drugs worldwide. Generic and trade names of the most commonly prescribed benzodiazepines are listed in Table 3.1. Dalmane, Halcion, and Restoril are used primarily to alleviate insomnia, whereas most of the other benzodiaepines are used as anxiolytics (i.e., tranquilizers). Two of the newer benzodiazepine-like agents used to treat insomnia are Ambien (zolpidem) and Sonata (zaleplon). Soma (carisoprodol), yet another benzodiazepine-like drug, is used as a muscle relaxant. A benzodiazepine not approved for prescription use in the United States, but available in other countries and here on the illicit drug market, is Rohypnol (flunitrazepam). This drug dissolves readily in carbonated beverages and is capable of inducing "blackouts" (anterograde amnesia) for many hours following its ingestion, similar to the effects of consuming large doses of alcohol (i.e., binge drinking). The use of Rohypnol to perpetrate sexual assault on unsuspecting women has led to its reputation as the "date rape" drug.

Like barbiturates, benzodiazepines were found to have more profound effects on cognitive and motor functions, more undesirable side effects, and higher potential for abuse and dependence than originally suspected. However, benzodiazepines are somewhat "safer" than barbiturates in terms of overdose potential. Benzodiazepines alone generally do not produce sufficient respiratory depression to cause death, but when combined with alcohol the potential for a lethal overdose reaction increases markedly.

An issue of ongoing controversy is whether benzodiazepines can ever be used safely in patients with SUDs. This issue arises frequently in regard to treating panic attacks and other anxiety disorders in patients who also have a history of significant alcohol problems. Many addiction therapists have noted that benzodiazepines can increase the rate of relapse in patients with a history of alcohol dependence. This should not be surprising, considering that alcohol and benzodiazepines have overlapping mechanisms of action in the brain and similar psychoactive effects. Benzodiazepines have been described as "solid-state" alcohol and the "driest of all martinis." Accordingly, there is concern that use of benzodiazepines or any other sedative agents by alcoholic patients is equivalent to controlled drinking and thus a setup for inevitable relapse. Even in patients with no history of SUDs, the risks of

TABLE 3.1. Commonly Prescribed Benzodiazepines

Generic name	Trade name
Alprazolam	Xanax
Chlordiazepoxide	Librium
Clonazepam	Klonopin
Flurazepam	Dalmane
Diazepam	Valium
Lorazepam	Ativan
Restoril	Temazepam
Triazolam	Halcion

long-term benzodiazepine use are seen as likely to outweigh the therapeutic benefits. Given the risks, it is prudent to reserve benzodiazepine use for situations in which pharmacological intervention to treat a severe anxiety disorder is truly needed and other interventions have failed.

Although the American Medical Association (AMA) acknowledges the potential risks of prescribing benzodiazepines to patients with alcohol use disorders, it does not take the position that benzodiazepines are contraindicated in all cases. Instead, physicians are urged by the AMA to use caution when giving benzodiazepines to patients with a history of alcohol problems. The American Society of Addiction Medicine, however, states that benzodiazepines should be avoided categorically in all patients with addiction histories and, where appropriate and indicated, alternative pharmacological treatments should be considered. For example, Buspar (buspirone), a nonsedative anxiolytic medication, is regarded as a safer alternative to any of the benzodiazepines, although the efficacy of this medication for treating anxiety disorders is questionable. Similarly, in treating insomnia, trazodone and some of the selective serotonin reuptake inhibitor antidepressants with significant sedative side effects appear to be safe and effective in patients with prior addiction histories. However, sedating antihistamines such as Benadryl (diphenhydramine) and similar over-the-counter medications are regarded by many addiction experts as more likely to contribute to alcoholic relapse. Although Ambien and Sonata have become extremely popular medications for alleviating sleep problems in the general population, the benzodiazepine-like characteristics of these drugs are seen as posing unnecessary hazards to patients with SUDs. Accordingly, many if not most clinicians in the addiction field advise patients to avoid these medications.

Patients with SUDs sometimes persuade unsuspecting physicians that their problems with anxiety and/or insomnia can be alleviated *only* by benzodiazepines. Some patients argue convincingly that benzodiazepines help not only to decrease their anxiety and/or insomnia, but also to decrease their desire to use alcohol or other drugs. A physician not experienced in dealing with SUDs may believe that prescribing benzodiazepines or similar medications may actually be therapeutic without realizing that these medications are likely to exacerbate rather than attenuate the patient's SUD. Even when the physician is aware of the patient's SUD, he or she may feel that alleviating an "underlying" anxiety disorder may help to remove some of the patient's motivation for self-medicating with alcohol and drugs and thus help the addiction to subside. Rarely, if ever, does this occur. What unsuspecting clinicians fail to realize is that problems with anxiety and insomnia are often induced by chronic use of sedative drugs and that these symptoms are among the most common features of sedative withdrawal. Accordingly, giving sedative-dependent patients more sedatives (except as part of a tapering procedure) is likely to perpetuate, not resolve, the problem. Intolerable anxiety is often the most prominent symptom of withdrawal from benzodiazepines, and its presence is often confused with the original symptoms of anxiety for which the medication was prescribed in the first place.

Stimulants

The category of central nervous system stimulants includes cocaine, methamphetamine, and a variety of prescription amphetamines such as methylphenidate (Ritalin) and dexedrine. The physiological effects of stimulant drugs include dose-dependent increases in heart rate, blood pressure, body temperature, and pupillary dilation. High doses of cocaine or methamphetamine may cause cardiac arrhythmia, seizure, respiratory failure, and death. Toxic psychosis can also develop, especially with chronic use of high doses. Even in the absence of a full-blown psychotic reaction, these drugs can induce paranoid delusions, visual and auditory hallucinations, and in extreme cases, volatile aggressive behavior.

Tolerance often develops to the euphorigenic and other psychoactive effects of these stimulant drugs, as evidenced by the need for higher and higher doses to achieve the same effects. As use escalates and continues, a point is often reached at which the user becomes refractory to the euphorigenic and other pleasurable psychoactive effects of these drugs no matter what quantity of drug is used. This leads to a phenomenon well known among cocaine and methamphetamine users as "chasing the high." Stimulant users caught in this vicious cycle experience a fleeting burst of drug-induced euphoria for no more than the first few seconds or minutes of a given episode of use and then find themselves ensnared in a futile attempt to recapture these feelings by compulsively readministering the drug again and again at shorter and shorter intervals, but the desired effects are rarely if ever recaptured.

It is important to note that while tolerance develops to the stimulant high, some users become sensitized rather than tolerant to certain physiological effects of stimulant drugs in ways that can be dangerous and even life-threatening. For example, with repeated use of a given dose of cocaine the user may experience a seizure even after the same or comparable dose taken previously had produced no such effect—a phenomenon known as reverse tolerance or "kindling."

Although progressive tolerance develops to the psychoactive effects of stimulants, there is no distinct withdrawal syndrome requiring gradual tapering or pharmacological detoxification following abrupt cessation of use. The potentially health-threatening period of stimulant use is limited mainly to the period of acute intoxication. Some addiction experts claim that the "crash," or immediate post-drug period (characterized by dysphoria, agitation, lethargy, cognitive dysfunction, prolonged sleep, and drug cravings), following a binge or "run" on cocaine or methamphetamine should be considered a withdrawal syndrome, but this does not seem consistent with the way in which withdrawal syndromes are typically defined. First, these post-drug symptoms are not relieved by further administration of the drug. To the contrary, taking more cocaine or methamphetamine during the post-drug crash usually makes the user feel worse, not better. Second, the crash subsides rather quickly on its own without medical intervention, except for the drug cravings, which may persist indefinitely. Crash symptoms are perhaps better understood as caused by repeated drug-induced alterations in brain chemistry (particularly in the dopamine system) rather than indicative of a withdrawal syndrome. Third, no pharmacological agents have been found to be effective in alleviating symptoms of stimulant "withdrawal." Often the best treatment for the post-stimulant crash is continued abstinence from all stimulant drugs. In light of these considerations, it appears that post-stimulant discomfort and dysphoria are best regarded as part of a post-drug rebound phenomenon rather than a withdrawal syndrome. This distinction is important, because stimulant users are often prescribed antidepressants, anxiolytics, and sleeping pills inappropriately in order to alleviate a supposed stimulant withdrawal syndrome.

In terms of acute psychoactive effects, cocaine and other stimulant drugs typically cause the user to feel euphoric, energetic, talkative, and more mentally alert. Some users find that these drugs help to increase their attention, motivation, and overall performance on various tasks. Others experience the opposite or no such effects. Still others report what appear to be paradoxical effects from stimulant drugs, particularly cocaine, consisting of feeling more relaxed and "mellow" rather than more energetic and stimulated. It should be noted, however, that rarely do these paradoxical effects point to the presence of an attention deficit disorder.

Whatever acute pleasurable or beneficial effects may be derived from short-term stimulant use, chronic or long-term use often yields the opposite effects. Thus, euphoria is typically replaced by irritability and mood disturbances; feeling energized is replaced by feeling lethargic; increased attention and mental alertness are replaced by distractibility and other cognitive deficits; and feeling more talkative and interactive is replaced by social avoidance and isolation.

The Linkage between Stimulant Drugs and Sexual Behavior

Many individuals report that cocaine and methamphetamine markedly enhance their sexuality by increasing libido, level of arousal, and fantasies. Although some users choose stimulant drugs deliberately and primarily for aphrodisiac effects, others do not experience heightened sexual arousal or interest by taking these drugs at all. Studies indicate that approximately 40–50% of male stimulant users derive enhanced sexuality from stimulant drugs, whereas fewer than 25% of female users experience this effect (Rawson,

Washton, Domier, & Reiber, 2002; Washton, 1989). The reasons for this gender discrepancy are unknown. It is also not known why some men and some women experience this aphrodisiac effect and others do not experience the effect at all. Stimulant users who do experience sexual-enhancing effects from a stimulant drug often do so almost from the first time they try the drug or upon increasing the dose beyond a certain threshold level that varies widely among individuals. In addition to experiencing increased sexual desire, they also report increased sexual fantasies coupled with decreased sexual inhibitions, sometimes including an enhanced desire or willingness to engage in sex acts that they either do not think about, find appealing, or are reluctant to try when not under the influence of stimulants. This may include indiscriminant sex with prostitutes, pickups, or other strangers who present increased risk of exposure to sexually transmitted diseases. Obsessive interest in pornography coupled with compulsive masturbation is often associated with stimulant drug use. It may also include cross-dressing, exhibitionism, and other paraphilias. A relatively little known phenomenon is that some overtly heterosexual men experience drug-induced homosexual fantasies and urges to engage in homosexual acts under the influence of cocaine and/or methamphetamine. Some of these men actually do have sex with men in the drug-altered state. When the drug high wears off, many of these men are repulsed and highly disturbed by their homosexual acts which may, in some cases, lead to intense suicidal ideation and even suicide attempts. For some individuals, the phenomenon of homosexual activity while using stimulant drugs may point to unresolved sexuality issues underlying such behavior. Many men (and women) with conflicts about their sexual orientation are able to express such feelings only while under the influence of drugs or alcohol and will often even use substances instrumentally in order to facilitate engagement in strongly desired but forbidden sexual behavior. Such issues need to be evaluated in the course of treatment, and psychotherapy dealing with sexuality and sexual orientation may be an essential part of recovery for many such individuals.

The link between stimulant drugs and sex can become extraordinarily powerful as usage increases. The most dramatic examples of this link can be seen in individuals who have a history of sexual acting-out behaviors or sexual compulsivity that predates their use of stimulant drugs. When such inclinations collide with cocaine and/or methamphetamine, the results are often overwhelming in the sense that these individuals' drug use escalates almost instantaneously into full-blown addiction that involves progressively intense, frequent, and hazardous sexual acting-out behaviors. Even individuals with no pre-drug history of sexual compulsivity can show an extraordinarily rapid progression from occasional to addictive drug use and an equally rapid progression from casual to compulsive drug-related sexual behavior.

Once the link between stimulant use and sex is firmly established, sexual activity of any kind acquires the ability to elicit marked cravings for drugs and increases the likelihood of relapse. Similarly, the use of drugs elicits marked cravings for the sexual experiences strongly associated with the drug use. This leads to a vicious cycle known as "reciprocal relapse" (Washton, 1989), in which drug use leads to sex and sex leads to drug use. Engaging in one behavior all but guarantees that the individual will engage in the other behavior. Clinicians need to be aware of this reciprocal relapse pattern because many stimulant users try to stop using the drug without discontinuing their previously drug-related sexual escapades—an effort that is doomed to fail because of the extraordinarily powerful conditioned associations that develop between drug use and sex. Individuals who have acted out sexually under the influence of stimulant drugs often feel extremely embarrassed, guilty, and reluctant to discuss it without the sensitive prompting of a knowledgeable, nonjudgmental therapist. Even then, it may require a few sessions to develop enough rapport and trust with the patient before that person is willing to engage with you in an open dialogue about it—especially for a male patient if the therapist is female.

What about the sexual dysfunction often caused by chronic cocaine or methamphetamine use? Whether or not an individual experiences any aphrodisiac effects from stimulant drugs, chronic increasing use of cocaine and/or methamphetamine will at some point impair sexual functioning reliably in both men and women. Erectile dysfunction and inability to achieve orgasm are the most common sexual side effects of chronic stimulant use. In recent years this has led to the increasing use of Viagra, Cialis, and similar medications by individuals who abuse stimulants and other drugs. In addition, many men and women completely lose their desire for sex as a result of using stimulant drugs in high doses and/or chronically. Glaring exceptions are individuals whose use of cocaine or methamphetamine is strongly associated with sex. Interestingly, as sexual performance in these individuals deteriorates as a result of their continuing use of stimulant drugs, their drug-related sexual acting-out behavior often intensifies, sometimes becoming increasingly bizarre in an attempt to override the tolerance that has developed to the drug's aphrodisiac effects. Often these individuals report that sex under the influence of the drugs no longer involves any physical stimulation or touching whatsoever. Instead, sex becomes an entirely mental or visual experience with no expectation of physical contact or of achieving orgasm.

Cocaine

Cocaine is a potent stimulant drug derived from the coca plant (*Erythroxylum coca*) grown primarily in Peru and Bolivia. Cocaine is generally available in the form of cocaine hydrochloride, a white crystalline powder that can be taken intranasally (i.e., by inhaling it up the nostrils). Snorting cocaine produces an onset of noticeable psychoactive drug effects approximately 10–15 minutes after inhalation, with peak effects occurring at 30–

60 minutes. Because the powder dissolves quite readily in water, a solution of cocaine hydrochloride can be drawn up in a syringe for intravenous injection. Some users mix cocaine and heroin in the same syringe, a drug cocktail known as a "speedball," aimed at smoothing out the undesirable side effects of each drug. A more popular combination is cocaine and alcohol. Most cocaine users drink alcohol together with their use of cocaine in order to prolong the cocaine high and to soften the unpleasant crash described previously. The combination of cocaine and alcohol produces a substance in the body known as cocaethylene, which mimics the psychoactive effects of cocaine but has a longer duration of action. Cocaine is classified by the U.S. Food and Drug Administration as a Schedule II controlled substance, meaning that it has a high abuse potential and limited medical usefulness. It is still sometimes used as a local anesthetic in nasal and eye surgery. Cocaine is the only drug known to be both a central nervous system stimulant and a local anesthetic. Other central nervous system stimulants, such as methamphetamine, have no local anesthetic properties, and other local anesthetics, such as novocaine and lidocaine, have no central nervous system stimulant properties. Cocaine purchased on the street is usually diluted or "cut" with various types of white powders including local anesthetics to inflate its volume, mimic the numbing effects of cocaine on the tongue and throat that experienced users expect, and thereby increase the dealer's profits.

Serious medical consequences associated with chronic cocaine use are relatively uncommon as compared with those of other psychoactive substances such as alcohol. Fatal reactions to cocaine, although rare, can and do occur, often resulting from adverse effects on cardiovascular function, from brain seizures, or from malignant hyperthermia. Chronic intranasal use of cocaine can lead to serious sinus infections, perforation of the nasal septum, and repeated nosebleeds. Smoking cocaine can lead to chronic chest congestion, lung infections, and impaired breathing capacity as a result of inhaling the hot vapors into the lungs. Intravenous injection of cocaine is often associated with abscesses at injection sites and may expose those who share injection apparatus to serious transmittable diseases such as HIV and various forms of hepatitis.

Cocaine freebase or "crack" is the smokeable form of cocaine. Cocaine hydrochloride powder cannot be efficiently smoked because most of the active drug in the powder decomposes when heated with a flame. Smoking a drug produces more rapid intoxication than nasal inhalation and even more rapid onset of effects than intravenous injection. Smoking, also known as pulmonary inhalation, is perhaps the fastest way to get a drug into the bloodstream and brain. Smoking crack produces a nearly instantaneous, extremely intense, but very brief high that lasts only several minutes after each "hit" or inhalation of the cocaine vapors from the crack pipe into the lungs. The rapid onset and offset of its intense euphoric effects contribute to the markedly increased addiction potential of smoking crack as compared with snorting co-caine powder. Another factor contributing to the rapid development of addic-tion with crack is the greater intensity of the crash following the drug-induced high. Intense euphoria, followed immediately by intense dysphoria and drug cravings, compels the crack smoker to return to the euphoric state as quickly as possible. Crack is not a stronger drug pharmacologically than cocaine powder; its greater impact is attributable entirely to the fact that it can be used by a more efficient route of drug administration—smoking. Smoking crack, as compared with snorting cocaine powder, not only is associated with more rapid progression from initial to full-blown addiction, but also leads to more severe disturbance in mood, mental state, and cognitive functioning, in-cluding drug-induced depression, paranoia, and attention deficits.

Intensive binge patterns of use are more common among crack smok-ers than cocaine snorters. Crack smokers may go on marathon binges last-ing several days, during which time they consume large quantities of the drug costing large sums of money, often in the hundreds or thousands of dollars. Usually the binge goes on until the user runs out of drug supplies or money or collapses from physical exhaustion. It is important to note that although the effects and consequences of smoking crack are often more dramatic than those of snorting cocaine powder, intranasal use of cocaine is by no means safe or self-limiting as previously thought prior to the emer-gence of the cocaine epidemic in the 1980s. Repeated cocaine use by any route of administration can lead to addiction and other adverse health and psychosocial consequences.

Methamphetamine

Commonly known on the street as speed, crank, crystal, or meth, metham-phetamine is a powerful stimulant drug made easily in clandestine labora-tories from relatively inexpensive and readily available over-the-counter ingredients. Use of methamphetamine was previously seen primarily on the West Coast and in Hawaii, but more recently has spread to the Midwest, South, and Northeast regions of the United States. Crystal methamphet-amine is significantly less expensive than cocaine, but its effects are longer lasting. It can be snorted, swallowed, or dissolved in water and injected intravenously. It can also be converted to a hard crystalline form known as "ice," which can be smoked. Like cocaine, methamphetamine causes the accumulation of the neurotransmitter dopamine in selected brain areas, which gives rise to the intense stimulation and feelings of euphoria experi-enced by the user. Unlike cocaine, which is quickly removed and almost completely metabolized in the body, methamphetamine has a much longer duration of action, and a larger percentage of the drug remains unchanged in the body, which ultimately leads to prolonged stimulant effects. Whereas 50% of cocaine is removed from the body within 1 hour, 50% of methamphetamine is removed within 12 hours. Smoking cocaine produces a high that lasts a number of minutes, but smoking methamphetamine produces a high lasting 6–8 hours. The effects of methamphetamine include increased activity, decreased appetite, and an agitated excitement that may resemble a manic episode. Chronic use can lead to stimulant-induced psychosis, marked agitation, and violent behavior. In terms of sexual effects, it has been noted that drug-induced hypersexuality is more intense and longer lasting with methamphetamine as compared with cocaine. In addition, tolerance to methamphetamine's aphrodisiac effects appears to develop more slowly, and in some cases not at all, as compared with such tolerance to cocaine, and impairment of sexual functioning is much less likely to occur as a result of chronic methamphetamine use. Accordingly, the extent of drug-related hypersexuality and sexual acting-out behaviors associated with methamphetamine use appear to be much greater than those associated with comparable levels of cocaine use.

Like cocaine, methamphetamine is often used in a "binge and crash" pattern, but the crash and rebound depression from methamphetamine is typically much more severe. Moreover, sleep following a binge of methamphetamine use can last for several days, and the drug-induced depression for several weeks. As with cocaine use, no pharmacologic interventions have been found to be effective in alleviating post-drug dysphoria or cravings following methamphetamine use. In light of methamphetamine's extraordinarily potent stimulant effects, its physiological impact and thus its potential medical consequences can be profound. Methamphetamine can cause a variety of cardiovascular problems. It markedly increases heart rate and blood pressure and can cause life-threatening cardiac arrhythmias and stroke-producing damage to small blood vessels in the brain. Hyperthermia (elevated body temperature) and convulsions can occur with methamphetamine overdoses, resulting in rapid death if not treated.

Prescription Stimulants

A variety of prescription stimulant drugs are available for treating medical conditions, including narcolepsy, obesity, and attention deficit disorder, and sometimes as adjunctive medication for treatment-resistant depressive disorders. Methylphenidate (Ritalin) is often the treatment of first choice for attention-deficit/hyperactivity disorder (ADHD). Dexedrine, dextroamphetamine (Adderall), and pemoline (Cylert) are more potent stimulants and thus used less often for treating ADHD, especially in children. The overprescribing of these medications for high school and college students has created a widespread illicit market for diverted supplies of various stimulant drugs on school campuses, especially Ritalin and Adderall.

Modafinil (Provigil) is used to improve wakefulness in individuals with narcolepsy. The use of stimulant drugs to treat depression and obesity remains controversial. Although the use of these medications does not lead inevitably to SUDs if managed properly by a responsible physician, stimulants are not likely to provide efficacious long-term treatment for either depression or obesity. Tolerance to their appetite suppressant effects develops very quickly. Often these medications provide time-limited benefits, which are eventually overshadowed by the risks.

The types of problems associated with repeated use of cocaine or methamphetamine can also occur with any of the aforementioned prescription stimulants, including tolerance, dependence, mood disorders, paranoia, cravings, psychotic symptoms, violent behavior, and medical consequences commonly associated with chronic use of stimulant drugs.

Caffeine

Caffeine is the most widely used central nervous system stimulant worldwide. Unlike the other stimulant drugs discussed thus far, caffeine is not associated with gross changes in behavior and affect and rarely causes significant impairment in psychosocial functioning except in individuals who are unusually sensitive to its effects. It is interesting to note that prior to its widespread acceptance, caffeine too was considered a dangerous habit-forming drug.

Caffeine diminishes drowsiness and fatigue and can sometimes increase mental acuity and performance on certain types of tasks. Large doses can produce excitement, restlessness, anxiety, and insomnia. Caffeine increases heart rate, blood pressure, and the force of contractions of the heart. Mild tolerance to caffeine develops at low doses. Significant tolerance and physical dependence can occur with repeated use of high doses (i.e., above 600 milligrams caffeine per day). The caffeine withdrawal syndrome is characterized by headache, irritability, restlessness, lethargy, and yawning.

Coffee contains 80–140 milligrams of caffeine per cup, as compared with 60–100 milligrams per cup for tea and 25–55 milligrams per glass for cola beverages and other caffeinated soft drinks. Nearly 100 different over-the-counter preparations contain caffeine-type stimulants. Other sources of caffeine include chocolate and a variety of prescription drugs.

Individuals with a history of addiction to stimulant drugs such as cocaine and methamphetamine are often encouraged by addiction counselors to refrain completely from consuming caffeine-containing beverages and foods. This recommendation is based on concerns that the stimulant effects of caffeine may elicit cravings for an individual's prior stimulant drug of choice. No empirical work has been done to confirm or refute this recommendation. Psychiatric contraindications for caffeine use include panic disorder and bipolar disorder. Medical contraindications include cardiovascular problems, particularly arrhythmias; prior stroke or ischemic attacks; gastrointestinal disorder and peptic ulcer disease.

Opioids (Narcotics)

Opiates are drugs derived directly from opium found in the poppy plant (*Papaver somniferum*). Morphine and codeine, for example, are opiates. Opioids is a more encompassing category that includes the opiates (i.e., opium derivatives) as well as (1) the semisynthetic narcotics such as diacetyl morphine (heroin), hydrocodone (Vicodin), and oxycodone (Percoset, OxyContin) which are produced by chemically altering the opiate derivates, and (2) the synthetic narcotics such as meperidine (Demerol), propoxyphene (Darvon), methadone (Dolophine), and fentanyl (Duragesic), which are synthesized entirely in the laboratory. All opioids produce a constellation of physiological and subjective effects similar to those of morphine. The most prominent pharmacological effect of opioids and the primary basis for the medical usefulness of these drugs is analgesia, or pain relief. They are also used medically as adjuncts to anesthesia and for cough suppression. The various opioids differ from one another in terms of oral absorption rates, lipid solubility, analgesic potency, duration of action, and rate of metabolism. Half-lives of opioids range from just a few minutes for heroin to as long as 30 hours for methadone.

Opioid use has been known to have occurred throughout recorded human history, dating back to references to "poppy juice" in the third century B.C. Smoking opium was widespread during the late part of the 19th century and early part of the 20th century in the United States among Chinese immigrants, but it was the invention of the hypodermic needle, combined with the use of morphine to treat wounded Civil War soldiers, that appears to have contributed most heavily to the eventual development of intravenous opioid addiction as a major public health problem in the United States.

Opioids are by far the most effective pain relieving agents. In fact, when taken in sufficient doses, these drugs provide extraordinary relief not only from somatic pain, but from emotional or psychic pain as well. People who become addicted to opioids often report being emotionally numb and unable to feel upset while on opioids, which appears to be the drug's primary reinforcing effect. Opioids produce feelings of euphoria or well-being, improved mood, decreased anxiety, and decreased anticipation, worry, and concern. Even when tolerance to the euphoria develops as use continues, the emotion-numbing effects of these drugs often remains intact. Interestingly, opioids can also have significant antipsychotic effects, although no opioid medication has ever been approved for this indication (Verebey, 1982).

The intensity of the opioid-induced euphoria or "rush" depends largely on the route of drug administration. As with other types of psychoactive drugs, the most intense rapid-onset euphoria is produced by intravenous administration and smoking, whereas intranasal and oral administration produce much slower and less intense effects. Heroin is usually administered intravenously, but it is the only opioid that also can be snorted or smoked—increasingly popular ways to use heroin that have increased the drug's popularity, especially among middle-class users who refuse to consider taking any drug by intravenous injection.

The acute physiological effects of opioids include papillary constriction (meiosis), slowed respiration, reduced gastrointestinal motility resulting in constipation, and in some cases nausea and vomiting. The mechanism of death caused by opioid overdose is respiratory arrest. Opioids can have opposite effects on energy level and mental state in different individuals. Whereas some individuals experience drowsiness, mental confusion, and lethargy, others experience increased energy, increased productivity, particularly in regard to performing tedious or unpleasant tasks (e.g., cleaning, paying bills), and difficulty in sleeping. Opioids are generally not toxic to the human body, and most of the major medical illnesses associated with chronic opioid use are attributable to lack of adequate self-care, including poor nutrition, unprotected sex, and the use of nonsterile injection apparatus, which contributes to the spread of HIV, hepatitis, and other serious infections.

As use continues, all opioids produce tolerance, requiring increasing doses to achieve the same effects, and physical dependence characterized by a well-defined withdrawal syndrome in the absence of the drug. The classic signs and symptoms of acute opioid withdrawal include runny nose (rhinorrhea), tearing eyes (lacrimation), dilated pupils (mydriasis), sweating (diaphoresis), yawning, "goose flesh" (piloerection), chills, diarrhea, vomiting, insomnia, stomach cramps, loss of appetite, low energy, irritability, and agitated restlessness. The acute symptoms of opioid withdrawal are often likened to having a flu. The onset and time course of the withdrawal syndrome depend to a large extent on the half-life of the particular opioid on which the individual is dependent. For example, heroin withdrawal begins within several hours after the last dose and reaches peak intensity within 36 hours, whereas methadone withdrawal does not begin until approximately 24 hours after the last dose and then peaks at approximately 72–96 hours. In addition to the acute withdrawal symptoms, which usually subside within a week or two, long-term opioid dependence often results in a variety of withdrawal symptoms that linger for many months, often referred to as the protracted or post-acute withdrawal syndrome (PAWS). These lingering symptoms may include low energy, insomnia, depressed mood, deep muscle aches and pains, irritability, and anhedonia. Such symptoms can make it very difficult to distinguish whether the patient is experiencing a protracted abstinence syndrome or a coexisting mood disorder, as discussed more fully in Chapter 5.

All opioids exhibit cross-tolerance. Accordingly, all drugs in the opioid class produce similar physiological effects and all can block the withdrawal syndrome if taken in equivalent doses. Medical detoxification or withdrawal from opioids is usually accomplished by switching patients from their opioid drug of choice to a longer-acting opioid (e.g., methadone or buprenophine) and then gradually tapering them off the substitute medication in order to minimize the intensity of the withdrawal syndrome. Patients with low levels of opioid dependence typically are not detoxified using methadone for fear of increasing rather than decreasing their levels of dependence with this potent opioid. Instead, they are more likely to be treated with clonidine, a non-opioid medication that reduces opioid withdrawal symptoms.

Pharmacological adjuncts used in treating opioid dependence include methadone and buprenorphine for opioid maintenance (substitution) therapy (discussed in Chapter 6) and naltrexone, an opioid antagonist, to help prevent relapse. Opioid antagonists are medications that block the effects of opioids at the level of the opioid receptor. When naltrexone molecules are attached to opioid receptors in the brain and other sites in the central nervous system, the effects of all morphine-like opioid drugs are completely blocked. Under these conditions, taking an opioid drug will not produce euphoria or any other opioid-like psychoactive effects, nor will it depress respiration or have any other opioid-like physiological effects. The short-acting opioid antagonist, naloxone, is used in emergency medicine to revive comatose patients from a narcotic overdose, whereas the longer-acting antagonist, naltrexone, is used to prevent relapse by maintaining the blockade of opioid effects following detoxification. A daily 50-milligram dose of naltrexone blocks opioid effects for approximately 24 hours. Naltrexone is not a cure or stand-alone treatment for opioid addiction, but it can be an extremely valuable component of a more comprehensive treatment approach that includes appropriate psychosocial interventions.

Marijuana and Other Cannabinoids

Marijuana and other cannabinoids are derived from the *Cannabis sativa* (hemp) plant. Most of the psychoactive effects of cannabinoids are due to the substance delta-9-tetrahydrocannabinol (THC), although other psychoactive chemicals also exist in the plant. The potency of various cannabinoids can vary widely. Marijuana has a THC content of 1–5%. Hashish, which is harvested from resin at the top of mature plants, can have a THC content of 10%. Hashish oil, a highly concentrated form of the drug, can have a THC content as high as 15–30%.

Marijuana is usually smoked, but can also be taken orally with diminished effects. Smoking marijuana produces fairly rapid changes in mood, time sense, memory, and other aspects of brain function. The most desired effects are a sense of euphoria, relaxation, and overall well-being. Many users experience enhanced sensations, including increased sensitivity to tastes, sounds (especially music), light, and colors. Other effects include giddiness and increased appetite, particularly for sweets (known as "the munchies"). Not surprisingly, weight gain is a common byproduct of chronic marijuana use. Short-term memory is impaired by marijuana. The most obvious evidence of this impairment occurs when a conversation between two marijuana smokers becomes disjointed because one or both people forget what they have been talking about in the middle of the conversation—a frequent stimulus for hysterical laughter. Marijuana also alters a person's sense of time. Time passes by more slowly; minutes may seem like hours. Some people experience severe thought disruption with hallucinations and delusions, although these effects are uncommon except at extremely high doses. Performance on simple motor tasks is generally unimpaired, but driving performance is noticeably impaired at high doses.

Some people experience profound dysphoria from marijuana, which may include panic anxiety with feelings of impending doom, paranoia, and a sense of unreality. Research evidence indicates that marijuana exacerbates depression in those who are prone to it. New users who experience these extremely unpleasant effects are not likely to continue using the drug. However, sometimes these effects occur in experienced users who had previously enjoyed the marijuana high. At present, there is no explanation for this apparent unexpected reversal of psychoactive effects.

Concern has grown over the years about deficits in attention and motivation associated with chronic marijuana use, especially in adolescents and young adults. These deficits may be both accompanied and exacerbated by marijuana-induced depression as evidenced by symptoms such as negative moods, pessimism, blunted affect, and social withdrawal.

The physiological effects of marijuana include tachycardia (rapid heartbeat), bloodshot eyes, dry mouth, and slightly elevated blood pressure. There is no scientific evidence supporting earlier claims that marijuana causes birth defects or suppresses immune function. There is conflicting evidence regarding marijuana's effects on sex hormones, sperm count/motility in males, and fertility in females. Chronic smoking of marijuana can impair pulmonary functioning, similar to chronic smoking of tobacco. Furthermore, the tar produced by marijuana smoking is known to be carcinogenic.

Two medical uses for marijuana have been identified, although there is still a good deal of controversy surrounding this issue. One medical use is to counteract the intense nausea caused by anticancer drugs used for chemotherapy. The other is to reduce intraocular pressure caused by glaucoma.

THC distributes rapidly into lipoid (fat) tissues throughout the body, followed by a much slower elimination phase. Because THC is excreted slowly from fat cells, it can be detected in urine for up to 40 days after last use in chronic users.

Tolerance to some of marijuana's effects develops with repeated use, although regular use of relatively low doses does not appear to diminish the euphoria and other desirable psychoactive effects. Long-term heavy use, however, leads to the development of substantial tolerance, requiring increasingly higher doses to achieve the same or similar effects. As with other psychoactive drugs, a point is often reached where the chronic user is unable to achieve the desired effects no matter how large a dose is used. A small but significant number of long-term heavy users experience withdrawal symptoms such as insomnia, irritability, and restlessness when use is discontinued abruptly. No medication is indicated for treating these symptoms, which usually subside without intervention in a few days. Interestingly, as compared with people using alcohol and/or other addictive drugs, relatively few marijuana users ever seek treatment. This may be due partly to the extraordinarily long latency that often occurs between initiation of marijuana use and the development of significant psychosocial impairment. Many people smoke marijuana for decades without exhibiting noticeable evidence of impairment. It may also be due to the fact that signs of marijuana intoxication and drug-altered behavior typically are not as dramatic as those of other drugs. Alcohol, for example, produces rather obvious signs of intoxication (slurred speech, unsteady gait, etc.) when taken in sufficient doses. The same can be said of other central nervous system depressants as well as cocaine and opioids. Marijuana users often "fly below the radar" in terms of showing detectible signs of intoxication and other changes in affect and/or behavior.

Therapists are often in a quandary about how to deal with marijuana-using patients they are treating for other types of mental health problems. For example, some patients report that they use marijuana infrequently or "recreationally" without the use of other substances. Others report that they use marijuana regularly but in a controlled manner, similar to the way some people drink moderate amounts of alcohol in the evening after work and/or in social situations on weekends. Still others report that when they use marijuana they are less likely to use other drugs that have caused them serious problems in the past. A common theme in all of these cases is that the individual views marijuana use as distinctly helpful rather than harmful and accordingly is likely to be highly reluctant or completely unwilling to give it up. As discussed in greater detail in subsequent chapters of this book, the therapist's first task is to conduct a thorough clinical assessment to determine the nature, extent, and related consequences of the patient's use of marijuana and other substances as a necessary step before deciding how best to intervene. Motivational interviewing and counseling techniques (also discussed latter in this book) can be especially helpful in dealing with marijuana users who express no desire to change their drug-using behavior. Sometimes the motivation for stopping or significantly curtailing marijuana use emanates from a recognition that marijuana actually exacerbates rather than alleviates the problems that led the patient to seek help in the first place. For example, the therapist can help patients suffering from depression to realize that even occasional use of marijuana can exacerbate depressive symptoms and counteract the therapeutic benefit of antidepressant medication.

LSD and Other Hallucinogens

LSD (lysergic acid diethylamide) is a hallucinogenic drug associated with the psychedelic culture of the 1960s. After fading from the drug scene for many years, LSD and other hallucinogens have made a strong comeback since the 1990s. Most users are white male adolescents and young adults. Other hallucinogens include mescaline, derived from Mexican cactus, and psilocybin, found in certain types of mushrooms. LSD is much more popular and readily available in the United States than either of these two other drugs.

LSD is ingested by chewing or eating a small tab of paper ("blotter acid") on which the drug has been sprayed. The effects of LSD appear within 30–40 minutes after ingestion of extremely small doses (50 micrograms or less). The effects of a single dose may last for 8–12 hours. Psychoactive effects include perceptual distortions, usually involving altered shapes and colors, disorientation of time sense, difficulty in focusing on specific stimuli, labile mood, depersonalization, and mild sedation. Despite its classification as a hallucinogen, LSD rarely if ever produces frank hallucinations in terms of causing the user to see or hear things that actually are not there. Perceptual distortions, rather than hallucinations, are common effects of LSD. Physiological effects are few and typically unremarkable. These may include mild to moderate increases in blood pressure, heart rate, and body temperature. Tolerance develops quickly with the use of LSD, but dissipates within a week or so without any withdrawal syndrome. Episodic use of LSD is much more common than daily use.

The adverse effects of LSD include panic anxiety, usually caused by intense fear that one has lost touch with reality and will never return to a normal mental state; LSD-induced psychosis, which may last even after the acute drug effects have subsided, and a phenomenon known as "flashbacks" or hallucinogen persisting perception disorder (HPPD), consisting of unexpected reoccurrences of LSD-like experiences (e.g., perceptual distortions) long after the drug was last used. There is evidence that LSD causes acute alterations in brain neurotransmitters, especially in serotonin, but more persistent or permanent changes have not been documented. Despite earlier claims that LSD causes genetic (chromosomal) damage and birth defects, there is no scientific evidence to support these claims.

"Club" Drugs, PCP, and Inhalants

The so-called "club" or "party" drugs include a wide variety of psychoactive agents, many of which have little in common with one another except for the particular circumstances under which they are used and, in some cases, the fact that they are volatile substances taken by inhalation. The term "club drugs" has been applied to several different drugs that are used most frequently at dance clubs, after-hours clubs, all-night dances, concerts, and bars. Most users of these drugs are adolescents and young adults, although age is not a barrier to use. MDMA (Ecstasy), GHB, and ketamine are some of the club drugs whose popularity has risen markedly in recent years. Because many of these drugs are manufactured illegally, their strength and purity are variable and unpredictable. The vast majority of people who use club drugs feel that these agents are nontoxic and nonaddictive. It is rare for them to seek treatment for problems related to these substances. Although tolerance and withdrawal phenomena have been observed in some users, the occurrence and intensity of such phenomena are highly variable between individuals. There is little doubt, however, that with increasing use of these drugs some individuals develop a strong need or compulsion to repeat the drug-induced experience, even when faced with increasingly negative effects.

MDMA (Ecstasy)

MDMA (3, 4-methylenedioxymethamphetamine) is similar in chemical structure to the central nervous system stimulant methamphetamine and to the hallucinogen mescaline. Accordingly, it can produce both stimulant and hallucinogenic effects. MDMA's hallucinogenic effects are reportedly much milder than those of LSD and mescaline. The drug is most often available in tablet form and ingested orally. The usual pattern of MDMA use is episodic and situation specific. Daily or compulsive use is rare, and there is no evidence that physical dependence develops with repeated use.

MDMA (Ecstasy) stimulates the release of serotonin from brain neurons, producing a drug-induced high that lasts from several minutes to hours. The drug's psychoactive effects vary with the individual taking it, the dose and purity of the drug, and the environment in which is taken. Combining MDMA with other drugs such as alcohol and/or cocaine can markedly alter both the nature and the intensity of the high. MDMA can produce stimulant effects such as an enhanced energy, self-confidence, and sociability. Other effects include feelings of closeness with others, peacefulness, and empathy. Adverse psychoactive effects include confusion, depression, insomnia, anxiety, and paranoia, which can last several days or weeks after taking the drug. Physiological effects include muscle tension, teeth clenching, nausea, blurred vision, faintness, chills, and sweating. MDMA-related deaths have been reported. These do not appear to be the direct result of the drug, but of poor ventilation and insufficient water intake in many dance club environments, leading to malignant hyperthermia. The stimulant effects of MDMA, which enable users to dance vigorously and incessantly for long periods of time, can lead to dehydration, hypertension, and heart or kidney failure, especially when combined with large amounts of alcohol. There is also evidence that MDMA can be neurotoxic, leading to long-lasting and perhaps permanent impairment of memory and other brain functions.

GHB (Gamma-Hydroxybutyrate)

GHB (gamma-hydroxybutyrate) is often called "G" or "liquid Ecstasy," although chemically it is unrelated to MDMA. The drug is used primarily by adolescents and young adults. GHB is often manufactured in homes according to recipes available on the Internet, using ingredients purchased through health food stores or available in dietary supplements. GHB can be produced as a clear liquid, white powder, tablet, or capsule. It is often combined with alcohol. GHB is a central nervous system depressant. At low to moderate doses it can relieve anxiety, produce relaxation, and increase sociability. However, as the dose increases, the sedative effects induce sleep and eventually lead to coma and death. Alcohol increases the likelihood of a fatal overdose reaction. The intoxicating effects of GHB begin 10–20 minutes after the drug is taken and typically last several hours, depending on the dose. It is cleared rapidly from the body, making it difficult to detect in blood or urine.

Ketamine

Known on the street as "Special K," ketamine is an injectable anesthetic drug that has been used medically in both humans and animals since the early 1970s. Most of the ketamine legally manufactured and sold in the United States is intended for veterinary use. Ketamine is produced legally in liquid form for injection and otherwise sold on the street as a white powder that is either snorted or smoked with tobacco or marijuana. At low to moderate doses, ketamine produces a euphoric feeling described by some users as "floating." It can also distort perceptions of sight and sound and produce a trance-like state of detachment or dissociation from the environment. At higher doses, it produces delirium, amnesia, agitation, and impaired motor coordination. Fatal overdose reactions can occur as a result of drug-induced respiratory failure.

PCP (Phencyclidine)

The effects of PCP (phencyclidine) are remarkably similar to those of ketamine, although PCP is much more potent and has a longer duration of action. Like ketamine, PCP is a dissociative anesthetic that induces a trance-like state and feelings of being "out of body" or detached from the environment. PCP has been used as an anesthetic in veterinary medicine, but never approved for use in humans because of the adverse reactions that arose during clinical trials, including extreme agitation and dysphoria experienced by patients emerging from anesthesia. Powdered PCP is illegally manufactured in laboratories and sold on the street by such names as "angel dust," "dust," "boat," and "rocket fuel." The powder is usually sprinkled on marijuana or tobacco and then smoked. The effects of PCP can be bizarre and volatile. Users report feelings of detachment from reality; distortions in time, space, and body image; and sometimes hallucinations, panic, and intense fear. Some report feelings of invulnerability and increased physical strength. PCP users may become severely disoriented, violent, or suicidal. Under the influence of PCP, speech is often sparse and garbled. Repeated use of PCP can produce dependence, characterized by cravings, inability to control use, and compulsive drug-seeking behavior. Many PCP users are brought to emergency rooms because of overdose reactions and/or the drug's dysphoric effects.

Considering the wide variety of psychoactive drugs available today, it is difficult to understand why some users choose PCP. Rarely if ever do users of PCP report experiencing a distinctly pleasant drug-induced euphoria. To the contrary, most report distinctly negative and even terrifying effects of PCP on their mood and mental state. Many users of PCP find their attraction to the drug difficult to understand and often are surprised by their compulsion to use the drug repeatedly. The reinforcing effects of PCP seem to consist mainly of the total escape into unreality and the "mind-numbing" effects caused by the drug.

Inhalants

Inhalants are volatile substances that produce chemical vapors that can be inhaled to induce psychoactive mood-altering effects. These drugs are rarely, if ever, taken by any route of administration other than inhalation. The use of inhalants is most prevalent among young people.

The category of inhalants encompasses a wide variety of chemicals with different pharmacological effects, including organic solvents and aerosol propellants found in household products, nitrites found in room deodorizers and anesthetics, and nitrous oxide gas. The wide disparity between drugs in this category foils attempts to generalize their pharmacological properties and effects. Most inhalants produce rapid onset of an intense but very brief burst of euphoria, often manifested as giddy intoxication. The most prevalent pharmacological effect of inhalant drugs is central nervous system depression. At low to moderate doses inhalant drugs typically evoke disinhibiting effects similar to those of alcohol, but of greater intensity and shorter duration inasmuch as inhaled chemicals are rapidly absorbed into the bloodstream and quickly distributed to the brain and other organs. Other alcohol-like effects may include slurred speech, dizziness, and impaired motor coordination. Because the intoxication lasts only a few minutes, inhalant users frequently seek to prolong the high by continuing to inhale repeatedly over the course of several hours, a very dangerous practice because of the increased risk of suffering loss of consciousness and death. After repeated doses of inhalants, users often feel drowsy for several hours and may experience a lingering headache. As with the club drugs described earlier, tolerance and withdrawal phenomena have been observed in some inhalant users, but the occurrence and intensity of these phenomena are highly variable between individuals. Similarly, with increasing use of inhalants some individuals develop a strong need or compulsion to repeat the drug-induced experience, sometimes despite increasingly adverse effects. No medications are indicated for treatment of inhalant abuse or dependence.

Nitrous oxide (also known as "laughing gas") is the most widely abused of the inhalant gases. It can be found in whipped cream dispensers fitted with cartridges containing pressurized nitrous oxide gas used as a propellant. These cartridges, known as "whippets," can be purchased in grocery and party supply stores. Typically, users discharge the pressurized gas from a cartridge into a balloon or plastic bag, from which the nitrous oxide is then inhaled. Nitrous oxide is used medically as a sedative and anesthetic in dental procedures and for minor surgery. Dentists and oral surgeons have easy access to supplies of nitrous oxide and administer it routinely to patients in the course of their daily work. Not surprisingly, many of these professionals experiment with nitrous oxide and some end up using it compulsively.

Nitrites are considered a special class of inhalants because, unlike other drugs in this category, they act directly on the central nervous system to dilate blood vessels and relax muscles. Whereas other inhalants are used primarily to induce euphoria, nitrates are used primarily as sexual enhancers. Use of these drugs is associated with unsafe sexual practices that can greatly increase the risk of contracting and spreading infections such as HIV and hepatitis. (Because nitrites relax the sphincter muscle, they are often used by gay men to facilitate anal intercourse.) Nitrites increase heart rate and produce a flushed sensation of heat, excitement, and lightheadedness that lasts several minutes. The most popular nitrites are amyl nitrite and butyl nitrite. These drugs can come packaged in small sealed glass tubes that are snapped open to release the drug vapors for inhalation. Accordingly, these drugs are often referred to as "snappers" or "poppers." They are more commonly available in liquid form sold in small bottles. The vapors from the liquid are inhaled directly and repeatedly from the bottle.

Nicotine

Nicotine is in a drug category by itself. The most important psychoactive chemical in tobacco, nicotine has psychoactive effects that are complex, subtle, variable, and thus difficult to characterize. Some people report that smoking helps them to concentrate and sustain attention. Others claim that it helps them to relax and feel less anxious. Tobacco use is not associated with slurred speech and other signs of intoxication commonly seen with alcohol and other sedative-type drugs. Similarly, tobacco does not induce the profound euphoria, elevation of mood, and increased alertness characteristic of stimulant drugs. However difficult it may be to characterize nicotine's psychoactive effects, it is clear that nicotine is addictive; an enormous number of people use tobacco products, and the health consequences of chronic tobacco use are staggering. Currently, an estimated 25% of adults in the United States smoke tobacco. Tobacco kills more than 430,000 U.S. citizens each year—more than alcohol, cocaine, heroin, homicide, suicide, car accidents, fire, and AIDS combined. Tobacco use is the leading preventable cause of death in the United States.

Nicotine, one of more than 4,000 chemicals found in the smoke from tobacco products such as cigarettes, cigars, and pipes, is the primary psychoactive substance in tobacco that acts on the brain. Smokeless tobacco products such as snuff and chewing tobacco also contain many toxins, as well as high levels of nicotine. Nicotine is recognized as one of the most frequently used addictive drugs; it is a naturally occurring colorless liquid that turns brown when burned and acquires the odor of tobacco when exposed to air. There are many species of tobacco plants; the *tabacum* species serves as the major source of tobacco products today. Since nicotine was first identified in the early 1800s, it has been studied extensively and shown to have a number of complex and sometimes unpredictable effects on the brain and the body.

Cigarette smoking is the most prevalent form of nicotine addiction in the United States. Most cigarettes in the U.S. market today contain 10 milligrams or more of nicotine. Through inhaling smoke, the average smoker takes in 1–2 milligrams of nicotine per cigarette. There have been substantial increases in the sale and consumption of smokeless tobacco products also, and more recently, in cigar sales.Nicotine is absorbed through the skin and mucosal lining of the mouth and nose or by inhalation in the lungs. Depending on how tobacco is taken, nicotine can reach peak levels in the bloodstream and brain rapidly. Cigarette smoking, for example, results in rapid distribution of nicotine throughout the body, reaching the brain within 10 seconds of inhalation.

Cigar and pipe smokers, however, typically do not inhale the smoke, so nicotine is absorbed more slowly through the mucosal membranes of their mouths. Nicotine from smokeless tobacco is also absorbed through the mucosal membranes.

Nicotine is unquestionably addictive. Most smokers use tobacco regularly because they are dependent on nicotine. Considering that addiction is characterized by compulsive drug-seeking and use, even in the face of negative health consequences, tobacco use certainly fits the description. It is well documented that most smokers identify tobacco as harmful and express a desire to reduce or stop using it, and nearly 35 million of them make a serious attempt to quit each year. Unfortunately, less than 7% of those who try to quit on their own achieve more than 1 year of abstinence; most relapse within a few days of attempting to quit. Other factors to consider in addition to nicotine's addictive properties include its high level of availability, the small number of legal and social consequences of tobacco use, and the sophisticated marketing and advertising methods used by tobacco companies. These factors, combined with nicotine's addictive properties, often serve as determinants for first use and, ultimately, addiction.

Traditionally, nicotine dependence has not been included in discussions about alcohol and other drug addictions. Like caffeine, nicotine is not associated with gross changes in behavior, personality, and affect. Nor has it been known to cause significant impairment of psychosocial, cognitive, or motor functioning. Not surprisingly, smoking cessation programs and other treatments for nicotine dependence have not been part of mainstream treatment for other chemical addictions. Similarly, mental health practitioners who specialize in treating alcohol and other drug addictions often have little or no experience in treating nicotine dependence. However, this situation has been changing in recent years with the growing recognition of a strong association between nicotine and other chemical addictions (Fertig & Allen, 1995). Tobacco dependence is especially common among people who abuse alcohol and other drugs. As compared with an estimated prevalence of 25% in the general adult population in the United States, the prevalence of nicotine dependence in substance-dependent patients has been reported to be upwards of 85%. Not only do alcohol-dependent persons smoke more heavily than their non-dependent counterparts, but they are also less likely to succeed in attempts to achieve abstinence from smoking. Tobacco-related illnesses are the leading cause of death in patients previously treated for alcohol and other drug addictions.

Despite an apparently strong association between nicotine and other drug dependencies, incorporating smoking cessation into substance abuse treatment programs has been slow at best and continues to be somewhat controversial. Addiction treatment programs have been reluctant to target patients' concurrent nicotine dependence owing to concerns that doing so would impose additional demands and discomfort on patients that could increase dropout rates and reduce treatment effectiveness. Many programs fear that asking patients to give up cigarettes at the same time as alcohol and drugs might be asking too much. There are also concerns that making smoking cessation a standard feature of substance abuse treatment programs could diminish the attractiveness of these programs to prospective patients, particularly those who are not ready to stop smoking. Despite these understandable concerns, however, several studies have demonstrated favorable patient acceptance and promising benefits of implementing concurrent interventions for tobacco use and other substance dependencies (Fiore et al., 2000).

FINAL COMMENT

Psychotherapists need to have both a clinical and an intuitive understanding of psychoactive drugs. This knowledge is essential not only for diagnosis and treatment planning, but also to establish credibility with patients. It is important for therapists to know more about the pharmacology and use of the various psychoactive drugs than their patients do. Psychoactive drugs are a unique class of chemical agents that affect brain function and behavior in complex ways. The mood-altering and other effects of these drugs are not absolute, but rather depend on a number of different variables. All drug effects are dose dependent and vary significantly, depending on route of administration, frequency and chronicity of use, presence of other substances, the physical and psychological state of the user, and the setting and circumstances in which use occurs. The different categories of psychoactive drugs discussed in this chapter have one fundamental feature in common: they all produce changes in mood and mental state experienced as reinforcing enough by large numbers of individuals to warrant repeating. Sometimes the reinforcing effects of these drugs are so powerful that they propel vulnerable users into patterns of habitual and compulsive use. The desire for chemical mood alteration is not *de facto*, pathological (Milkman & Sunderwirth, 1987). Rather, it appears to be fundamentally human as evidenced by the fact that use of psychoactive substances (derived mainly from plants) has existed in virtually all cultures throughout recorded human history (Siegel, 1989). Drug abuse and addiction are not inevitable outcomes of experimenting with psychoactive substances. Certain historical developments have contributed to increasing prevalence of these problems worldwide. Chief among these are the appearance of purified and artificially synthesized drugs many times more potent than the naturally occurring varieties; rapid methods for delivering drugs to the brain (e.g., intravenous injection), and, certain cultural influences that heighten the appeal of a "quick fix" escape from the unpleasant realities of daily life (Washton & Boundy, 1989). The drive to change one's mood instantly regardless of the qualitative nature of that change from the pre-drug state appears more potent than the desire to experience euphoria per se. This is clearly evidenced by the compulsive repetitive use of dissociative hallucinogens such as PCP and ketamine which often induce delusions and hallucinations that terrify the user.

CHAPTER 4

Ingredients of the Integrated Approach

Doing What Works

Our integrated approach to treating SUDs has evolved over many years of working with patients in both institutional settings and office practice. Although studies on the treatment of SUDs have demonstrated convincingly that no one method of treatment is better than all others, the addiction field continues to be split into opposing factions, each claiming superiority of its own approach. Our clinical experiences have taught us to steer clear of any dogmatic approach claiming to be the single best method for treating SUDs. We are by no means the first to acknowledge or write about the importance of a more flexible, integrated approach (e.g., Kaufman, 1994; Margolis & Zweben, 1998; Shaffer & Gambino, 1990), but the addiction treatment system at large has been slow to move beyond rigid adherence to the disease model and heavy reliance on confrontational tactics. Although in recent years motivational and other client-centered approaches have been incorporated increasingly into addiction treatment programs in both the public and private sectors, a welcomed change indeed, many individuals who make contact with traditional treatment programs still encounter an inflexible, "one size fits all" approach.

The integrated approach described here neither requires nor recommends adherence to one conceptual model or method of treatment. To the contrary, this approach is nondogmatic and encourages clinicians to exercise creativity, flexibility, and reasonableness in treating SUDs as they would in addressing other types of mental health problems. The approach is integrated in the sense that it blends together many seemingly disparate and competing treatment approaches, including 12-step oriented addiction counseling, supportive psychotherapy, cognitive-behavioral therapy, Rogerian client-centered therapy, psychodynamic insight-oriented therapy, motivation enhancement therapy, harm reduction therapy, interpersonal therapy, patient education, and pharmacotherapy—all of which are brought together to meet the individual and changing needs of patients at different stages of treatment.

We view abstinence as the preferred treatment goal, especially for patients whose pattern of substance use provides clear evidence of impaired control and poses significant risk of serious harm if use continues. Nonetheless, we do not mandate abstinence or make it a precondition for patients to receive our help. And we do not convey disappointment or disapproval to those who do not choose abstinence as their goal. Developing individualized treatment goals as part of engaging patients "where they are" is an essential aspect of the integrated approach, as discussed more fully in Chapter 8.

In the discussion that follows we describe certain ingredients and distinguishing features of the integrated approach: (1) the centrality of the therapeutic relationship; (2) application of the stages-of-change model to enhance patient–treatment matching; (3) application of motivational interviewing techniques to engage patients and enhance readiness for change; (4) dividing treatment into successive stages focusing on specific tasks and goals; (5) using the self-medication hypothesis to understand and address certain psychodynamic aspects of the addiction; (6) using aspects of the disease model to justify a request for total abstinence; (7) using on-site urine drug testing as a clinical tool to support and reinforce behavior change; (8) facilitating patient engagement in self-help programs; (9) avoiding certain therapeutic traps and dilemmas.

CENTRALITY OF THE THERAPEUTIC RELATIONSHIP

A central overriding feature of the integrated approach is its pervasive emphasis on the therapeutic relationship between patient and therapist. Of particular value in this regard are motivation-enhancement techniques (described in a later section of this chapter) that are designed to facilitate patient engagement and enhance readiness for change. Regardless of what particular issues or tasks are being addressed during a given phase of treatment, the therapist's style, stance, and overall attitude toward the patient are often the most critical determinants of treatment engagement, retention, and outcome. Unfailing respect for the patient's autonomy and freedom of choice is essential. The therapist must maintain vigilant self-awareness, especially in regard to controlling behaviors and other counter-transference reactions that can alienate patients and lead them to drop out of treatment. Aggressive confrontation and not giving patients the benefit of the doubt, the mainstay of traditional addiction counseling, are seen as counterproductive and antithetical to the integrated approach. It is essential for therapists to maintain unfailing respect for the patient's autonomy, sensitivities, defenses, and personal strengths. And clinicians must remain ever mindful of the power of the therapeutic relationship to engender both benefit and harm. The therapeutic relationship is by far the most important ingredient of the integrated approach and, as in all other forms of good psychotherapy, it is the primary vehicle for facilitating positive change.

PHASES OF TREATMENT

Treatment within the integrated model is divided into different phases, each focusing on a specific set of tasks and goals. There are no rigid or clear-cut dividing lines between the different phases, as they often blend gradually and sometimes imperceptibly from one to the next. Moreover, not all patients necessarily progress in linear or stepwise fashion through the different phases. Patients can and do enter treatment at different phases, progress through them at different rates, and move back and forth between phases or straddle more than one phase at a given point in time.

Assessment

The primary tasks of the assessment phase are to engage the patient in a therapeutic relationship and to perform a multidimensional assessment of the patient's substance use and related problems. This is often the most critical phase because it sets the tone for just about everything that follows and has a profound impact on whether the patient becomes engaged in the therapeutic process or drops out. Effecting a positive outcome rests heavily on creating a safe environment in which patients feel they can be open, honest, and forthcoming with you about the details of their substance use and related difficulties without fear of being judged or rejected. The assessment explores in detail the nature and extent of the patient's past and present substance use, negative consequences associated with use, its functional role and significance in the person's life, including how it may continue to serve some positive function, and the patient's motivation and readiness for change. Techniques for conducting a multidimensional assessment of substance use are discussed in Chapter 7.

Individualized Goal Setting and Treatment Planning

Completing a multidimensional assessment paves the way for establishing individualized treatment goals and collaboratively developing a treatment plan with your patients to help them work toward achieving those goals. An essential ingredient of this process is to match treatment interventions to the patient's level of motivation and stage of readiness for change. The stages-of-change (SOC) model informs and guides the process of finding the "best fit" between where the patient is and what the therapist should be doing to endgender positive change at each stage of the process (Connors, Donovan, & DiClemente, 2001; DiClemente, 2003; Prochaska, DiClemente, & Norcross, 1992).

Taking Action

This phase focuses on helping patients change their substance use behavior and achieve their initial treatment goals of reducing or stopping their alcohol and drug use. Although this phase focuses primarily on changing substance use behavior, other presenting problems and ongoing issues also are addressed.

Preventing Relapse

This phase concentrates primarily on doing what is necessary to maintain and solidify positive gains and prevent relapse to the former pattern of substance use. The development of relapse prevention strategies emanates from recognition that the types of clinical interventions needed to initiate changes in substance use behavior differ from those needed to maintain these changes and prevent relapse over the longer term (Marlatt, 1985; Marlatt & Gordon, 1985). A wide variety of relapse prevention strategies are discussed in Chapter 10.

Psychotherapy in Ongoing and Later-Stage Recovery

This is not a specific treatment phase, but a thread that runs throughout the treatment, with the focus and timing of psychotherapeutic interventions based on individual needs. The types of issues that need to be addressed at any given point in therapy are difficult to specify in advance for all patients because of the wide variation among individuals in regard to how and why they present for treatment and the complex psychological and sociological context within which alcohol and drug problems are often embedded. For example, some patients who present with alcohol and drug problems want to focus immediately on some of the psychological issues (e.g., poor self-esteem, relationship conflicts and failures, etc.) that they feel are connected to their ongoing substance use, whereas other patients want to focus only on changing their substance use behavior whether or not they are aware of other psychological factors that may be present.

THE STAGES-OF-CHANGE MODEL

Coming to grips with a serious problem and taking the necessary steps to resolve it is a process, not an instantaneous event. Recent research shows that people progress through a series of different stages along the way toward overcoming problem behaviors such as alcohol and drug abuse, and that for treatment to be effective it must be carefully matched to the particular stage of the process in which the person happens to be at the time. The stages-of-change (SOC) model (Prochaska & DiClemente, 1986) describes not only the stages of change that individuals move through as they attempt to modify or overcome problem behaviors such as substance abuse, but also the types of interventions most likely to be effective within each stage and to promote movement onto the next stage. The five stages of change in this model are precontemplation, contemplation, preparation, action, and maintenance.

The Five Stages of Change

Precontemplation is the stage in which the problem is evident to others, but not to the individual with the problem. Patients in this stage are generally unaware or underaware of their problem and do not understand why others are so worried about it. The more strongly they are confronted or badgered about the problem, the more likely they are to dig in their heels and argue that the problem does not exist or that it is not serious enough to warrant doing anything about it. For example, because those in the precontemplation stage are generally unaware that the behavior in question is a "problem" or that it may be contributing to other problems, they invest no energy into thinking about or attempting to change. Patients in precontemplation do not ordinarily seek treatment unless propelled to do so by negative consequences such as an arrest, DWI, or the threat of losing a marriage or other valued relationship. Although these individuals may enter treatment convinced that their only problem was getting caught, this situation presents an opportunity to increase their awareness and, it is hoped, their motivation to change.

In the contemplation stage, individuals begin to experience ambivalence or conflict about the behavior that is now perceived as possibly a problem, but they take no action inasmuch as it is not yet entirely clear to them that the problem is serious enough to warrant doing anything about it. The contemplator may vacillate, thinking about whether or not to do something about the problem, which reflects the ambivalence and motivational conflicts that characterize this stage. Individuals in this stage weigh the difficulties of living with the problem against the challenges created by the prospect of making changes. An individual with a serious alcohol problem may, for example, dread trying to participate in social activities with heavy-drinking friends without drinking himself, but fear the decline in health warned of by his physician if his drinking continues. At this point, disengaging from his social network is not perceived to be a viable option. People can remain in contemplation for very long periods of time or return to it on the heels of relapse after periods of extended abstinence.

In the preparation stage the balance tips in favor of change, and individuals decide to take some type of action but have not yet decided what method to employ or exactly how to go about making such a change. Moreover, they have not yet committed themselves to specific goals or to a truly effective course of action (such as getting outside help), although they intend to do so in the near future. They may experiment with reducing the number of drinks they have in a given day or the number of days per week they use cocaine, but are not quite ready to stop completely. In typically human fashion, most people in this stage hope to find the fastest, easiest, and most painless way to accomplish the desired change and may feel frustrated and discouraged when faced with the reality that no such method exists. This is essentially a warm-up stage; behavior changes are in the making, but the person has not yet reached the point of taking definitive action.

The action stage begins when the person has committed to specific goals, has chosen a definitive method for achieving those goals, and has begun in earnest to do something about the problem behavior. People in this stage make significant changes to reach a clearly defined goal such as abstinence or a significant reduction in use. They make committed efforts to change and take effective goal-oriented action, either on their own or with professional assistance. For example, actively working toward a goal of reducing alcohol consumption by 50% within 2 weeks, achieving 30 days of total abstinence, attending a few AA meetings, and/or seeking professional help from a therapist or program are indicative of individuals in the action stage. In this stage, the person typically takes definitive action to break the habitual pattern of alcohol and drug use, such as changing daily routines and avoiding people, places, and things associated with prior use. This change is visible to others and often elicits considerable support. This period may also include managing physiological withdrawal. Although people can and do navigate this stage successfully without professional intervention, there is much that a knowledgeable therapist can do to facilitate and guide the process, including teaching early recovery skills based on cognitive-behavioral therapy techniques.

In the maintenance stage the primary goal is relapse prevention, that is, to maintain progress and prevent backsliding or relapse. An addictive behavior is often easier to stop initially than to keep it stopped over the long term. The types of behaviors necessary to initiate change are different from those needed to maintain it, and so the maintenance stage is one of solidification, in which the patient makes more extensive changes and learns new coping patterns for emotions and relationships. A wide variety of relapse prevention techniques are useful in this stage to help patients maintain abstinence.

Relapse in the SOC model is defined not only as a return to the former pattern of alcohol and drug use, but more broadly as regression (i.e., movement backward) from any given stage of change to an earlier one. For example, when a vacillating patient in the contemplation stage encounters aggressive confrontation by a counselor who sees the patient as "resistant" and "unmotivated," the patient may regress (i.e., relapse) back to the precontemplation stage because such negative feedback diminishes rather than enhances the person's motivation and readiness for change. Sometimes relapse is a byproduct of success when a patient feels dramatically better after a sustained period of abstinence and begins to believe that occasional or controlled use is possible again without losing other gains. It can also occur when a patient loses respect for the power of relapse triggers, such as certain situations and activities where alcohol and drugs may be present. For example, a patient may continue to attend sporting events with friends who drink as part of the ritual. The patient may manage to remain abstinent for a period of time, but is likely to relapse at some point in the face of repeated exposure to these triggers. The patient may reject self-help participation and succeed for a while, but eventually conclude that this type of recovery support network is indeed essential to maintain progress. Relapse is common and offers an opportunity for new and deeper learning about addiction and recovery, but the therapist must avoid sounding complacent about alcohol and drug use while working to reduce shame and promote learning from the experience. No matter how successful a patient has been, it is always possible for motivation to wane. Patients then cycle back through earlier stages of change and lose their foothold in the recovery process. Although some patients show linear progress in recovery without relapse, it is more realistic to expect some backsliding, even if the treatment is clearly effective in producing positive change.

Clinical Value of the Stages-of-Change Model

The clinical value of the SOC model is the framework it provides for matching treatment interventions to the particular stage of the change process the patient happens to be in. Treatment techniques that work well with patients in one stage may be ineffective or countertherapeutic, or may seriously backfire, with those in another stage. Knowing which stage the patient is in provides important clues about what will work and what will not. A patient and therapist working at different stages (a therapeutic mismatch or misalliance) is one of the most common sources of patient resistance and premature dropout from treatment. Interventions mismatched to the patient's stage of readiness for change are likely to be unhelpful and may even be harmful.

For example, when a therapist insists on immediate action, such as stopping all substance use and going to AA meetings, with a patient who is in the precontemplation stage, the patient is likely to experience the therapist as insensitive and controlling, like a parent pressuring for change when the person is not yet convinced that change is really needed. Similarly, patients who believe that developing social supports and taking other concrete measures will make it easier for them to give up alcohol are likely to resist spending time talking with a therapist about their self-esteem problems or childhood (Connors et al., 2001). A common mismatch occurs when patients in the contemplation stage collide with therapists or treatment programs that expect them to be in the action stage. This mismatch is likely to result in failure to engage the patient in treatment. The therapist or program expects the patient to comply with requests for immediate behavior change, such as stopping all substance use without further delay, while the patient is not at all convinced that this type of action is really necessary. The more the clinician insists on change, the more reluctant and resistant the patient becomes. These types of mismatches can and often do degenerate into no-win power struggles. The therapist increasingly confronts the patient's "denial" while the patient digs in her heels, insisting that no such problem exists. Typically, this misalliance and impasse are blamed on the patient, as the clinician concludes that the patient was "resistant," "in denial," and "just not ready to change" in the first place.

Certain types of treatment interventions are best suited for patients in each of the five different stages of change, and choosing interventions properly matched to the patient's stage of change is among the therapist's most important tasks in the integrated approach. For example, motivational interviewing and other engagement strategies that start "where the patient is" are most appropriate for patients in the early stages of precontemplation and contemplation. Interventions such as discussing various treatment options and negotiating a treatment plan are most appropriate for patients in the preparation stage. Specific behavior change strategies for establishing abstinence or curtailing use are best suited for those in the action stage, whereas relapse prevention strategies are most appropriate for those in the maintenance stage.

MOTIVATIONAL INTERVIEWING TECHNIQUES

In recent years a significant advance in the adaptation of psychotherapeutic approaches to treating SUDs has been the development of motivational interviewing techniques (Miller & Rollnick, 1991). These techniques have provided a new way to conceptualize and deal more effectively with the problems of patient resistance and poor motivation. Within the framework of the stages-of-change model, motivational interviewing techniques combine Rogerian principles of patient-centered therapy with a variety of cognitive-behavioral interventions designed to reduce patient resistance and enhance motivation and readiness to change. This approach has helped to focus long-overdue attention on the need for effective strategies to deal with ambivalent, resistant patients who are in the early stages of change (i.e., precontemplation, contemplation, and preparation). Motivational interviewing represents a major departure from the standard confrontational approach that has dominated the addiction treatment field for several decades (see Miller & Rollnick, 1991, pp. 52–54, for detailed comparison of motivational interviewing vs. confrontation-of-denial approaches). Motivational interviewing is a noncoercive, nonauthoritarian approach intended to help patients free up their own motivations and mobilize their internal resources so they can move forward in the process of change. It gives clinicians an effective way to reconceptualize their approach to "resistant" and "unmotivated" patients and defines the critical role of the clinician in helping patients move from one stage of change to the next.

In motivational interviewing, patients' reluctance or inability to acknowledge having an alcohol or drug problem is seen not as resistance, denial, or lack of motivation, but rather as an outgrowth of an individual's ambivalence and conflicted attachment to the substances. Individuals who have developed SUDs often want to stop using alcohol and drugs, but at the same time they do not want to or do not feel ready to stop using. Painful ambivalence, including fears about facing reality without the chemical buffer provided by alcohol and drugs, drives them to suppress and selectively ignore negative aspects of their substance use. Instead of facing reality, they rationalize and minimize substance-related consequences while trying to convince themselves and others that the problem either does not exist or is just not serious enough to warrant concern.

The task of clinicians encountering patients embroiled in this dilemma is to help them reduce their ambivalence and tip the balance in favor of change. Motivational interviewing techniques are designed to do just that—to increase the chances that substance-abusing patients will recognize and actually do something about their alcohol and drug problems. Motivation, like ambivalence, is seen not as an immutable characteristic of people who have alcohol and drug problems, but as a fluctuating state of readiness or willingness to change that can be influenced by situational factors and certain types of interpersonal interactions. In the motivational interviewing approach, a therapeutic patient-centered relationship between clinician and patient is considered the primary vehicle for moving the patient along the path to positive change. Patients are given permission and expected to resist, they are encouraged to explore their ambivalence about changing and consider various options to resolve their dilemma while the clinician acts as facilitator. Patient resistance is taken not as an indicator of poor motivation but as a signal that the clinician is pressing too hard, prematurely, or in the wrong direction (i.e., out of sync with where the patient happens to be at the moment). Some of the basic principles of and techniques of motivational interviewing are:

1. *Express empathy for your patients' plight.* Look beyond their substance-using behavior and recognize the fears and difficulties involved in changing what are often long-standing and deeply ingrained patterns of living. Remain tolerant of the range of patients' reactions to receiving objective feedback about their alcohol and drug use, including anger, denial, astonishment, arrogance, shame, embarrassment, reticence, and the like.

2. *Avoid arguments.* Do not argue or debate with patients about whether or not they have an alcohol and drug problem and what to do about it. Patients are not adversaries to be defeated.

3. *Roll with resistance.* When patients show signs of resistance, the clinician should back off. Resistance is a sign that whatever you are trying to do is not working and it would be better to try something else. When you encounter resistance from patients, avoid the temptation to regard this as a challenge to your authority or to react with frustration or annoyance. Stay in the role of compassionate clinician and expert who can advise and guide patients in making good decisions for themselves.

4. *Avoid coercive or pressuring tactics.* The responsibility for change rests solely with the patient and not with the therapist. The therapist should assume the role of change facilitator, not authoritarian, dictator, or controller. Convey your willingness to work with substance-abusing patients in a mutually cooperative partnership to define and address the problem.

5. *Be positive and reassuring.* Let patients know that alcohol and drug problems are not the result of character flaws or moral deficiency, but disorders that can be treated successfully.

6. *Express interest, concern, and curiosity.* Simple expressions of interest and caring by the therapist can go a long way toward creating a trusting atmosphere that encourages truthful self-revelation.

7. *Ask open-ended questions.* When interviewing patients about their alcohol and drug use, it is best to ask open-ended questions rather than yes/no questions. Open-ended questions elicit relevant details rather than simple yes/no answers. For example, rather than ask "Have you ever felt that

your alcohol and drug use was a problem?" which can be responded to with a simple "yes" or "no," it would be better to pose an open-ended question such as "Tell me about your alcohol and drug use over the past year and to what extent you have ever felt it to be a problem."

8. *"Start where the patient is,"* not where you want him to be. Match your treatment interventions to the patient's stage of readiness for change, as discussed earlier. Don't jump too far ahead by pressing for changes that patients are not yet ready to make.

Miller and Rollnick (1991) have outlined eight essential building blocks of motivational strategies summarized by the mnemonic "ABCDEFGH" (pp. 20–28):

1. *Give ADVICE.* When properly timed and delivered, simple advice offered by a knowledgeable, caring professional can be motivating and empowering.

2. *Remove BARRIERS.* Patients need help in overcoming practical, emotional, and attitudinal barriers to change. This may include assisting patients with transportation or child care problems, offering flexible appointment times, and pairing up newcomers with supportive peers who can "show them the ropes."

3. *Provide CHOICES.* This is based on the belief that intrinsic motivation is enhanced by giving the person a voluntary choice between different courses of action without subjecting him to external pressure or coercion. Few people like to be told what to do and resist or recoil when presented with no choice. The patient's personal investment in treatment is enhanced when offered a choice among a number of alternatives.

4. *Decrease DESIRABILITY.* In-depth assessment of pros versus cons of a person's substance use may reveal a variety of unrecognized or unappreciated consequences, as well as distorted notions about the presumed necessity or benefits of alcohol and drug use. Interventions that provide objective, realistic feedback about substance-related problems and consequences can help to tip the balance in favor of change.

5. *Practice EMPATHY.* An empathic therapist style is associated with low levels of patient resistance and greater receptivity to change. This includes empathic and reflective listening as well as conveying warmth, respect, supportiveness, and active interest.

6. *Provide FEEDBACK.* An important motivational task is to provide clear feedback about a patient's situation, behavior, and consequences. Accurate knowledge of the present situation is an essential ingredient in developing motivation for change.

7. *Clarify GOALS.* An essential task is to help the patient clarify, define, and set goals that are realistic, desirable, and attainable. This involves helping patients define where they are now as compared with

where they would like to be. Seeing a large gap or discrepancy between one's current status and desired goals can be motivating, but only if the person believes that the goals are actually attainable and can see a clear path for achieving them.

8. *Actively HELP.* Clinicians must be active, optimistic, involved, and empowering. Their role encompasses that of teacher, coach, guide, and supporter. Giving advice, offering recommendations, and alerting the patients to potential obstacles or pitfalls are all essential parts of the clinician's role.

CLINICAL USE OF THE DISEASE MODEL

The disease model has long been the foundation of traditional approaches to treating addiction, but it continues to be a topic of controversy and debate among mental health professionals and the public at large. Many people question the legitimacy of viewing addiction as a disease and are concerned that doing so dangerously absolves drug- and alcohol-addicted individuals of personal responsibility for their excessive substance use and related irresponsible behaviors. However, most concerns about the disease model stem from misinterpretations and misunderstandings based on lack of accurate information. For example, the notion of addiction as a disease does not absolve individuals of personal responsibility for their behavior, but it does reduce the paralyzing shame and guilt that impairs their ability to acknowledge and address the problem. Although individuals who become addicted to alcohol and drugs are not responsible for having the disease, which can be viewed as a biochemical "brain allergy" to psychoactive substances (whether substance induced, inherited, or both) associated with pathological thinking and behavior when these substances enter the brains of affected individuals, they most certainly *are* responsible for remaining abstinent and making the requisite behavioral and lifestyle changes necessary to prevent relapse. They are also fully responsible for any harm done to others while under the influence of intoxicants. Individuals who have the disease, regardless of etiology, respond differently to psychoactive substances than those who do not have the disease. Not only do they experience difficulty in controlling the quantity and frequency of their use, but they also become obsessed and preoccupied with using these substances and continue to use them despite life-damaging consequences. It is difficult to understand the habitual, self-destructive tendency of the addicted person who resorts repeatedly to excessive alcohol and drug use, even in the face of severe life-damaging consequences, as anything but pathological.

Certain tenets of the disease model have enormous therapeutic value and can be utilized for patients' benefit regardless of your theoretical orientation. You need not wholly accept or believe in all aspects of this model in order to utilize selected pieces of the approach to help your patients deal with their alcohol and drug problems. According to an AA slogan, when questioning the value of the program you are advised to "take what you need and leave the rest." The model is not only an extremely useful clinical tool, guiding the clinician's therapeutic stance on a variety of important treatment issues, but it also aids in lifting the paralyzing shame, guilt, and self-recrimination that interfere with addressing addictive disorders in constructive ways.

Among the most useful tenets of the disease model is the importance of total abstinence from all intoxicants as the most reliable way for individuals who have the disease to avoid relapse and ensure the widest margin of safety. From a clinical perspective, there are several reasons for this. First, there is the often observed phenomenon of drug substitution in which individuals develop addictive patterns with other substances that they may or may not have abused in the past. For example, it is quite common for patients in recovery from cocaine or opioid addiction to develop problems with alcohol that sometimes progress into full-blown alcohol dependence. Especially for those with no pre-drug history of alcohol problems, resumption of normal drinking patterns seems entirely doable to them and they find it hard to justify why they have to deprive themselves of a glass or two of wine with dinner or a bottle of beer or two while watching a sporting event. Actually, it appears that some individuals can accomplish this safely, but it is impossible to predict who they are. The risks of trying this experiment with social drinking can be considerable for those with the more severe forms of the disorder, and sometimes only after experiencing further alcohol-related harm do they decide that controlled or responsible drinking is for them simply not attainable.

A second reason for total abstinence is the role that other substances can and often do play in precipitating relapse to a person's drug of choice. For example, people addicted to cocaine often have difficulty accepting the idea that alcohol or marijuana can reduce their ability to refuse offers of cocaine and may actually stimulate cravings for cocaine. Addiction specialists have long noted that resumption of cocaine use is frequently preceded by use of these other substances, particularly alcohol, and recent empirical evidence supports these clinical observations (Rawson, Obert, McCann, Smith, & Ling, 1990).

The clinical value of the disease model notwithstanding, it must be recognized that not everyone with an alcohol or drug problem has the disease of addiction and applying this model too broadly or indiscriminately can reduce its clinical utility and produce unwanted results. For example, individuals who meet DSM-IV criteria for a diagnosis of abuse but not dependence may or may not have the disease of addiction. Whether or not these individuals are merely in the early stages a disease process that is moving them from abuse toward full-blown addiction (which is impossible to predict reliably), they are not likely to see the disease model as applicable to their current pattern of substance use and attempts to force them into this mold are likely to be unproductive and diminish the therapist's credibility. Even those who unequivocally meet the criteria for a diagnosis of substance dependence often have difficulty in accepting the disease model as applicable to their problems. In general, the more severe an individual's addiction, the more likely it is to conform to the disease model.

Furthermore, despite the clinical utility of the disease model, when patients hesitate or refuse to embrace this model unequivocally you should not construe this as evidence of resistance, denial, or unwillingness to "surrender" or use it to justify confrontational tactics. Helping patients see the potential value of the disease model in facilitating their recovery should be approached therapeutically within the framework of the stages-of-change model and motivational interviewing techniques discussed earlier. Keep in mind that it is not necessary for patients to accept the disease model and the identity of "addict" or "alcoholic" in order to address their substance abuse problem and begin the recovery process in earnest.

CLINICAL VALUE OF THE SELF-MEDICATION HYPOTHESIS

The self-medication hypothesis adds a clinically valuable psychodynamic perspective and understanding to the treatment of patients with SUDs. This perspective is especially useful because it provides a basis for explaining some of the subjective and experiential aspects of the meaning and function of psychoactive substances in an individual's life. It also helps to explain the characteristics of people who come to rely on substances and provides a basis for conceptualizing substance use as serving the function of self-medication in an attempt to cope with certain types of deficits and problems (Murphy & Khantzian, 1995). Essentially, the self-medication hypothesis holds that substance-dependent individuals are predisposed to use and become dependent on psychoactive substances largely as a result of ego impairments and deficits in their sense of self. These deficits result in self-regulation disturbances in the critical areas of affect management, self-esteem maintenance, capacity for self-care, and self–other relations (Dodes & Khantzian, 1991). The most frequently described function of substance use within this framework is the management of intolerable and overwhelming affects. Connections between certain affect states and the use of certain substances have been noted: for example, the use of opioids to manage anger, rage, and loneliness; the use of cocaine and other stimulants to manage depression, boredom, anhedonia, and feelings of emptiness or to instill a sense of omnipotence or grandeur; and the use of alcohol to manage anxiety, social awkwardness, and sexual inhibitions. On a more general level, psychoactive substances may be used to compensate for a defective stimulus barrier that leads to affective flooding and as a way of self-soothing that cannot be achieved by ordinary means (Krystal, 1988). Deficits in the capacity to be aware of and appropriately label one's internal affect states, a condition known as "alexithymia," has also been noted as a distinguishing feature of people who become addicted to mood-altering substances.

In light of these observations, an important part of ongoing psychotherapy for patients with SUDs is to help them identify, understand, and overcome their self-regulation vulnerabilities and deficits, as discussed in Chapter 11.

ENCOURAGING INVOLVEMENT IN SELF-HELP PROGRAMS

The self-help system is an invaluable resource to the therapist treating substance use and to those who are in recovery. It is important for you to facilitate the use of these programs without assuming that they eliminate the need for you to address a patient's substance use at all stages of the recovery process. In self-help group meetings, your patient will see repeatedly that she is not alone in the self-destructive behaviors she views as isolating her from humankind. Confession can bring some relief from the overpowering feelings of shame, particularly when others share similar experiences. Your patient will be exposed to a wide variety of role models for recovery, hear strategies for achieving and maintaining abstinence, and have an opportunity to participate in a social structure that does not involve drinking and using.

The self-help groups available today are growing in number and variety, but by far the most comprehensive support structure is offered in the 12-step system. "Twelve-step programs" is the generic name for the many descendents of AA. AA started in 1935, and currently more than 2 million people call themselves members. The only requirement for membership is a desire to stop drinking. Other variants of the organization developed around illicit drugs and grew in membership, particularly in urban communities. Narcotics Anonymous, or NA, is a common choice for drug users and includes those who use stimulants, opioids, and other substances. Although the basic steps of recovery are the same, it is important for people in the early stages to hear "their story," and thus they may get a better start in a drug-specific meeting. As their involvement in recovery deepens, many seek out meetings in which there are participants with long-term sobriety, and these are most plentiful in AA. Gradually, more NA meetings have become available with participants who have achieved many years of recovery.

Resistance to 12-step program attendance is to be expected and should be handled as a clinical issue. You can make it clear that you will not immediately insist on meeting attendance, but the patient's objections are a fruitful topic for ongoing exploration. The issue of attendance at self-help meetings can provide a mirror that will reveal your patient's conflicts about addiction and many other issues as well. The opening ritual, "I am Josie, I am an addict" is an opportunity for patients to look inside and check out their willingness to acknowledge their addiction. Patients in the early stages may detest this part of the ritual, and exploration often reveals their ambivalence about viewing themselves as addicted. On the behavioral level, you can let the patients know that they can introduce themselves by name only, as a guest, or by some other designation of their choosing. However, it is important to ask them to listen to that inner voice that rebels at the phrase "I am an alcoholic/addict." Thus, you can work on the behavioral and emotional levels concurrently, conveying that at some point it is important to give the self-help system a fair try.

A growing list of research studies document that those who become involved in the self-help system show improvements in many domains of functioning (Ouimette, Moos, & Finney, 1998; Polcin, Prindle, & Bostrom, 2002; Tonigan, Toscove, & Miller, 1996). There are several ways of facilitating the use of these programs. "Stranger anxiety" and discomfort at being an outsider are early obstacles to participation. Connecting your patient with someone to accompany him to a meeting is a good way to begin. The central office (listed in the Yellow Pages of the phone book under Alcoholics Anonymous, Narcotics Anonymous, etc.) can usually help arrange this. You can also suggest that your patient ask a recovering friend or colleague to assist. If it is impractical to arrange for someone to accompany your patient, you can nonetheless discuss how to cope with the awkwardness and provide encouragement to proceed. Eliciting patients' ideas of what goes on in meetings and what they fear is a valuable way to correct misconceptions and explore charged issues. Give plenty of permission to be ambivalent, and stress that having mixed feelings doesn't mean that they cannot benefit from continuing attendance. Those who object to "that religious stuff" can be encouraged to "take what you need and leave the rest" and can also be informed that many of the early participants of AA were atheists and agnostics. Social isolates can be assured that it is usually possible to regulate the distance between themselves and others, particularly if they avoid small meetings that tend to pull for everyone to participate. You can also role-play how to set boundaries if the friendliness of meeting participants is experienced as too intrusive.

Sometimes patients are immovable in their unwillingness to attend 12-step meetings but are open to other possibilities. LifeRing, Moderation

Management, Women for Sobriety, and SMART Recovery are examples of alternatives with enthusiastic supporters. Information about these groups can be found on the Internet, and meeting schedules are frequently available online. The main drawback is the relative paucity of meetings, so you may need to find other ways to generate the level of support required by each particular patient.

It is important to avoid a power struggle if patients refuse self-help participation, while continuing to explore the relevant issues. Reframing the discussion to focus on the underlying principles is a productive approach. Self-help programs offer two essential ingredients that promote success: (1) a subculture that supports recovery and (2) a process for personal development that has no financial barriers. You can ask your patient to consider how to achieve those goals and track their progress. It is necessary to maintain a long-term perspective. Many patients do well initially, then fall into regular relapse patterns because they changed their substance use but nothing else. It is tempting but unwise to assume professional therapy will fill all the gaps and provide all the necessary learning. Social support has repeatedly been shown to be a key factor in a solid recovery, and it is important to promote the requisite lifestyle changes in whatever ways are possible.

AVOIDING CERTAIN THERAPEUTIC TRAPS
AND DILEMMAS

There are a variety of ways for therapists to become ensnared in resistance. Most patients come to us in distress, and it is easy to dwell on the obvious negative consequences of alcohol and drug use as soon as we spot them. The patient may acknowledge negative consequences in the course of the interview, tempting you to make recommendations immediately. Often the patient then expresses ambivalence about whether the problem is "really that serious," or whether your unexpected recommendations are warranted. This is particularly likely to happen when the patient is seeking help for other issues. The patient can perceive you as unwilling to focus on the areas of primary concern, and a power struggle then ensues. The struggle is compounded if the therapist falls into the trap of engaging in a game of cat and mouse, in which the therapist pounces on every indication that alcohol and drugs are a problem and uses every example to "make the case." The distinction between the cat and mouse game and providing feedback on negative consequences is frequently one of tone. It is important to remain forthright and utilize opportunities to explore resistance in a calm and constructive manner. You should remain aware of signs of overinvolvement within yourself, or of a savior trap in which you become more invested than the patient in addressing her substance use.

It is desirable to monitor patients' receptiveness carefully at the initial stages. Some secretly view their alcohol and drug use as a serious problem, are frightened about it, and relieved when you articulate concern. Others are only beginning to grasp the seriousness of their problem and need time to digest new information and adjust their perspective. If you can allow the patient to talk about the benefits of drinking and/or using while listening without judgment, the patient is more likely to perceive you as one who can understand the complexity and allow him to move at a manageable pace. At the same time, you should carefully note the perceived benefits of substance use or the positive functions it still serves, as these will have to be addressed in the course of treatment. For example, if your patient uses alcohol to initiate communication with her husband on difficult issues, you might acknowledge this benefit of drinking and offer to help her address these issues in other ways.

Some therapists are prone to making certain types of therapeutic errors with substance-abusing patients. When patients feel that reducing or giving up their alcohol and drug use will only make things worse, not better, some therapists may accept this view without challenge and decide that addressing a patient's problematic alcohol and drug use should wait until other problems are sufficiently resolved. But the more knowledgeable you are about the insidious effects of different drugs, the more easily you can make the case that although substance use may bring short-term relief, it can delay or undermine making other therapeutic gains. For example, it is common for patients to tout the enhanced mood they get briefly from marijuana and be unaware that regular use actually exacerbates depression (Bovasso, 2001). Similarly, alcohol elevates a person's mood for a short while before the central nervous system depressant effects take over. Regular drinking worsens depression over time. It is almost always possible to provide a psychological explanation for substance use, but such insights are usually more helpful once the compulsive use of alcohol and drugs is no longer clouding the clinical picture.

Although aggressive confrontation is not a recommended strategy, some therapists err in the direction of passivity. It is in the nature of serious alcohol and drug problems that the individual with the problem is often unable to acknowledge and see it clearly. This is partly because of a lack of understanding about the potential negative consequences of use, and partly because these consequences often develop insidiously over time in barely perceptible steps. It is your responsibility to bring these problems into focus. Waiting for the patient to bring up a problem can lead inadvertently to serious consequences and puts the therapist at risk of failure to meet the standard of professional care. It is not necessary to convince a patient that he is a drug- or alcohol-dependent person in order to recommend a change in behavior. Some therapists assume that acceptance of such a label is essential, but in many cases it is a stumbling block that evokes resistance. Such labels are highly stigmatized, and often your patient can agree that some change needs to be made long before he can digest the implications of what the potential benefits of recovery might be. We discuss how to navigate these various obstacles in chapters that follow.

FINAL COMMENT

In this chapter we described the essential ingredients of an integrated approach to treating patients with SUDs. Our treatment model embodies diversity and flexibility: differing theories are drawn upon to understand and treat patients, and differing interventions are woven together as they move through different stages of recovery. Various elements are integrated in a way that allows treatment to operate on several different planes at once, moving freely among different theoretical orientations, treatment approaches, and techniques. The integrated model encourages therapists, as well as patients, to remain open-minded and flexible, recognizing the true complexity of SUDs and the need to become versatile in managing the broad array of issues that arise with patients who abuse alcohol and drugs. Above all, we do not take a doctrinaire approach, as we believe strongly that patients with SUDs require treatment that is individualized and able to adapt to their changing needs.

Being fundamentally pragmatic, the guiding principles of the integrated approach are:

1. Start where your patients are, not where you or others want them to be.
2. Give your patients permission to resist so that you can dance, not wrestle with them.
3. The first and foremost goal of treatment is not abstinence, but to engage and encourage patients so they come back.
4. Establishing a solid therapeutic relationship with your patients takes precedence over everything else, except their safety.
5. Do what works and be open-minded, flexible, and humble enough to change what you are doing if it is not yielding the desired results.
6. Above all, do no harm!

CHAPTER 5

Considerations in Addressing Concurrent Psychiatric and Substance Use Disorders

The incidence of psychiatric disorders and other mental health problems is notoriously high among people with SUDs. Of particular relevance for the present discussion are the Axis I mood and anxiety disorders. There is also a large population of substance-abusing patients with Axis I psychotic disorders (including schizophrenia and schizoaffective disorders) and other forms of severe debilitating mental illness (Drake et al., 2001; Minkoff & Drake, 1991; Minkoff, Zweben, Rosenthal, & Ries, 2003).

Co-occurring Axis II personality disorders among patients with SUDs generally fall into the categories of antisocial, borderline, and narcissistic disturbances, although the incidence of these problems is considerably lower than common stereotypes of these patients would suggest. In particular, antisocial personality disorder is frequently overdiagnosed in this population owing to the failure to assess antisocial behaviors independently of active substance use. Chronic drug use frequently causes changes in personality, behavior, and personal values that violate societal expectations and norms. Compulsive lying, emotional detachment, social isolation, impulsive and manipulative behaviors, and disregard for the negative impact of one's behavior on others often are sequelae of the deterioration of ego functioning and emotional dysregulation caused by chronic addiction.

We focus here primarily on the Axis I mood and anxiety disorders, as these are the most common forms of psychiatric illness found among functional patients with SUDs seen in office-based psychotherapy practice. Discussion of specific psychotherapeutic and behavioral interventions for treating each type of psychiatric disorder that may accompany alcohol and drug abuse is beyond the scope of this book. We focus here instead on some of the important factors that therapists should consider when assessing and treating patients who present with SUDs and coexisting psychiatric complaints. Our overall clinical approach takes seriously the notion that when both types of disorders are present, they are coexisting coprimary independent conditions worthy of equal clinical attention. It recognizes that the SUD may not have caused, although may exacerbate, the psychiatric illness, and vice versa. These separate illnesses interact with one another in complex ways that require coordinated simultaneous treatment. However, the first task is to determine whether these are enduring psychiatric symptoms that represent an actual coexisting disorder or are merely temporary symptoms induced by the chronic drug use itself.

CONSIDERATIONS IN ASSESSMENT

The evaluation and diagnosis of patients with co-occurring psychiatric and substance use disorders can be quite complex. Clinicians are faced with the difficult task of distinguishing whether the patient's presenting signs and symptoms are due to an underlying psychiatric disorder or to the consequences of drug intoxication, toxicity, or withdrawal. Making this distinction can be difficult because the effects of chronic alcohol and drug use can mask underlying mental illness and can also mimic actual psychiatric syndromes. Nonetheless, doing so is important not only from the standpoint of accurate diagnosis, but also for selecting appropriate treatment interventions.

The assessment problem stems from the fact that both acute and chronic effects of psychoactive substances can produce dramatic changes in an individual's mood, mental state, personality, behavior, and overall level of psychosocial functioning. During periods of chronic intoxication as well as acute and protracted withdrawal, many individuals manifest symptoms of mood and/or anxiety disorders. In addition to depressed or labile mood, patients report sleep and appetite disturbances, diminished libido, pessimism, low energy, apathy, anhedonia, shame and guilt, and sometimes suicidal ideation. Difficulty in concentrating, irritability, restlessness, generalized anxiety, panic attacks, and low frustration tolerance are also common complaints. Moreover, in some individuals these signs and symptoms persist for weeks or months after cessation of alcohol and drug use, which further complicates the diagnostic picture. Lingering symptoms may be indicative of a concurrent psychiatric disorder (e.g., atypical depression or dysthymia), but they may also be due to drug-induced disruptions in brain neurotransmitters that require prolonged periods of abstinence before normalization of mood and mental state can occur. For example, in chronic cocaine users who present with concurrent symptoms of depression, it is often difficult to determine whether the depressive symptoms are due to cocaine-induced changes in brain chemistry, an expectable response to the dopamine depletion caused by cocaine use, or to a primary mood disorder that may have preceded and perhaps contributed etiologically to the development of the drug problem. The clinical picture is further complicated when patients are using multiple substances, as is so often the case. For example, cocaine users frequently drink large quantities of alcohol to counteract the unpleasant side effects or aftereffects of high-dose cocaine use. This combined use of a stimulant and a depressant can create dramatic swings in mood, affect, and behavior that closely mimic symptoms of bipolar disorders.

Interestingly, the broad array of psychiatric signs and symptoms caused by chronic alcohol and drug use do not appear to be very substance specific in the later stages of use. During the stage of acute intoxication, each type of substance produces its own characteristic profile of psychoactive effects, but as use continues and leads to increasing tolerance and dependence, the chronic effects of most substances on an individual's mood and mental state become more and more alike. For example, chronic use of depressants, stimulants, or opioids leaves users with a complex of symptoms that looks like depression, including sleep and appetite disturbances, fatigue, anxiety, and irritability.

It is important to recognize that chronic substance use not only can and often does cause severe disruption to mood and mental state, but can also destabilize and diminish an individual's sense of self, injecting chaos into interpersonal relationships and causing deterioration in the person's overall level of psychosocial functioning. Clinicians must be careful not to draw premature conclusions about an individual's level of psychiatric disturbance without having an opportunity to see how that person functions after a sustained period of abstinence. For example, marital relationships often are profoundly affected by a individual's alcohol and drug use, and it can be quite difficult to discern whether severe marital problems have contributed to development of the SUD, have resulted from consequences of the SUD, or both. The same may apply to an individual's interaction with coworkers, parents, children, siblings, and others, creating a clinical impression of psychosocial dysfunction that may be largely substance induced. Similarly, substance abuse can also cause or exacerbate certain types of behaviors and interaction styles (including being hostile, demanding, and manipulative) that mimic features of antisocial, borderline, and/or narcissistic personality disorders.

Considering the complexities involved in evaluating substance-abusing patients who present with concurrent psychiatric symptoms, how can an accurate assessment and differential diagnosis be accomplished? One approach is to take a detailed history to evaluate the temporal relationship between the emergence of psychiatric symptoms and the use of psychoactive substances, even though it may not be possible to arrive at a definitive conclusion based on this information alone. It is important to assess, for example, whether the psychiatric symptoms existed before the onset of substance use, and if so, to what extent the problem initially improved and then worsened as the substance use continued. It is also important to assess whether during any prior periods of sustained abstinence from alcohol and drugs, the psychiatric symptoms continued to exist or became increasingly severe. A history of responding positively to psychotropic medication during prior periods of abstinence is another important clue, as well as a family history of psychiatric illness. However, because patients often are not good historians and the assessment interview often takes place during a period of active addiction or shortly thereafter, history alone rarely provides definitive answers.

Most clinicians rely on their own clinical observations of the patient's functioning and symptomatology during the first few weeks of treatment to see whether the patient's status improves or worsens with abstinence. The length of alcohol- and drug-free time needed to allow drug-induced symptoms to resolve sufficiently to unmask the patient's true mood and mental status cannot be predicted with certainty in any given case and depends on a variety of factors, such as the types of substances that were used as well as the intensity and longevity of the use. By a conservative estimate, a period of at least 4–6 weeks is necessary in most cases before a reasonably accurate picture of the patient's baseline functioning is revealed. If a patient's psychiatric symptoms persist beyond this point, they are probably due to true psychiatric illness rather than to drug toxicity or withdrawal. Conversely, if by this point the patient's psychiatric symptoms subside, they were most likely byproducts of chronic drug use and not indicative of a concurrent psychiatric condition. Thus, a longitudinal approach to assessment is usually necessary, with repeated observations to distinguish between drug-induced symptoms and psychopathology.

Although premature diagnosis of a psychiatric disorder before the patient has achieved a period of sustained abstinence can cloud the diagnostic picture and lead to erroneous conclusions, there are instances when, from a purely practical standpoint, more immediate action must be taken. For example, when patients continue to complain during the early stages of abstinence of intolerable depression and/or anxiety that impairs their ability to function and precludes their ability to participate in treatment and/or benefit from it, there is no reason to delay consideration of a trial on appropriate psychotropic medication. In some cases, short-term psychiatric hospitalization may be required to stabilize a patient's mood and/or manage suicide risk.

CONSIDERATIONS IN TREATMENT

Psychotropic Medication

Pharmacological treatment for co-occurring psychiatric disorders, where indicated, can substantially improve treatment outcomes in patients with SUDs. In general, psychotropic medications alone are not effective in alleviating mood disorders that are induced by the substance use itself or in reducing cravings and urges to use alcohol and drugs repeatedly. Placing patients on these medications prematurely can cloud the diagnostic picture, making it more difficult to determine whether an independent coexisting psychiatric disorder is actually present, but in some cases immediate pharmacological intervention is required to help manage psychiatric risk, especially when suicidality and/or psychotic symptoms are present. Chapter 6 addresses issues regarding use of psychotropic medications in greater detail.

Prioritizing Tasks and Goals

The first treatment goal with patients suffering from concurrent SUDs and psychiatric disorders is remission in both problem areas with resulting stabilization of psychosocial functioning. The agenda includes the tasks of establishing abstinence and reducing psychiatric symptoms. The first priority is to help the patient establish abstinence, without which little clinical progress can be made. Abstinence from all psychoactive substances is the first step in preventing further decline in the patient's psychiatric status and providing an opportunity to formulate a reasonably accurate psychiatric diagnosis. Although the specific techniques for helping these patients establish abstinence are virtually the same as with other chemically dependent patients (as discussed in Chapter 9), an important considerations to keep in mind is that patients with coexisting psychiatric conditions, particularly severe mood disorders, deeply fear that giving up alcohol and drugs will make them feel worse, not better. Often they are afraid that giving up alcohol and drugs will leave them in an intolerable state of helplessness and unpredictability, at the mercy of painful affects with no ability to manage them. Many of these patients are misled when their alcohol and drug use alleviate uncomfortable feeling states for a short while, but then leave them feeling worse when the effects wear off. Sometimes the substance use does not really alleviate emotional discomfort, but only shifts the patient from one uncomfortable state to another, which may be different but not better. Consider the following case:

> David, a divorced 48-year-old businessman, had been drinking 9 ounces of vodka per day and smoking marijuana daily for the 2 years prior to seeking treatment for addiction. Describing himself as "severely anx-

ious, neurotic, and depressed since childhood," he had been in classical psychoanalysis for the past 10 years with a psychiatrist who was also maintaining him on four different medications—an antidepressant, a mood stabilizer, an anxiolytic, and a sedative for sleep. As David's drinking progressed steadily on the heels of his divorce 2 years earlier, he noticed that the various medications stopped working and his anxiety and depression worsened. Alcohol and marijuana gave him a brief respite from emotional discomfort, but tolerance developed and his consumption levels increased progressively. David felt trapped in a vicious cycle of increasingly unmanageable addiction and intolerable emotional pain that was moving him closer and closer to potential suicide, at which point he sought the help of an addiction psychologist. Despite recognizing that alcohol and marijuana were contributing to his problems, he was terrified by the thought of giving them up. He could not imagine how he would be able to get through a single evening at home alone without using these substances to get some relief, even though whatever relief he got was minimal and short-lived. His fears prevented him from seeing this situation realistically, as indicated by his question during the initial interview: "Tell me, Doc, do you *really* think that my drinking and pot smoking are so serious that I have to give them up completely? I've been depressed and anxious my entire life, long before I ever used alcohol and drugs. I'm frightened that stopping them altogether will make me feel worse, not better."

David's case illustrates a variety of issues, including the use of alcohol and drugs to self-medicate psychiatric symptoms; the ineffectiveness of psychotherapy that does not address a serious alcohol and drug problem; the diminishing effectiveness of psychotropic medications and deterioration of a person's mental status in the face of chronic alcohol and drug abuse; and a patient's paralyzing fear that giving up alcohol and drugs will not help, but actually make things worse.

It is important to educate patients who fear changing their alcohol and drug use so they can see that although these substances may provide some relief from distress initially, over time they are likely to backfire and make everything worse. They must also understand that the effects of most psychoactive substances are biphasic. For example, alcohol initially enhances mood and may produce euphoria, but because it is fundamentally a central nervous system depressant and has that effect on the brain each and every time it is used, its overall effect is to lower stress tolerance and exacerbate negative mood states. Similarly, although cocaine acutely uplifts mood and boosts energy level, over time it depletes dopamine levels in selected brain areas, resulting in worsening depressive symptoms that override and overshadow a continuously shrinking period of cocaine-induced euphoria. The therapist must skillfully chip away at the patient's conviction (tacit or stated) that the alcohol or drug use is helping and point to facts that support the opposing view, that the substance use is actually diminishing, not enhancing, how she feels. A therapeutic alliance can be formed around the idea of an trying an "experiment with abstinence" (discussed more fully in Chapter 8), in which the patient will have an opportunity to explore whether abstinence actually makes things better. The therapist should point out that although abstinence from alcohol and drugs will not fix everything, using these substances undermines a person's ability to deal with problems in ways that can be revealed only after abstinence has been established for a while. Another important consideration is that alcohol and drug use tend to diminish the effectiveness of most psychotropic medications used to treat coexisting psychiatric disorders (Schuckit, 1996, 2000).

The willingness of patients with concurrent psychiatric disorders to accept an experiment with abstinence or, alternatively, a significant reduction in use as an initial treatment goal often depends substantially on the nature of the therapeutic relationship at that point. Establishing rapport and trust as quickly as possible is a priority in working with all patients, but is perhaps even more important with these individuals. Some patients will agree to accept your recommendations on faith combined with their confidence in your clinical judgment if a good working alliance has been established. When patients indicate a readiness to either stop using completely or cut down substantially, a clear plan for doing so should be developed that includes appropriate medical and psychological interventions. Patients should be reassured that the therapist will be available for frequent contact to provide needed encouragement and support as painful feelings inevitably surface. Giving patients permission to contact you outside normal working hours, if needed, can be extremely reassuring and often helps to reduce levels of anxiety and anticipation even if they never exercise this option.

Preparing Patients for Participation in Self-Help Programs

Twelve-step programs (e.g., AA, NA) provide an invaluable recovery network for learning and peer support, and patients should be routinely encouraged to attend. But therapists must make a special effort to offset potential problems and prepare patients with coexisting psychiatric conditions for participation in self-help meetings. One problem that can arise in meetings, as mentioned earlier, is the tendency of some members with an anti-medication bias to pressure others into discontinuing prescribed medications, based on the mistaken presumption that recovery does not count unless one is entirely drug free, with no exceptions. You must assure your patients that no member of AA is authorized to play doctor and that prohibiting appropriately prescribed medication is not embodied or even suggested in the AA program or philosophy, no matter what some members might argue to the contrary.

"Double trouble" AA meetings are available in many cities, at which patients with both disorders may feel more comfortable. These meetings typically are more welcoming and encouraging to patients with psychiatric conditions, not only because of the absence of an antimedication bias, but also because patients who have suffered from comparing their own recovery unfavorably with that of others in AA who do not have these conditions, find that these meetings provide them with a better reference point for gauging their progress and feeling better about themselves. In regular AA meetings, where discussion focuses almost exclusively on issues directly related to recovery from alcohol and drug use, there sometimes is little tolerance for people with mental health problems, who may be misunderstood and mischaracterized as "too needy," "too whiny," or "wallowing in self pity." Rejection or failure to connect with others in these meetings may serve only to further reinforce a patient's poor self-esteem, lack of optimism and hope, and social anxiety. Similarly, many patients with serious psychiatric problems are often accused of resistance or lack of motivation because their psychiatric symptoms are not recognized or seen as legitimate complaints.

The Roles of Individual and Group Psychotherapy

Generally speaking, patients with coexisting psychiatric disorders will require more individual attention from a therapist than do others being treated for SUDs, especially until their psychiatric symptoms have been substantially reduced. Patients with psychiatric disorders require closer monitoring and more frequent contact, which may include brief "check-in" visits interspersed with longer therapy sessions that focus primarily on establishing abstinence and managing painful affects and unstable mood states. Patients should be seen individually no less than twice a week during the early phase of treatment. Regular individual sessions should be continued with all patients, including those who may enter group therapy or a structured treatment program. Ongoing individual therapy is critically important with these patients because, in our view, it provides indispensable ballast for the therapeutic work. More so than with other patients, the therapist assumes a place of special importance with those suffering with psychiatric illness. Their transferential relationship with the therapist can be extremely intense. The initial work with these patients consists mainly of a pragmatic "how to" approach that establishes a holding environment and supplies the necessary encouragement and support for establishing abstinence and containing painful affects. The ego-strengthening value of this approach facilitates patients' motivation to change and reinforces small gains within the framework of taking "one step at a time." Avoiding intensive uncovering therapy and focusing instead on reality-oriented issues and supportive problem solving is essential for all patients in the early phases of addiction treatment, but is even more important for patients suffering from concurrent psychiatric disorders, in order to minimize exacerbation of their anxiety and other painful affects before they have had a chance to acquire the skills necessary to manage their emotional discomfort more effectively.

Many addicted patients are haunted by traumatic experiences such as incest or family violence and raise these issues early in treatment. Often painful or overwhelming affects associated with these memories surface for the first time in patients' lives once they are abstinent for a brief while and the chemical blanket of alcohol and drug use no longer masks these feelings and keeps them out of conscious awareness (Evans & Sullivan, 1995; Sullivan & Evans, 1994; Young, 1995). Certainly, the therapist should not give short shrift to these memories and associated affects or convey a message that these issues are inappropriate to discuss, but it is important to keep the focus primarily on the initial goal of helping the patient to express and deal with uncomfortable feelings without resorting to alcohol and drug use. As treatment progresses, ongoing therapeutic work aimed more pointedly at addressing these issues can be undertaken with appropriate cautions.

Although group therapy is the principal treatment modality in addiction treatment programs, it often must be used more selectively with patients who have coexisting psychiatric disorders. Group therapy can be very effective with these patients, but only after their psychiatric status has stabilized for a while and they have been prepared adequately by the therapist for entering a group. Inevitably, some patients are not clinically appropriate for group treatment owing to severe impairment in object relations, and others flatly refuse to enter a group despite the therapist's encouragement to give it a try. Sometimes patients with personality disorders that preclude their ability to participate appropriately and derive benefit from group therapy, do well in AA and other 12-step programs. They seem better able to accept feedback from peers in the more informal "non-therapy" setting of AA meetings and appear to benefit especially from tenets of the 12-step program that emphasize taking personal responsibility for one's behavior and its negative impact on others, taking advice and guidance from others who have "been there," and, perhaps most important, identifying and working to overcome one's "character defects."

Most patients with mood and anxiety disorders whose symptoms are under reasonably good control can be mainstreamed into a regular addiction recovery group. In fact, group therapy (discussed more fully in Chapter 12) can be extremely beneficial to these patients in conjunction with concurrent individual therapy, especially when the same therapist provides both modalities of treatment. As a patient's problems reveal themselves naturally in the group as a result of the ongoing group process and interaction between group members, the therapist is in an ideal position to point out in real time when the patient's maladaptive defenses and problems in regulating his feelings are called into play. The therapist can draw connections between these behaviors/affects and the patient's prior use of alcohol and drugs as an attempt to cope with these problems (Khantzian, 1981; Murphy & Khantzian, 1995). The group process also serves to diffuse and dilute transference issues that can undermine individual therapy.

RECIPROCAL RELAPSE

It is important to keep in mind that relapse to a co-occurring psychiatric condition is likely to precipitate a relapse to using alcohol and drugs. Indeed, a reciprocal relapse pattern in which relapse to one problem precipitates relapse to another is common. For example, Janice enjoyed an extended period of sobriety once her mood was normalized on antidepressants. Without mentioning it to her therapist, she concluded that she was "cured" and discontinued her antidepressant medication. Her mood gradually worsened, and 5 weeks later she resumed drinking. Thus, it is useful for your patients to identify early relapse warning signs in relation to a psychiatric condition as well as to their alcohol and other drug use.

ADDRESSING SUICIDE RISK

The frequency of both suicide attempts and completed suicides is substantially higher among people with SUDs than in the general population. Surveys report that between 20 and 30% of patients entering addiction treatment programs have made at least one suicide attempt, and the incidence of completed suicide is probably three to four times that found in the general population (Mirin & Weiss, 1991). Not surprisingly, the presence of depressive disorders in individuals who also abuse alcohol and drugs increases the risk of suicide as compared with such risk in either disorder alone. In addition to the direct biochemical effects of alcohol and drugs on the brain that may increase the likelihood of suicide, the array of negative psychosocial consequences (e.g., job loss, disrupted relationships, alienation of friends and family, etc.) often associated with chronic substance use can contribute to a profound sense of hopelessness and helplessness that may further heighten an individual's suicide risk. Moreover, individuals with serious SUDs, particularly those who have concurrent psychiatric conditions, tend to have low frustration tolerance and display impulsivity and poor judgment, particularly in response to stressful situations. Not only are these often premorbid characteristics that predate an individual's substance dependence, but often they become even more exaggerated during periods of active substance use. Patients with a history of previous suicide attempts are often at elevated risk for another suicide attempt if they relapse to alcohol and drugs after a period of abstinence. Their resulting sense of failure, shame, hopelessness, and self-loathing can become so intolerable that suicide appears as the only escape route from the pain and the ultimate "solution" to their problems. Consider the following case:

> George, a 45-year-old physician, had been completely abstinent while in treatment for addiction for approximately 1 year when he relapsed to cocaine after having several glasses of wine at a friend's wedding. When George initially came into treatment, he was put on notice by the licensing board that one more relapse would result in suspension of his medical license for a minimum of 2 years. As a teenager, he had made a suicide attempt after a homosexual encounter with an older man. This event left him with a legacy of fear and shame about his sexuality, but neither these feelings nor his earlier suicide attempt were addressed during treatment for his cocaine addiction, which focused almost exclusively on establishing and maintaining abstinence. George presented originally with depressive symptoms that remitted successfully with antidepressant medication, but denied any current or recent suicidal ideation or intent. His pattern of cocaine use had involved marathon binges of smoking crack cocaine during which he had multiple sexual encounters with male prostitutes. He identified himself as heterosexual and felt extremely conflicted by the sexual encounters with men, which he said occurred only when he was under the influence of cocaine. He was married, with two children, but his family knew nothing about his sexual escapades on cocaine. Apparently, after his drinking wine at the friend's wedding, George went out on another all-night cocaine and sex binge with male prostitutes. He called his wife in the middle of the night from a hotel room to say that he was profoundly depressed and did not feel that he could go on. Not only was he demoralized by the relapse, but feeling desperate and overwhelmed with shame and guilt and facing the prospect of losing his medical license, George took his own life. He was found the next morning dead by hanging in a hotel room a few miles from his home with a lengthy suicide note on the floor beneath him.

This case underscores several important points: the need to assess patients carefully at the beginning of treatment for past and present suicidal ideation and behaviors, to repeatedly assess suicide risk through all stages of treatment, and to work toward resolving issues that may keep the patient at increased risk for suicide.

FINAL COMMENT

Among patients with SUDs presenting for treatment, a substantial minority are also found to be suffering from one or more concurrent psychiatric disorders. The presence of psychiatric symptoms complicates the tasks of clinical assessment and diagnosis because the acute and chronic effects of alcohol and drugs can mimic the symptoms of nearly every type of psychiatric disorder. Conducting an accurate assessment and formulating a psychiatric diagnosis is best done, ideally, only after the patient has been abstinent for a period of 4–6 weeks, but this is often neither possible nor practical. Clinicians are encouraged to rely on their clinical judgment and take a longitudinal approach to assessment, with repeated observations, in trying to distinguish between drug-induced symptoms and true psychopathology. Therapists have an important role to play in making sure that their patients with coexisting SUDs and psychiatric illness are not only properly diagnosed, but that these patients receive appropriate treatment that addresses both disorders effectively. This usually requires working cooperatively with a psychiatrist or other physician who can prescribe psychotropic medication, when indicated. Therapists should help to foster patient compliance with prescribed medication regimens and educate patients about the interaction between the two types of disorders and how to manage both of them. Therapists should also prepare patients with coexisting psychiatric disorders for involvement in self-help programs and help them anticipate and cope with potential obstacles they may encounter. A combination of individual and group therapy, delivered by the same therapist where possible, is often the most effective strategy for maximizing patient retention and therapeutic gains. Clinicians must address proactively the heightened suicide risk often found among patients with coexisting SUDs and psychiatric disorders.

CHAPTER 6

The Role of Medications

It is essential for nonmedical therapists to recognize the value and appropriate use of pharmacological interventions in treating patients with SUDs. Because certain types of medications can be very helpful, it is important for therapists to work cooperatively with physicians to ensure that medications, when indicated, provide patients with maximum therapeutic benefit. Interdisciplinary cooperation is vital to an integrative approach. Therapists are in an excellent position to monitor and encourage medication compliance and to help patients work through obstacles and concerns about taking medication when these issues arise. Many patients are too hesitant, confused, or distracted to ask pointed questions and express their concerns when meeting with a prescribing physician, and, realistically, many physicians do not have time during tightly scheduled office visits to engage patients in lengthy discussions about medication or to help them work through these issues. Therapists can help substantially in this regard by orienting patients to the expected benefits of medication, fostering their adherence to the prescribed regimen, and encouraging them tolerate transient side effects. They should also help patients acquire a realistic perspective on the relative roles of medication and psychosocial interventions. For example, patients should be informed that when pharmacotherapy is clearly indicated, the combination of medication and therapy is almost always more effective than either of these interventions alone. Not surprisingly, patients with addiction histories often are enamored with pharmacological solutions to problems and may attribute almost magical qualities to medications. Ironically, many others are suspicious, mistrustful, and rejecting of prescribed medications despite having self-administered street drugs of unknown composition and purity possibly thousands of times. Some patients reject medication partly owing to a strong antimedication bias they encounter from others in recovery who maintain an unreasonable and potentially harmful all-or-nothing stance toward cessation of drugs, even when the prescribed medication is nonaddictive, not acutely mood altering, medically indicated, and monitored by a physician and therapist who are fully familiar with the patient's SUD.

The types of medications used in treating SUDs fall generally into four categories: (1) medications to manage detoxification and withdrawal, (2) medications to facilitate relapse prevention, (3) medications to treat coexisting psychiatric conditions, and (4) opioid agonist medications as maintenance/substitution therapy.

MEDICATIONS USED TO MANAGE WITHDRAWAL

Medications used to manage withdrawal, when indicated, differ according to the type of drug the patient is being withdrawn from. Withdrawal from depressant or sedative-type substances (e.g., alcohol, barbiturates, benzodiazepines) is managed with substitute drugs that fall within the same class, but using agents that have a longer duration of action than the patient's drug of choice. For example, withdrawal from alcohol is often accomplished by substituting diazepam (Valium) or lorazepam (Ativan), both of which have substantially longer half-lives than alcohol. The longer half-life allows for a smoother withdrawal because blood levels of these medications do not drop as quickly as do blood levels of alcohol. The first goal is to stabilize the patient on a sufficient does of the substitute medication to prevent the emergence of dangerous or intolerable withdrawal symptoms. Then the substitute medication is tapered gradually over the course of several days or weeks, as clinically required, and ultimately discontinued completely. A similar procedure is used to withdraw patients from opioids such as heroin, codeine, and oxycodone. Typically, the patient is stabilized on a longer-acting opioid such as methadone, buprenorphine, or propoxyphene (Darvon), and then gradually tapered off this medication in a way that minimizes withdrawal discomfort. Sometimes when the patient's starting level of opioid dependence is low, no opioid substitute medication is given because of a concern that it may actually increase rather than decrease the patient's level of pharmacological dependence. In these cases, non-opioid medications such as clonidine and/or mild sedatives are more likely to be used to manage withdrawal symptoms.

MEDICATIONS USED TO FACILITATE
RELAPSE PREVENTION

Naltrexone (Trexan or ReVia) is a medication used to prevent a relapse to opioid use and to attenuate the reinforcing effects of alcohol. It is an opioid blocker or antagonist that occupies opioid receptor sites, so that if patients use any opioids while on naltrexone, they do not produce drug-induced euphoria or physical dependence. Using opioids while on naltrexone is not reinforcing and there is no unpleasant reaction. Naltrexone is neither psychoactive nor addictive. Three factors limit the clinical usefulness of naltrexone: (1) the necessity for patients to be completely detoxified from opioids and remain opioid free for at least several days after their last use of any opioid before they can take a first dose of naltrexone safely without experiencing a severe withdrawal reaction; (2) poor patient compliance in taking naltrexone following opioid detoxification (Greenstein, Arendt, McLellan, O'Brien, & Evans, 1984; Resnick, Schuyten-Resnick, & Washton, 1979, 1980; Resnick & Washton, 1978; Resnick, Washton, Thomas, & Kestenbaum, 1978); and (3) lack of familiarity with naltrexone by physicians and other clinicians. Naltrexone is most effective when used in conjunction with psychosocial interventions (Resnick & Washton, 1978) and has been shown to be a highly effective treatment for opioid-dependent physicians and other medical professionals in that it allows them to return to work environments where they protected against the risk of relapse in the face of having easy access to prescription opioids (Washton, Gold, & Pottash, 1984a, 1984b, 1985).

When used to prevent a relapse to alcohol use, naltrexone does not completely block the effects of alcohol but appears to modify reward pathways so that drinking is less reinforcing or less pleasurable; accordingly, patients are somewhat less likely to return to out-of-control drinking patterns while taking naltrexone (Volpicelli, Altterman, Hayashida, & O'Brien, 1992). Here too, naltrexone is most effective when used in combination with psychosocial interventions such as cognitive-behavioral therapy (O'Malley et al., 1992).

By far the most widely known medication for preventing a relapse to using alcohol is disulfiram (Antabuse). Like naltrexone, disulfram is neither psychoactive nor addictive. It works by blocking enzymes involved in the metabolism of alcohol, so that a person's ingestion of alcohol while on this medication causes a severely unpleasant (and potentially health-threatening) physical reaction. Disulfram works best when patients choose to take it as a deterrent for impulsive drinking. Except for atypical reactions, the medication is inactive unless the patient consumes alcohol. It is the expectation of a severely unpleasant reaction that attenuates the desire to drink. Patients on disulfram who plan to drink must discontinue taking the medication for a number of days before taking a first drink. Many patients report that it was life saving; it "bought" them enough time to develop alternative coping mechanisms. Interestingly, many also report that their cravings are minimal when they are on disulfuram. This is not a medication effect; disulfuram does nothing to suppress craving. Patients report that relief comes from the feeling that once they take their daily pill, they have made the decision not to drink and the struggle is eliminated. Many describe this as quite freeing. However, there are patients who are so impulsive that they will drink while they are on disulfuram, in which case it can be dangerous for them to take it.

As with other medications used to facilitate relapse prevention, disulfuram is most effective when used in combination with psychosocial interventions. Unfortunately, it is often prescribed by a physician who is disconnected from the rest of the treatment process. Disulfuram is useful only insofar as it protects the patient while he is mastering key stressors and learning new coping skills.

Acamprosate (Campral), a medication extensively studied and used in Europe, has been approved recently for prescription use in the United States for treating alcohol dependence. It is an amino acid derivative affecting neurotransmitter systems in a manner that reduces relapse rates. A recent systematic review and meta-analysis indicates that acamprosate appears to be especially useful in promoting abstinence from alcohol, in contrast to naltrexone, which appears more effective in reducing alcohol consumption (Bouza, Magro, Munoz, & Amate, 2004). Studies also suggest that the combination of acamprosate and naltrexone taken together is more effective in preventing alcohol relapse than either medication taken alone (Kiefer et al., 2003). Although both naltrexone and acamprosate are safe and reasonably well tolerated, compliance is a problem requiring attention.

MEDICATIONS USED TO TREAT CO-OCCURRING PSYCHIATRIC CONDITIONS

As discussed in Chapter 5, pharmacological treatment for co-occurring psychiatric disorders, when indicated, improves treatment outcomes in patients with SUDs. In general, psychotropic medications aimed at treating a co-occurring psychiatric disorder are not effective in alleviating substance-induced mood disorders and or in breaking the cycle of compulsive alcohol and drug use. Placing patients on these medications too early in the treatment process can cloud the diagnostic picture, making it more difficult to determine whether an independent coexisting psychiatric disorder is actually present. Nonetheless, psychotropic medication may be required immediately in some cases to manage psychiatric risk, especially when suicidality and/or psychotic symptoms are present.

Medication compliance and development of realistic expectations about the potential benefits and limitations of medication are key issues for patients who suffer with co-occurring psychiatric disorders and SUDs. Some patients appear for the initial interview already receiving psychotropic medication prescribed by a psychiatrist or other physician. In addition to inquiring about the type(s) of medications patients may be taking, as well as particulars regarding dosages, side effects, and perceived beneficial effects, it is equally important to assess patients' understanding of why they are taking the medications. It is essential to clarify for patients that medication given to treat the psychiatric disorder will not, by itself, prevent a relapse to using alcohol and drugs. This unrealistic expectation is encountered most frequently in patients whose psychiatric disorder predated their substance abuse. Their history has led them, quite understandably, to believe that once the psychiatric symptoms are alleviated, they either will no longer have a desire to self-medicate with alcohol and drugs or will be better able to moderate their use of these substances and not lose control. Although it is true that when psychiatric symptoms are in remission the desire to self-medicate with alcohol and drugs may be somewhat reduced, this belief ignores the fact that once an addiction has developed it continues to exist independently of the psychiatric disorder and actually has a life of its own. Apart from the psychiatric condition, countless triggers and other conditioned cues associated with prior substance use can set off cravings and drug-seeking behavior. Moreover, the lack of adequate coping skills common to nearly all people who become addicted to alcohol and drugs can also rekindle the desire to self-medicate in an attempt to deal with significant life stressors, whether or not there is a coexisting psychiatric disorder.

Another key issue in regard to medication compliance is the nature of the patient's interaction with the prescribing physician and the level of cooperation and communication between the nonmedical therapist and the physician. Ideally, the patient will have good rapport with the clinicians and both clinicians will have good rapport with each another. Regrettably, this is not always the case, and nonmedical therapists may have to "shop around" to find a psychiatrist or other physician who has the clinical expertise and therapeutic style conducive to working effectively with addicted patients as part of a team. As nonmedical therapists become increasingly knowledgeable and sophisticated about psychotropic medications, clinical partnerships between psychotherapists (particularly psychologists) and primary care physicians are becoming increasingly common, especially in geographic areas where psychiatrists are in short supply. The idea of taking psychotropic medication often elicits so much anxiety and concern in some patients that any therapist working with these patients should be prepared to orient them appropriately and respond to questions about the workings, benefits, and potential side effects of different types of psychotropic medications and to address patients' common fears such as, "Are these medications addictive?" "Does taking these medications mean that I'm really crazy?" "Do I have to take them forever?" and "How will I know when I don't need them any more?" The issue of medication should be approached as a joint decision made with the active participation of the patient, the therapist, and the prescribing physician.

Many patients with SUDs complain of depression, anxiety, and labile moods, and effective management requires a high level of attentiveness. Your most challenging treatment dilemma is to gauge the proper balance between psychosocial and pharmacological interventions. It is certainly plausible to assume that among individuals who have become dependent on alcohol and drugs, coping skills have declined or perhaps never developed adequately in the first place, and that treatment should address these deficits. A wide variety of cognitive-behavioral strategies are available to enhance such efforts. However, it is easy to underestimate the severity of the depression and anxiety your patient is experiencing and to discourage medication intervention as undermining "real therapy." It is best to be pragmatic and help the patient explore both sides of the issue and make decisions collaboratively. For example, tolerable levels of anxiety have signal value that can initiate and guide adaptive behaviors, but patients cannot approach problems and learn new coping skills when their anxiety is chronically overwhelming and debilitating.

Benzodiazepines (e.g., Valium, Ativan, Xanax, etc.) are excellent anxiolytics (antianxiety agents) but are often considered inappropriate for people with SUDs, particularly those with histories of abusing alcohol or other sedative-type drugs. All benzodiazepines are cross-tolerant with alcohol, and thus may be subject to abuse themselves, or may precipitate a relapse to alcohol use by stimulating similar reward pathways in the brain. Most addiction-savvy physicians prefer to avoid prescribing benzodiazepines to people with a history of alcohol abuse or other SUDs. Selective serotonin reuptake inhibitors (SSRIs) are often the medications of first choice for managing anxiety and work safely and effectively for many patients. However, it is advisable to remain pragmatic, as episodes of overwhelming anxiety over a period of time are virtually guaranteed to lead to an eventual relapse to alcohol and drug use. The recommendation to avoid benzodiazepines has been accepted for a long time, but there are actually few careful studies that explore this issue. Some physicians have employed these medications selectively and infrequently and report good results with specific patients. A recent study by a highly regarded group of researchers concluded that patients with posttraumatic stress disorder, with and without SUDs, who were prescribed benzodiazepines, did not in fact relapse to substance use at higher rates and showed reduced need for health care utilization (Kosten, Fontana, Sernyak, & Rosenheck, 2000). Thus, it may be that carefully prescribed and monitored benzodiazepine use may not undermine recovery efforts in some cases, but may in fact promote it. Nonetheless, the risk–benefit ratio of using benzodiazepines should be considered very carefully before these medications are prescribed to patients with SUDs. Furthermore, patients who do receive these medications should be monitored closely. They should be given judicious doses and small supplies, requiring regular contact with the prescribing physician for refills; they should be placed on a regular schedule of drug and alcohol testing; and their care should be carefully coordinated via ongoing contact between the prescribing physician and the nonmedical therapist.

OPIOID AGONIST MEDICATIONS:
METHADONE AND BUPRENORPHINE

Psychotherapists have new opportunities for collaborating with physicians as a result of the recent approval of an opioid agonist medication that can be used in private practice settings to treat opioid addiction. The approval of two forms of buprenorphine (Subutex and Suboxone) in 2002 created an opportunity for physicians and therapists to team up to provide comprehensive care for opioid users, stemming from well-documented findings that medication combined with psychosocial interventions produces the best clinical outcomes. Methadone maintenance is the best studied and most widely available form of agonist treatment in the United States. It is provided only in specially licensed facilities, in combination with counseling and other ancillary services. Many of the physicians in office practice who may prescribe buprenorphine are primary care physicians (not psychiatrists), who generally neither want nor have the clinical expertise to provide these other services. Therapists wishing to provide these other services must be knowledgeable about opioid addiction and the research on effective treatment. Many patients who have engaged in a long and discouraging struggle to remain opioid free show significant improvement when one of these medications is added. However, a medication alone is rarely sufficient for a condition that has so many behavioral manifestations.

Most therapists lack specific knowledge about opioid addiction and often share the stereotype that most heroin users are indigent, criminally involved, and unemployed. In fact, employed middle-class heroin users are rarely studied, but research indicates that there is a surprisingly large insured population that has problems with heroin (Eisenhandler & Drucker, 1993). Accurate data on prescription opioid use are remarkably difficult to obtain. The Drug Abuse Warning Network (DAWN) reports offer a glimpse through its data on emergency room visits related to the abuse of narcotic analgesics (Substance Abuse and Mental Health Services Administration, 2003). These medications include hydrocodone (e.g., Vicodin), oxycodone (OxyContin, Percoset), meperidine (Demerol), and propoxyphene (Darvon). According to the 2003 DAWN report, the incidence of opioid-related emergency room visits has been increasing since the mid-1990s and more than doubled between 1994 and 2001. Since 1999 oxycodone use has increased the most rapidly. Reliable data on problematic users who remain below the radar of sentinel or epidemiological studies are difficult to obtain.

Until recently patients on opioid agonist pharmacotherapy, such as methadone, could be treated only in clinics with special licenses, and most private practitioners were unfamiliar with the rationale and appropriate use of methadone as a maintenance medication during and after psychosocial interventions were provided. The Drug Addiction Treatment Act that went into effect in 2002 permitted the prescribing of a partial agonist, bu-prenorphine, by specially trained and certified physicians in private offices. Aside from receiving training, the physicians prescribing beprenorphine must certify that they have the ability to refer patients for the necessary ancillary services. Inasmuch as the scientific data base consistently supports the importance of psychosocial services in conjunction with medication, physicians who attend the specialized buprenorphine training are urged to arrange such services through collaboration with other caregivers if they cannot provide the needed services themselves. Psychotherapists participating in this collaboration must not only understand basic principles of addiction treatment, but must have specific knowledge about opioid addiction and agonist treatment as well.

Stereotypes and misunderstandings about heroin addiction and opioid agonist medication abound, even among experienced clinicians. For many reasons, agonist medication is neither necessary nor currently possible for treating addiction to non-opioid substances such as alcohol or cocaine. However, many studies support the view that abnormal brain chemistry is part of the vulnerability to heroin addiction, a consequence of regular use, or both (Payte, Zweben, & Martin, 2003). Such abnormalities have been described as "receptor system dysfunction" by Vincent Dole, the physician who conducted the early research that made methadone available for clinical use (Dole, 1988). Dole stated that brain function could be corrected, though not cured, by ongoing methadone maintenance, in much the same way that thyroid dysfunction is corrected by maintenance medication. Although ideologically unpalatable to some, an extensive research data base demonstrates poor long-term outcomes for chronic heroin users who are not on methadone maintenance, despite numerous treatment efforts. A 33-year follow-up study of a large cohort of heroin users, most of whom were not on methadone, indicated high death rates and poor psychosocial outcomes for the majority of those who survived (Hser, Hoffman, Grella, & Anglin, 2001). Although members of this study cohort were not socially advantaged, clinical experience indicates that many middle-class opioid users who substitute other drugs end up in treatment or deteriorate through the use of alcohol or prescription drugs. Heroin and prescribed opioids have the same effect on the brain receptors for opioids and can induce physical dependence and addictive behaviors. Both have relatively high abuse potential, especially in vulnerable users, who may begin their trajectory with legitimate use for medical problems. A social cushion offers some protection, but it is common to see lost productivity, impaired relationships, and poor health consequences in many former opioid users who made a variety of drug substitutions. The stigma against methadone has made it unacceptable to many middle-class patients, and many prestigious addiction treatment centers refuse to offer it or insist that it be discontinued in order for a person to participate in their programs. This practice persists despite its being a violation of the Americans with Disabilities Act. Opioid users who do poorly with psychosocial treatment alone can always be described as insufficiently motivated, unwilling to attend enough 12-step meetings, or otherwise uncooperative about doing what it takes to maintain "true recovery." Treatment providers of all persuasions have sophisticated ways of explaining their failures without questioning basic assumptions.

Rationale for Treatment with Opioid Agonists

The use of opioid agonists as a maintenance pharmacotherapy was initiated by Vincent Dole and Marie Nyswander, physicians who studied methadone in the 1960s (Dole & Nyswander, 1965, 1967). They held the view that there was something unique about the condition of opioid addiction that made it difficult for heroin users to remain drug free for extended periods of time. They were unwilling to attribute this categorically to lack of sufficient patient motivation, and their hypothesis concerning neurotransmitter abnormalities was supported and elaborated by decades of subsequent research. Their original notion that opioid addiction involves a "metabolic defect" evolved to the concept of "receptor system dysfunction," and research suggesting that abnormalities may be pre-existing (e.g., genetic vulnerability) or the result of chronic opioid use itself. They hypothesized that opioid maintenance pharmacotherapy restores the neurotransmitter balance. In the case of methadone, it is usually not difficult to find the therapeutic window in which the patient does not crave opioids and is not oversedated. Once this is accomplished, the patient is much better able to make use of psychosocial interventions. Studies examining the relative influence of psychosocial interventions conclude that patients on an appropriate dose of methadone show much better outcomes when adequate or enhanced psychosocial interventions are included in the first 6 months of treatment (McLellan, Arndt, Metzger, Woody, & O'Brien, 1993). Conversely, even high-quality psychosocial services do not produce good outcomes in the absence of adequate and stable doses of medication (Sees et al., 2000).

   In the case of methadone, it is difficult to overstate the role of stigma in shaping policy and clinical practice. For practical purposes, it is similar to using thyroid medication to normalize hormone levels, but from the outset the use of methadone was heavily influenced by the antipathy toward therapeutic use of opioid agonists, particularly for ongoing maintenance. Initial regulations required that methadone be viewed as a transitional medication to help addicted individuals achieve a "drug-free" lifestyle with improved psychosocial functioning. Because of its addictive properties, methadone was considered a "drug," not a medication, and time limits were placed on its use. For patients, this policy did not produce lasting gains. Studies supported Dole and Nyswander's original premise that methadone corrected but did not cure dysfunction, and that gains would be lost when the medication was stopped. It was found that fewer than 20% of chronic opioid users would remain free of illicit drugs by the end of 1 year if they discontinued their methadone. Short-term success (e.g., 6 months) occurred, but follow-up studies showed increasing relapse rates. Although 20% appear to be able to discontinue methadone and preserve their gains, no one is able to predict who those individuals will be. Although it is essential for patients to address inner and outer risk factors, such as management of emotions and participation in social groups that do not use drugs or engage in criminal activity, this alone is not sufficient to produce success. Fortunately, research scrutiny has been intense for three decades, and the knowledgeable professional community has concluded that indefinite maintenance is likely necessary for the majority of chronic users. This view is supported by two major scientific bodies that examined the evidence in the early 1990s and concluded that the treatment is effective and barriers need to be reduced (National Consensus Development Panel on Effective Medical Treatment of Opioid Addiction, 1998; Rettig & Yarmolinsky, 1995).

Contributing to the long-standing stigma associated with opioid maintenance or substitution therapies like methadone is the tendency to equate physical dependency on a medication with the addiction syndrome and associated antisocial behaviors. Early models of addiction were organized around a pharmacology model, based on opioids and alcohol, which have defined indications of tolerance and withdrawal. The cocaine epidemic stimulated a reformulation of addictive disorders into behavioral terms. This is reflected in the DSM-IV, in which criteria for substance dependence can be met even if there is no physical dependence. Over time, addiction specialists and others have begun to emphasize the distinction between physical dependence and the addiction syndrome. They note that physical dependence can occur with medications that clearly improve rather than impair patient functioning. This concept includes the woman on benzodiazepines for anxiety disorder who does not escalate her dose, does not engage in drug-seeking behavior, and has crippling anxiety symptoms without the medication even when the physical withdrawal period has passed. It includes the patient with chronic pain whose functioning is somewhat affected by opioid use, but who is able to maintain a higher level of functioning when his pain is adequately controlled. Confusion of physical dependence with an addictive disorder is part of what creates undermedication of pain, even in patients with terminal illness. This is an issue that is finally being addressed in the licensing requirements of medical providers.

Addiction treatment professionals are increasingly distinguishing between physical dependence and addictive disorders. Methadone treatment providers define a patient as abstinent if he is not drinking alcohol or using illicit drugs and is using legal ones as prescribed. In many localities, the field as a whole uses "abstinence-based" or "drug-free" to describe programs outside the methadone treatment system, but this has become increasingly untenable in an era when co-occurring addiction and other medical disorders are recognized as the norm and many patients are on psychotropic medication. It becomes awkward to explain why patients on antidepressants are abstinent but patients on methadone or buprenorphine are not. Increasingly, medication is viewed as quite compatible with recovery if the patient is not drinking or using illicit drugs. Some of the insurance-funded treatment programs are endorsing buprenorphine while forbidding methadone, using creative logical contortions to explain why one is acceptable but the other is not. In the end, the methadone issue cannot be avoided, because many patients will only partially improve on buprenorphine because of the dose ceiling. In a rational medical practice—still in the future in our country—such patients will be switched to methadone as easily as they are switched between antidepressants. At present, this is impeded by both regulation and stigma.

Buprenorphine

Although the stigma associated with methadone lessened considerably, it became clear that wide acceptance would be achieved slowly, despite the fact that the medication is safe, effective, and inexpensive. As buprenorphine was investigated as a treatment for opioid addiction, efforts were successful in not imposing on this medication many of the regulatory obstacles that burdened and limited the use of methadone. The Drug Addiction Treatment Act of 2000 (DATA 2000) allows qualified physicians to acquire the privilege to prescribe buprenorphine by completing educational requirements and applying for a waiver of the special registration requirements defined in the Controlled Substances Act. The primary goal of these actions is to expand the clinical context of medication-assisted treatment by making buprenorphine available in office-based medical practice, outside of public clinics and treatment programs.

Buprenorphine is a partial opioid agonist commonly used as an injectible analgesic in hospital care. It is also available as tablets that dissolve under the tongue (sublingual). This partial agonist has the significant advantage of a considerable margin of safety with little chance of a lethal overdose. One disadvantage is that patients with a high tolerance may find that its agonist properties are not sufficient to control their symptoms, and there is a dose ceiling that may limit its usefulness in these individuals Methadone maintenance patients on doses higher than 50–60 milligrams are likely to fall into this category. The average dose of methadone in U.S. opiod treatment programs is between 80 and 120 milligrams. Some patients who are doing well on methadone may wish to transfer to buprenorphine in order to change the treatment venue to an office practice and away from regulation-laden clinic care. Transfer to buprenorphine is possible when doses are reduced to 30 milligrams or below. If patients try to reduce their methadone doses in order to switch medications, the period of dose reduction may be unbearable without relapse. Even when patients try to reduce their methadone doses and switch to buprenorphine, and succeed for a period of time, some remain vulnerable and relapse in the face of stressors or temptations. It is as if patients have a "set point" in opioid tolerance that is adjustable only within a specific range. Reducing one's tolerance is only part of what is involved in determining an adequate dose of medication. In a nutshell, motivation is important but brain chemistry influences long-term prospects. Those who are able to taper off the medication often experience an easier transition to a medication-free state. Some patients report a positive effect on anxiety or mood. Buprenorphine may be a good choice if depression is a prominent part of the clinical picture.

The stigma attached to methadone has meant that working and middle-class patients who are insured may receive poor recommendations from the privately funded treatment system. You may see patients who have used illicit heroin or prescription opioids for years, achieved periods of abstinence, and repeatedly relapsed. These patients are criticized for inconsistent motivation and failure to participate regularly in the self-help system or make other behavioral changes. For some, antidepressants result in some improvement, but remission is incomplete. Over time their losses accumulate and their feelings of failure and hopelessness increase. They blame themselves for failure, and this is reinforced by their encounters with professionals with little specific understanding of opioid addiction.

> Dr. Daniels, a 45-year-old cardiologist, was referred to treatment by a colleague who became aware of the patient's pattern of self-prescribing various opioid drugs. For approximately 1 year, Dr. Daniels used hydrocodone cough syrup at least three to four times per week. He managed to avoid becoming physically dependent on the drug, but then switched from hydrocodone syrup to oxycodone tablets. At that point, his use increased substantially and several colleagues in the hospital noted that he was not acting "normal." His initial treatment consisted of inpatient opioid detoxification with methadone, followed by participation in an aftercare recovery group and attendance at AA and NA meetings. He voluntarily joined the physicians' health program administered by the state medical society where he practiced, and he was placed immediately on random forensic urine testing. Dr. Daniels remained abstinent for 3 months and then relapsed to taking hydrocodone syrup daily. This time he was obtaining the drug by calling in prescriptions to several pharmacies for fictitious patients under another physician's name and license number. When a suspicious pharmacist

reported this activity to the state medical board, the patient's license to practice medicine was suspended for 3 months. Thereafter, his medical license was restored, but several months after returning to practice he was again caught self-prescribing opioids (this time OxyContin). The board then suspended his license for a year with the admonition that if he relapsed again, his medical license would be revoked, perhaps permanently.

Dr. Daniels remained drug free again for less than 3 months and relapsed again to opioid use upon learning of his mother's death. The patient finally became aware of his use of opioids as self-medication to alleviate overwhelming feelings of anxiety, depression, and anger stimulated by a wide range of events and circumstances in both his personal and professional life. It was suggested that Dr. Daniels be given a trial on buprenorphine, rather than his attempting again to remain abstinent, in light of his repeated failure to do so successfully and the grave consequences to his medical career that would befall him if he relapsed again. The patient was placed on daily doses of buprenorphine and almost immediately felt "normal." He reported no euphoria from the medication, and there was no evidence of any drug-induced impairment in his cognitive functioning, affect, or psychomotor skills. The medical board gave him one final chance to return to medical practice when presented with a treatment plan that included buprenorphine maintenance in combination with appropriate monitoring and psychosocial treatment. As of this writing, the patient has remained stable on buprenorphine and abstinent from all other drugs for approximately 24 months. He has returned to medical practice and appears to be dealing well with the stressors in his life that previously led to his multiple relapses.

High-prestige treatment institutions may be the least likely to raise the possibility of using an opioid agonist, despite clear indication that a patient is floundering. It is always possible to point to some motivational or psychodynamic defect in the patient to explain why a treatment is failing. Methadone treatment is so stigmatized that it can be unthinkable to even consider referring a patient. Because an office-based physician can prescribe buprenorphine, it may be seen as a more acceptable option. Ironically, patients may get more appropriate recommendations in the methadone treatment system that primarily treats those who are indigent or nearly so. Yet patients who have experienced methadone, often through short-term detoxification, are keenly aware that it produced an improved sense of well-being, a feeling of being normal.

Your job in such circumstances is to give permission to consider opioid agonists as a potentially key tool in sustained improvement. Recommendation to a physician familiar with these medications is the best way to define a course of action. In general, a history of opioid use greater than 1 year, with multiple attempts to discontinue and repeated relapse, is an indication that agonist medication is appropriate. A knowledgeable physician, familiar with the extensive evidence base and not influenced by stigma, is in the best position to make recommendations.

The transition to buprenorphine from dependence on other opioids can be stressful, and it is important to provide adequate support. Patients are asked to wait until they experience definitive signs of withdrawal before buprenorphine is started, as induction goes more smoothly and there is less chance that the first dose of buprenorphine will induce a more severe withdrawal syndrome. This can be difficult for some patients, because of both the actual physical discomfort and the fears of unbearable discomfort based on past experiences. It is important to ask the patient to plan realistically. You need to ask questions about arrangements such as a ride to and from the physician's office or clinic during the first 24 hours of medication treatment, as well as encourage or intervene to promote a calm and supportive home environment. Family members should be asked to refrain from trying to work on difficult issues until the patient is more stable. Reassurance and frequent contact are important during this period.

If the patient is using a short-acting opioid like heroin, the onset of withdrawal occurs 6–12 hours after the last ingestion. Most prescription drugs are short acting unless they are given in a sustained-release formulation. Methadone is long acting, and withdrawal may not ensue for 36–72 hours, depending on the patient's metabolism of the drug.

Table 6.1 presents the signs and symptoms of opioid withdrawal.

TABLE 6.1. Signs and Symptoms of Opioid Withdrawal

Early to moderate	Moderate to advanced
Anorexia	Abdominal cramps
Anxiety	Hot or cold flashes
Irritability	Increased blood pressure
Craving	Increased pulse
Dysphoria	Insomnia
Restlessness	Low-grade fever
Fatigue	Muscle and bone pain
Headache	Muscle spasm
Increased respiratory rate	Mydriasis (with dilated, fixed pupils at
Lacrimation	peak)
Mydriasis (pupil dilation, mild)	Nausea and vomiting
Piloerection (gooseflesh)	
Rhinorrhea	
Yawning	

A stable dose of buprenorphine can often be reached by the 3rd or 4th day after the first dose, with no withdrawal and no craving or desire to use. However, it can take many months for body systems to adjust—for example, for stress hormones and menstrual cycles to become normal. You should encourage patients to reduce or modify work commitments for the first 3–4 days to allow time for adjustment to the medication.

Once the patient is maintained on buprenorphine, you should have an agreement with the prescribing physician about methods and frequency of communication, indications of serious concerns, and intervals to review and update the treatment plan. Many patients wish to discontinue prematurely. Once they feel better, they conclude they are "cured" and are eager to taper off the medication. This should be discouraged, as it takes 6–12 months for a gradual normalization of the body and often longer than that to complete the lifestyle changes that will promote enduring recovery.

If, after a few weeks, the patient is still experiencing objective or subjective symptoms of withdrawal, it may be that the ceiling for buprenorphine is not high enough and you should support the patient in considering methadone. First, explore the possibility that the discomforts are psychological. Does the patient miss getting high? Is she expecting too much? Buprenorphine, unlike heroin, leaves patients with the normal stresses and miseries of everyday life. Is she resenting family responsibilities, such as dealing with children's homework? Is the patient expecting to feel "loaded" or sedated? You may need to educate the patient about what is "normal" and the need to let go of the "abnormal normality" of a partially intoxicated state. The benefit of opioid agonist medications is that they allow the patient to function in the normal range, without euphoria or oversedation.

If the patient is avoiding drug triggers and is still experiencing craving, closer scrutiny is needed. You can ask your patient to list all his triggers, such as drug-using buddies or environments, physicians' offices, particular pharmacies, or stressful parts of the day or week. Patients should be encouraged to avoid or modify triggers as best they can and develop a coping strategy for the rest. Patients who remove themselves from triggers may be able to remain abstinent and comfortable on lower doses of opioid agonists. If the reasonable lifestyle changes have occurred and the patient is still distressed, it is time to reconsider which medication is appropriate. It is important for you to emphasize that individuals process drugs very differently and that an inability to progress on buprenorphine is not a personal failure. You may need to bring in family members at this time as well, to address their disappointment and other negative feelings. Ideally, such a meeting includes the prescribing physician, but over time you can become knowledgeable enough to handle the questions and issues that arise. Keep in mind that effective psychoeducation relies on a good sense of timing in both giving information and exploring areas of misunderstanding and resistance.

At the time of this writing, it is illegal for a physician to use methadone to treat addiction in an office-based practice unless that physician obtains the same type of license required for clinics. If your patient being treated with buprenorphine has had previous experience in being on methadone, she may have a good basis for comparing the relief obtained by both medications. Be sure to inquire if the patient had a period of at least several months on a stabilized dose of methadone without the confounding influence of heroin or other drug use. If the patient has had no experience with methadone, it may be important to encourage her to consider it. You can expect strong resistance to becoming involved with a licensed clinic and its often oppressive regulations. Fortunately, there has been strong federal leadership in the last decade to reduce this type of barrier, and patients who do well can obtain 30 days of take-home medication if no state regulations or clinic rules preclude this. You may need to support your patient in enduring the demands and restrictions, in the interest of interrupting the downhill trajectory that occurs with illicit opioid use.

PRINCIPLES OF COLLABORATION BETWEEN PHYSICIANS AND NONMEDICAL THERAPISTS

Good collaboration takes as much skill as good therapeutic intervention, and you and the prescribing physician will create your teamwork as you work together. You can offer a comprehensive psychosocial assessment and treatment plan, tasks that require much more time than most physicians have available. You should establish communication pathways and procedures for collaboration on routine as well as urgent matters. You and the physician should clarify roles in the formulation and implementation of the treatment plan. It is important to specify indications that the current plan is not working and to define a process for revising it.

TRAINING

The more you know about treating addiction in general and opioid dependence in particular, the more effective you will be. The Center for Substance Abuse Treatment (CSAT) offers a free online course for counselors working with patients on buprenorphine, and information is available on its buprenorphine website (www.buprenorphine.samhsa.gov) as well. Taking the required physicians' course is invaluable, as it will increase your knowledge and sense of comfort with the medication. It will also give you a clear picture of the constraints and options of the physician and will help you work out an effective collaboration. There is also an online version of the physicians' 8-hour course offered by the American Academy of Addiction Psychiatrists (AAAP; www.aaap.org).

FINAL COMMENT

An essential component of treating SUDs effectively in many patients, appropriate and well-timed pharmacological intervention requires close collaboration between the treating therapist and the prescribing physician. Therapists need to have a basic understanding of the indications, characteristics, limitations, and appropriate uses of the pharmacological interventions that are used to facilitate detoxification, to reduce relapse rates, to treat co-occurring psychiatric conditions, and to provide opioid maintenance therapy. Medications can enhance the recovery process in a variety of ways. It is important to keep in mind that medications are not a substitute for the work of recovery, but where indicated they can augment the success of patients' efforts. Regular inquiry about adherence to prescribed regimens, recommended intervals for check-in visits with the prescribing physician, and feelings about taking medication are important issues to address in the therapy. Therapists usually have a greater opportunity to explore with patients the charged issues around medication than physicians whose contact with patients is often restricted to brief follow-up visits.

PART II

Clinical Strategies and Techniques

CHAPTER 7

Assessment

An assessment should focus on many different dimensions of a patient's substance use and related issues. The various components of a multidimensional assessment are presented here in a particular sequence that can be used to structure the interview process. However, decisions about exactly what issues you need to address at what point in the interview (or in subsequent sessions) and how deeply you should delve into each issue are largely matters of clinician judgment. Suffice it to say at this point that an assessment is not intended to proceed in linear fashion, follow the same template for all patients, or obtain information at the expense of developing rapport, trust, and a working therapeutic relationship with the patient.

The clinical function and importance of assessment should not be underestimated, considering that treatment inevitably takes place concurrently with assessment. Assessment is best viewed as the beginning phase of treatment and a clinical intervention that sets the tone for everything that follows. Assessment serves three distinct, but interrelated, functions: (1) to develop rapport with the patient and initiate a therapeutic relationship, (2) to determine the nature and extent of the patient's substance use and related consequences and identify factors that initiate and maintain the use, (3) to provide objective feedback based on the assessment results and determine the patient's stage of readiness for change in preparation for developing an initial treatment plan.

THERAPEUTIC APPROACH TO ASSESSMENT

Obtaining accurate information about your patients' substance use depends heavily on creating a safe environment that fosters their openness, honesty, and a willingness to be forthcoming with you about the details of their use and related issues without fearing that you will judge or reject them. Accordingly, your clinical stance must be devoid of presumptions and preconceptions about the nature, extent, and severity of a patient's substance use, as this information should emerge from the assessment process.

Conducting a comprehensive assessment for SUDs requires the same breadth and depth of clinical inquiry needed for any other type of mental health problem. Assessment is where the therapeutic process starts, and too often where it comes to an abrupt end, with patients who abuse alcohol and drugs. This is especially true for individuals who are not seeking your help for an alcohol or drug problem and those who are coerced or mandated by others to come to see you (discussed in a later section). Conveying empathy, nonjudgmental acceptance, and a warm, caring attitude yields much better results than aggressive confrontation. The assessment interview sets the tone for what follows and provides both patient and therapist with important clues about their ability to work together. Patients should come away from the assessment feeling that they have been heard and understood and with a sense of optimism about coming back.

The importance of the patient's early impressions and rapport with the interviewer should not be underestimated. Patients frequently hark back to the first interview as a critical turning point in coming to grips with their alcohol or drug problem. The interviewer's accepting, nonjudgmental attitude is often mentioned as a critical factor in helping them feel comfortable enough to disclose the truth about the nature and extent of their substance use. Inaccurate reporting about alcohol and drug use can result not only from patients' denial of the problem, but also from what they perceive the consequences of providing full disclosure might be. This is an issue that presents itself most clearly with mandated patients, but can also appear with those seeking treatment "voluntarily" in response to pressure from family members and significant others. Patients are more likely to withhold information about their substance use when threatened by real or imagined consequences. It is a grave mistake for clinicians to presume that all people with alcohol and drug problems are liars, manipulators, and sociopaths.

It is also important to recognize that although it is ostensibly the patient who is being evaluated, the interview is always a two-way process. Both you and the patient inevitably give and receive information about each other during the course of the interview. Patients with serious alcohol and drug problems often harbor a great deal of shame and guilt about their behavior, which heightens their sensitivity and reactivity to any hint of negativity the interviewer might express inadvertently, whether in body language, facial expressions, voice intonation, or choice of words. This exquisite sensitivity makes it especially critical for the interviewer to convey an empathic, nonjudgmental, accepting attitude toward patients with SUDs. Patients who use illicit drugs are especially keen on assessing whether the interviewer is familiar with the particulars of drug use. When they encounter clinicians who appear to know less than they do about drugs, they are usually willing to accept this limitation as long as the clinician is nonjudgmental and empathic. Although all clinicians need a working knowledge of psychoactive drugs and relevant clinical phenomena, they should not hesitate to ask patients to educate them about aspects of drug use that are beyond the scope of their current knowledge.

Recognizing the therapist's behavior as critical factor that profoundly influences the course and outcome of the assessment is a departure from traditional approaches that blame substance-abusing patients for creating any and all obstacles to engaging in the helping process. The assessment affords a unique opportunity to enhance patients' motivation for change and increase their willingness to engage in treatment. Using motivational strategies throughout the assessment is crucial, because patients' ambivalence and mistrust are often highest when they first appear for treatment. Some patients are reluctant to provide details about their alcohol or drug use or acknowledge that their use is a problem, let alone agree to accept anyone's treatment recommendations. The best rule to follow during the assessment is "Go slowly at first for the sake of getting things going at all."

BROACHING THE SUBJECT OF ALCOHOL
AND DRUG USE

When substance abuse is not a presenting complaint or among the reasons that the patient has come to see you, you must make a strategic decision about when and how to raise the issue of alcohol and drug use in the course of an initial interview. If you focus prematurely or spend an inordinate amount of time on this issue without first addressing patients' presenting complaints, they may bristle and feel misunderstood. They may perceive you (perhaps rightly so) as needing to control the agenda of the interview too tightly or even as having a personal axe to grind about alcohol and drug use. It is a delicate balancing act to engage your patients in collaborative exploration of their substance use in a way that does not provoke reactance or stimulate defensiveness. It can be helpful to mention to patients that because alcohol and drug problems are so highly prevalent in society at large, and especially among people seeking professional help for other types of life problems, it is considered good clinical practice for all health care professionals to routinely ask their patients about alcohol and drug use.

It is generally best to ask about alcohol and prescription drug use before inquiring about illicit drug use. This gives you a chance to establish initial rapport with the patient before addressing the potentially more sensitive topic of illicit drugs. When a patient does acknowledge use of alcohol or drug(s), you should be careful not to put the patient on the defensive. Avoid taking an aggressive or adversarial stance in which you assume that the patient's substance use is problematic until proven otherwise. The interview must not turn into a cat and mouse game of trying to corner the patient into admitting that he really does have an alcohol or drug problem. You should also avoid suggesting that you routinely exclude patients with SUDs from your clinical practice. This will stimulate mistrust and give patients reason to downplay or completely omit certain aspects of their substance use history.

Questions regarding substance use should be posed in a nonjudgmental, low-key manner that encourages open and honest self-disclosure. Despite initial reluctance, most patients respond openly to questions about their substance use if you address it in a routine manner, conveying an attitude of acceptance, respect, and genuine concern. Your interviewing style is of critical importance here: a matter-of-fact, friendly, curious, nonconfrontational approach definitely works best. You must be careful not to respond negatively to patients who are reluctant to discuss the details of their alcohol and drug use at the first interview. It is essential to honor the edict "Do no harm." You must categorically avoid taking an authoritarian stance, as well as body language and voice intonation, that may alienate patients and preclude an opportunity to establish good rapport.

ASSESSMENT TOOLS

An extensive collection of alcohol and drug abuse assessment instruments (e.g., the Michigan Alcoholism Screening Test, Drug Abuse Screening Test, CAGE, Alcohol Use Disorders Identification Test, etc.), including those used most frequently in addiction treatment programs and research studies, are readily available from government publications and websites (Allen & Columbus, 1995). However, most of these instruments are not well suited for use in office-based psychotherapy practice. Some are simply too lengthy and time-consuming, given the time constraints of a busy office practice. Others are too brief (as few as four questions) and focus mainly on signs of severe problems, leaving less serious and earlier-stage problems prone to being overlooked. Most of the available instruments deal only with alcohol use, only a few deal with specifically with drug use, and except for most lengthy instruments, few address the full spectrum of psychoactive substances. Regardless of how extensive, no screening instrument by itself can accurately determine the nature and extent of an SUD or provide a definitive diagnosis and cannot take the place of a focused clinical interview.

Self-Administered Substance Use Questionnaire

The questionnaire shown in Appendix 1 is designed to be self-administered by patients and to be used as a guide for conducting a focused assessment interview. This instrument can save a great deal of time because it provides you with a wealth of clinical information prior to the interview itself. Instead of taking copious notes during the interview, you can spend more time establishing a therapeutic relationship with the patient. The questionnaire is divided into several sections, each addressing a different aspect of the patient's substance use.

   • *History of Substance Use.* This section contains an extensive list of the different types of psychoactive drugs, in which patients indicate for each substance whether they ever have used that substance even once in their lifetime, whether they have ever viewed their use of that substance as a "problem," and the longest time able to remain abstinent from that substance when trying deliberately to stop. It also asks patients to list what substances (if any) they have used on each of the past 7 days and to indicate the specific amounts used on each of those days.
   • *Substance Use Profile.* This section contains 13 yes/no questions addressing various aspects of the patient's substance use and related consequences. The seven DSM-IV diagnostic criteria for substance dependence are embedded within these questions.
   • *Consequences of Alcohol and Drug Use.* This section contains an extensive checklist of psychosocial problems commonly associated with substance abuse.
   • *Treatment History.* This section asks about prior treatment for SUDs.
   • *Positive Effects of Substance Use.* This section contains a checklist of perceived positive benefits of alcohol and drug use.
   • *Physical Problems Related to Substance Use.* This section asks about signs of physical dependence on alcohol and drugs and medical complications that may have occurred during previous attempts to stop using.
   • *Sexual Behaviors and Substance Use.* This section of the questionnaire asks about various types of sexual problems and behaviors associated with alcohol and other drug use, including stimulant-related hypersexuality and other sexual acting-out behaviors.

Reasons for Seeking Help: Why Now?

It is important to ask the person seeking help for an alcohol or drug problem why he is doing so at this particular point in time. The patient's response to the question "Why now?" can provide useful information about internal and external factors that have led him to come to see you.

Without asking, you have no way of knowing whether the person views his substance use as a problem or has any intentions of changing it.

The following are some questions to ask patients who come voluntarily seeking your help for an alcohol or drug problem:

- "What recent events led to your making the appointment to come here today?"
- "Is there a serious crisis that we need to address today?"
- "Are other people encouraging or pressuring you to do something about your alcohol or drug use?"
- "What would have to happen here today for you to feel that this visit is worthwhile?"
- "How do you view your alcohol or drug use and what, if anything, are you hoping to do about it?

The following are some questions to ask patients who are being pressured or coerced into seeking your help for an alcohol or drug problem:

- "Whose idea was it for you to come see me today?"
- "What have they seen that makes them think that you need to be here?"
- "Do you agree with their reasons for wanting you to be here?"
- "What exactly would have to happen for them to be satisfied with what we do here?"
- "What will happen if they see you are taking steps to deal with your alcohol or drug use?"
- "How will that help you?"
- "What will happen if they see that you are not dealing seriously with your substance use?"
- "What problems or consequences will that cause for you?

In all cases it is important to know whether and to what extent the patient may be responding to a recent crisis and/or external pressure from others. Often it is an acute crisis or emergency demanding immediate attention that prompts people to seek help for alcohol and drug problems. Often the crisis has been generated by consequences resulting directly from the person's alcohol or drug use (e.g., a job in jeopardy, financial problems, marital problems, etc.). Sometimes the first session must be devoted entirely to dealing with the immediate crisis and the assessment must be deferred until the next visit. First priority must always be given to protecting the patient's safety and alleviating the immediate crisis, even if the crisis is directly related to the patient's alcohol or drug use. The therapist's rule of thumb here, as with all patients in distress, is to address and stabilize the most dangerous situations first and establish a safety net to protect the patient as much as possible from experiencing harm, before addressing factors that may have contributed to the current situation or attempting interventions that may cause more psychological stress. For example, the first thing to do with a cocaine-dependent patient who is experiencing paranoia and suicidal ideation is to manage her psychiatric risk before addressing her cocaine problem.

Coerced and Mandated Patients

Many individuals with alcohol and drug problems appear for treatment only in response to external pressure. Some state begrudgingly that their only reason for coming to the appointment is to comply with the wishes of a family member or significant other. Others are there to satisfy a mandate issued by a court, regulatory agency, licensing board, motor vehicle bureau, or other outside agency. In all such cases it is essential to determine the patients' understanding of exactly what they are being asked to do and specifically what consequences are likely to occur if they do not comply with these requests or mandates. Mandated patients pose a formidable challenge for any interviewer: How can you conduct an accurate, thorough substance use assessment with someone who comes to the interview with reason to actively withhold and/or falsify information? First, it is essential that the therapist fully expect and be mindful of the fact that mandated and coerced patients are likely to both feel and act angry, mistrustful, resentful, controlled, infantilized, humiliated, fearful, anxious, defensive, and suspicious. Accepting this reality can help in finding an effective way to "start where the patient is."

Berg and Miller (1992) propose several techniques for approaching mandated patients: (1) Be sympathetic to the patient's plight and validate his appropriately negative feelings in light of the unpleasant circumstances that brought him to your door; (2) accept without challenge that the individual's likely goal for the interview is to get the coercing agent off his back; (3) compliment the patient for recognizing the importance of at least showing up for the interview; (4) emphasize that showing up for the interview was a matter of personal choice and a positive indication of caring about oneself, as it was entirely possible to not show up and face the self-destructive consequences of that choice; (5) detach yourself from the coercing person or agency by stating clearly that your goal is not to coerce this individual into doing anything, but rather to help him achieve an accurate assessment and understanding of the nature of his involvement with psychoactive substances. If you are, in fact, required to issue an assessment report and treatment recommendations to the coercing person/agent, it is essential for you to say so very clearly and straightforwardly at the outset of the interview while underscoring that your task is to help the patient comply with the mandate and thereby avoid unnecessary consequences.

Intoxicated Patients

It is impossible to conduct a meaningful clinical interview with someone who is actively intoxicated. When patients do report having used alcohol and/or other drugs in the hours immediately preceding the interview but show no overt signs of impairment, a brief interview can be attempted, but the full assessment should be deferred until the patient is not under the influence of any psychoactive substances. If, however, the patient exhibits significant, observable signs of substance-induced cognitive, affective, or motor impairment (e.g., slurred speech, stumbling gait, inappropriate affect, or impaired responsiveness), you should defer the interview and take appropriate measures to protect the patient's safety. You can ask an intoxicated patient to give you her car keys and request permission to reach a family member or significant other who can come to your office to escort or drive the patient home. Alternatively, you can encourage the patient to remain in your office until she is sober enough to leave safely. In cases of severe intoxication and possible overdose reactions (e.g., patient lapses in and out of consciousness, exhibits seizures, or shows signs of labored breathing), you should call 911 immediately for emergency assistance.

Substance Use Profile

Types of Substances Used

The nature and extent of a patient's involvement with psychoactive substances should be explored in detail. Your inquiry should cover the full range of substances that fall within the various categories described earlier: alcohol and sedatives–hypnotics, stimulants, opioids, hallucinogens, cannabinoids, inhalants, and club drugs. In addition to the use of these substances, use of holistic preparations including vitamins, homeopathic or herbal remedies, and nutritional supplements should be explored. Many of these preparations contain ingredients that produce psychoactive effects of their own and/or potentiate the effects of other psychoactive substances. Certain herbal products, for example, mimic the effects of Ecstasy, a mild hallucinogen. Others contain the stimulant ephedrine, which can mimic or enhance the effects of other stimulants such as cocaine and amphetamine. There are also over-the-counter products that can cause changes in steroid and hormone levels, leading to disturbances in mood and personality.

When asking about the patient's substance use, do so with an attitude of curiosity and interest—not as an interrogation. Ideally, you will already have some idea about the patient's alcohol or drug history from the self-administered questionnaire. Begin by asking about current alcohol or drug use, focusing initially on specific aspects of use (i.e., types, amounts, and frequency) over the past 30–90 days, and then elicit similar information for the most recent use during each of the past several days. Pay attention to how patients describe their alcohol or drug use: their affect, voice intonation, body language, choice of words, level of detail, what is emphasized, what is de-emphasized, and how troubled or untroubled they appear to be about their substance use overall. It is also important to note how alcohol or drug use fits into their lives in terms of setting and circumstances of use, as well as positive and negative effects (as discussed in greater detail in later sections). The interview should also cover the past history of substance use, including the initiation of use and how the person's use of each substance progressed and evolved over time. It is helpful to know what substances the person ever tried, what he liked or disliked about each substance's effects, which substances became a problem, and why at various points in the patient's history of use certain substances were given up and others were initiated.

Regarding controlled substances prescribed for legitimate medical purposes (e.g., opioid analgesics for pain, benzodiazepines for insomnia or severe anxiety), it is important to evaluate whether these drugs are taken only for the prescribed purpose, only in the prescribed dose, and only for the prescribed duration. Patients who abuse prescribed drugs often obtain prescriptions from two or more physicians and fill them at two or more pharmacies to avoid raising suspicions about abuse and to maintain an uninterrupted drug supply. Rarely are any of the prescribing physicians aware that the patient is receiving prescriptions simultaneously from other physicians as well.

Because polysubstance use is so prevalent, it is essential to ask all patients about simultaneous and sequential use of different substances. For example, many people use alcohol before, during, and after cocaine to potentiate the high from cocaine and to alleviate a rebound syndrome of unpleasant aftereffects such as dysphoric mood, insomnia, paranoia, and extreme restlessness, commonly known as the "cocaine crash." Accordingly, you should ask all cocaine users, "How often and how much alcohol do you use before, during, or after cocaine?" Similarly, heavy drinkers often supplement or alternate their alcohol consumption with other depressants and/or sedatives–hypnotics such as benzodiazepines for their synergistic effects. In cases of polysubstance use it is extremely important not to overlook or downplay the clinical significance of the patient's use of secondary substances even when this use does not appear to be excessive or problematic. As is often the case with combining cocaine and alcohol, one drug can become a powerful cue or trigger for using another.

Route of Drug Administration

It is important to know specifically by what method or route of administration the patient has used each substance. As discussed in Chapter 3, this information is important not only because different routes are associated with different types of medical problems, but also because rapid drug delivery methods (e.g., smoking and intravenous injection) produce more rapid progression from initial to compulsive use patterns and more serious drug-related medical and psychosocial consequences.

Amount, Frequency, and Pattern of Use

The amount and frequency of alcohol or drug use are important variables in determining the level of a person's involvement with psychoactive substances. It is essential to know exactly how much of each substance the person consumes on a regular basis or during a typical episode of use. Ask first about the extremes. For example: "During the past 90 days or so, what was the maximum number of days in a given week that you used alcohol and drugs and what was the maximum amount you used in a single day?" Similarly, ask about the minimum number of days in a given week and the minimum amount used in a single day. Then ask about the average or most typical amount and frequency of use per week and per day in the past 90 days.

Determining the amount of substance use is straightforward with legally manufactured substances such as alcohol or prescription drugs, but more difficult to decipher with illicit (street) drugs. Alcohol use is typically measured according to how many ounces of each type of alcoholic beverage is consumed (e.g., beer, wine, or distilled spirits). A standard "drink unit" is defined as a beverage containing 13.6 grams of ethyl alcohol. Accordingly, a standard drink unit is equivalent to one 5-ounce glass of wine, one 12-ounce bottle of beer, or one 1.5-ounce glass of distilled spirits. When a person says, "I don't have a problem with alcohol; I drink only beer or wine, I never touch hard liquor," keep in mind that it is the total amount (dose) of alcohol consumed in a given time period, not the particular type of alcoholic beverage one drinks, that determines its effects. The impact of alcohol on an individual's brain function and behavior is determined by the dose of alcohol that actually reaches the brain, irrespective of the particular type of alcoholic beverage that is ingested into the stomach.

For illicit drugs such as cocaine, heroin, and marijuana, an accurate measure of consumption is difficult to discern because of the wide variations in street price, purity, and packaging. Often one has to rely on the patient's report of the amount of money he is spending on drugs as the best indicator of consumption level. Money spent on drugs may reveal less about the exact amount consumed than about the relative value of drugs to the user. It is important to know, for example, what proportion of the patient's income or savings is being spent on drugs and whether it has become necessary to borrow money in order to support the drug use. Are there depleted bank accounts, overdue bills, large credit card debts, or other unmet financial obligations due to drug use? This information provides at least some indication of the strength of an individual's attachment to the drug and the level of priority it has achieved in his life. But for people who are capable of supporting their substance use without financial hardship, evidence of the drug's priority in their lives must be identified by its impact on other areas of their functioning. A diagnosis of addiction should not depend on the patient's income or socioeconomic status.

Assessing amount and cost of an individual's illicit drug use requires familiarity with certain street terms. Heroin is typically sold in $5 ("nickel") and $10 ("dime") bags. People who inject heroin intravenously typically use between 3 and 10 bags a day. The weight and purity of heroin in a given bag are so highly variable that it is all but impossible to specify drug doses. As mentioned earlier, ascertaining the total amount of money spent on heroin per day or per episode of use is probably the best way to quantify the level of a person's heroin use. Crack cocaine is commonly sold on the street in plastic vials containing one to three tiny pea-size pellets or "rocks" at a price of $5–30 per vial, depending on the number and size of the rocks. Each rock provides no more than three to five inhalations (puffs) of cocaine vapor, and each puff provides an intense but short-lived euphoria lasting only a few minutes. The euphoria is followed by a rebound dysphoria or "crash" and then cravings for more cocaine. It is not difficult to see how this drives the development of compulsive use patterns. Cocaine powder is sold by the gram, the ounce (28 grams), the "quarter" (one-quarter ounce or 7 grams), or the "eight ball" (one-eighth ounce or 3.5 grams). Prices may vary anywhere from $30 to $50 per gram. Marijuana is typically sold in the form of individually rolled cigarettes (known as "joints" or "reefers") for a few dollars each, in dime bags that contain a quantity of loose plant material sufficient to roll two or three marijuana cigarettes, or by the ounce.

In addition to amount and frequency of use, the specific pattern of use should be explored. Patterns can range from occasional use, to intensive marathon binges separated by a number of days/weeks, to continuous use every single day. Binge patterns can create confusion in arriving at an accurate diagnosis. It is often assumed that patients who do not use substances every day could not possibly be dependent, especially if they are able to refrain from using for several days or weeks at a time. But binge patterns are in fact among the most difficult to break and often result in problems as severe as those associated with daily usage at lower doses. Binge patterns are very common with alcohol and stimulants such as cocaine and methamphetamine. During a typical binge lasting 2 or 3 days, the user may consume several hundreds or thousands of dollars' worth of the cocaine or methamphetamine. Typically, the binge comes to end when the person collapses from physical exhaustion or runs out of money, whichever occurs first. Similarly, alcohol binge patterns are quite common, as is often seen in patients who drink little if any alcohol during the work week, but then drink themselves into oblivion on weekends. Binge use is unusual with heroin, especially among intravenous users, because the increasing tolerance and physical dependence that develops with repeated use creates a growing demand for using larger amounts of the drug at shorter and shorter intervals to stave off withdrawal.

Setting, Circumstances, and Antecedents of Use

The assessment should also include a functional analysis of the individual's substance use that attempts to identify specific antecedents of the alcohol or drug use (i.e., the particular circumstances, events, and mood/affect states that most reliably precede and possibly elicit or "trigger" substance use) and the particular contexts or settings in which the use most often occurs. The patient should be asked to describe the people, places, and things most reliably associated with his substance use as well as any particular moods, emotional states, and other activities associated with use. For example, to what extent does the substance use occur at work, at home, at bars/clubs, when the person is alone, with dealers, with friends, or with coworkers? Who else in the person's household uses alcohol and drugs? To what extent does the patient's alcohol or drug use occur on the heels of experiencing intensely negative feelings? If there have been previous periods of abstinence, what events and circumstances preceded resumption of use? For some individuals, substance use occurs reliably on certain occasions, both positive and negative. These may include holidays, birthdays, job promotions, and financial successes, as well as anniversaries associated with unpleasant events such as the death of a loved one or the breakup of a significant relationship.

Inability to Control Use

An important variable in determining the nature and severity of an SUD is a cluster of behavioral symptoms indicating the degree to which substance use is no longer under the individual's volitional control. Indicators of control problems include (1) repeated lack of success in attempts to deliberately curtail or discontinue use, (2) inability to predict or limit how much one uses or how long an episode of use lasts once it has begun, (3) repeated drug cravings and irresistible compulsions or urges to use, (4) preoccupation or obsession with substance use, (5) increasing urgency or inordinate priority given to substance use, (6) rapidly escalating patterns of use after a period of abstinence; and (7) continued use despite increasingly severe and life-damaging consequences. Asking about the particulars of previous attempts to stop or curtail use alone or with outside help can be informative. In the Self-Administered Patient Questionnaire (Appendix 1), the section "The Substance Use Profile" asks several questions related to loss of control.

Keep in mind that loss of control over alcohol or drug use is neither instantaneous nor absolute. Loss of control does not necessarily imply that there is complete or total lack of control each and every time a person uses alcohol and drugs. For many people, including those who clearly meet the criteria for a substance *dependence* diagnosis, loss of control is intermittent. For example, a patient may drink on two or three occasions with no evidence of losing control or experiencing negative consequences. On the next occasion, however, the patient may drink uncontrollably, failing to show up for work the next day and getting arrested for driving while intoxicated. Often loss of control develops gradually over an extended period of time. Typically, when the invisible line is crossed from controlled to addictive use the individual is not aware that this transition is happening and is thus often unable to pinpoint retrospectively exactly when control over substance use may have been lost.

Switching from a less intensive to a more intensive route of drug administration often greatly accelerates the process of losing control. For example, cocaine users who switch from snorting cocaine powder to smoking crack cocaine often report an almost immediate loss of control over their ability to limit the amount and frequency of use. The same is often true of individuals who switch from snorting to either smoking or injecting heroin.

Pattern of Self-Medication with Alcohol and Drugs

You should carefully assess to what extent patients use psychoactive substances as self-medication to pharmacologically adjust, attenuate, or obliterate unpleasant thoughts, feelings, and moods. The association between negative affects and substance use may not be obvious to you or to the patient at first. There are many instances when alcohol or drug use does not occur when the person is actively experiencing emotional distress. Substance use is often a delayed reaction to accumulating and ultimately intolerable affects that kindle the desire for self-medication. Even when the connection between patients' substance use and intolerable thoughts/feelings appears quite obvious to the therapist, it is quite remarkable how often patients remain unaware of this connection until it is brought to their attention.

A pattern of self-medication with alcohol and drugs can be identified with a series of questions such as: To what extent does your alcohol or drug use occur when you are feeling anxious, fatigued, depressed, frustrated, angry, lonely, sexually aroused? Do you ever use alcohol and drugs to relieve depression, anxiety, or other negative feelings? To what extent does such use occur on the heels of conflict with your mate, boss, parent, or significant others? It is also important to ask about substance use in the past as compared with the present and how the pattern of use may have changed over time. This may reveal patterns of substance use linked to significant life events. For example, you might ask, "How did your alcohol or drug use change [while you were going through a divorce] [as a result of your father's death] [as you were becoming increasingly dissatisfied with your work]?"

Increased Tolerance

Pharmacological tolerance can be assessed by asking several pointed questions:

1. "Do you find that you need to drink or use more now than you did in the past to achieve the same effects?"
2. "Do you find that the amount of alcohol or drugs you currently use would have given you a much stronger effect in the past?"
3. "Can you now handle substantially more alcohol or drugs than you used to?"
4. "Do you keep drinking or using well beyond the point where previously you would have stopped?"
5. "Are you drinking or using more now but showing it less?"

Blackouts

Blackouts are episodes of amnesia or memory gaps induced by heavy consumption of alcohol and/or other sedative (depressant) drugs. The amount of alcohol required to produce a blackout can vary greatly from one individual to the next and may be impossible to predict. In most cases, however, blackouts result from consuming quantities of alcohol that markedly exceed the individual's current level of pharmacological tolerance as evidenced by signs of severe intoxication. The likelihood of experiencing a blackout is increased substantially by using alcohol and sedative drugs in combination with one another. Certain types of sedative drugs such as Rohypnol (the "date rape" drug) are well known for their ability to induce amnesia. Similarly, medazolam (Versed, a benzodiazepine) is used in clinical settings to sedate patients and deliberately induce amnesia for painful medical procedures (e.g., colonoscopy).

Many patients assume incorrectly that when you ask about blackouts you are referring to loss of consciousness rather than loss of memory induced by alcohol. It is essential, therefore, to phrase questions about blackouts carefully. For example, ask patients, "Do you sometimes find that after an episode of drinking you have trouble remembering what you were doing, who you were with, or where you where?" You should also ask, "Have you ever woken up somewhere after heavy drinking with no idea of how you got there or had someone tell you about something you said or did while intoxicated that you had no memory of?"

Positive Effects of Substance Use

One way to avoid eliciting patients' defensiveness about substance use and invite open discussion is to ask first about the positive effects before focusing on negative consequences. It is important to recognize that people become regular users only of substances that produce positive effects in the early stages of use. Psychoactive drugs induce pleasurable mood states and for some people enhance certain aspects of their functioning. It is simplistic to view all psychoactive drug use as a hedonistic pursuit aimed only at getting "high." From a clinical standpoint, it is much more useful to examine the functional and "self-medication" aspects of a person's substance use by exploring how substance use helps her than to focus only on how it causes her problems. This is consistent with the notion that for many people who eventually become addicted to psychoactive substances, their use in the early stages serves an adaptive function before the negative effects intensify and ultimately overshadow whatever positive benefits they were deriving from the substance use.

Accordingly, it is crucial for you to explore nonjudgmentally and without challenge the patient's view about the positive effects of substance use. You gain credibility and trust when you acknowledge the patient's reality that substance use can and often does provide benefits such as enhanced performance in certain tasks and increased ability to cope with certain types of stressful circumstances. Ask patients about what attracted them to the particular substances in the first place and what positive effects or benefits they still get from using these substances.

Negative Consequences of Substance Use

Doing a careful, detailed assessment of substance-related consequences to the patient's health and psychosocial functioning serves at least two critical functions: (1) it can help to identify problems that need to be addressed, and (2) it can enhance motivation for change by heightening the patient's awareness of problems or "costs" associated with his substance use.

Medical Consequences

Alcohol and other drug use can adversely affect a person's physical health in both obvious and not so obvious ways. For this reason, it is essential to inquire routinely about health problems often associated with abuse of alcohol and other drugs. For example, excessive alcohol use can (1) directly cause liver, gastrointestinal, and other internal organ dysfunction, (2) exacerbate a wide range of existing medical conditions, and (3) interfere with or nullify the therapeutic action of medications being prescribed for other medical or psychiatric conditions. Serious medical problems are more likely to be associated with abuse of alcohol than with other types of drugs. Cocaine and methamphetamine can cause cardiovascular problems, including arrhythmias (irregular heartbeat), myocardial infarction (heart attack), and sudden death; these problems are rare, considering the large number of people using such drugs. Most medical problems related to heroin use are secondary to contaminants in the drug and to use of nonsterile needles and syringes. The gastrointestinal and liver problems seen in patients using large quantities of prescription opioids are caused by the acetaminophen or ibuprofen contained in these compounds.

No matter what substances patients may be using, everyone with a significant history of substance abuse should be evaluated by a physician, preferably a practitioner with expertise in addiction medicine. Physical examination by itself is a relatively insensitive assessment procedure and a late indicator of serious alcohol or drug problems. Signs of substance dependence detectible by physical examination often do not appear until the problem has existed for many years, and even then these signs are often unreliable indicators. Similarly, clinical laboratory tests tend to be late-stage indicators. Certain blood tests, specifically gamma-glutamyltransferase (GGT), aspartate aminotransferase (AST), and alanine aminotransferase (ALT), are biochemical markers of liver tissue damage. Elevation of all three test values is strongly indicative of alcohol- or drug-related impairment of liver functioning, but can be caused by other disease processes such as infectious hepatitis. Of these three tests, GGT is perhaps the most sensitive indicator of alcohol-related liver problems. Serial GGT tests are sometimes used as markers of relapse. Elevations in mean corpuscular volume (MCV) and triglycerides are also associated with chronic and/or excessive alcohol consumption. Laboratory tests are not recommended for routine use, but can serve as adjuncts in selected cases to confirm or support a diagnosis, to establish a baseline for follow-up, and to monitor clinical progress. Positive test results suggesting impairment of internal organ function are sometimes strong motivators for patients who were previously reluctant to do anything about their alcohol or drug use. Urine drug testing is a potentially valuable assessment tool, as discussed in Chapter 9.

ASSESSING PHYSICAL DEPENDENCE THAT MAY REQUIRE MEDICALLY MANAGED WITHDRAWAL

It is essential to determine whether a patient is physically dependent on any substances and possibly in need of medically managed withdrawal. Medical treatment for withdrawal involves the use of medications under the care of a physician who knows how to properly manage withdrawal to ensure that the transition from active addiction to initial abstinence is achieved without harm or unnecessary discomfort. Abrupt cessation of chronic use of alcohol, barbiturates, benzodiazepines, and other sedatives can be health threatening or even fatal. Consumption of sedatives in daily dosages exceeding roughly three times the therapeutic dose range may require management in a hospital. In some cases, outpatient detoxification from sedatives is a viable alternative if the patient carefully adheres to prescribed medication regimens and shows up reliably for scheduled office visits with the physician who is managing the withdrawal. Similarly, alcohol withdrawal can often be managed safely on an outpatient basis with compliant patients when there is no history of medical complications (e.g., convulsions, delirium tremens) during previous detoxification attempts. Withdrawal from heroin and other opioids is distressing and uncomfortable, but rarely fatal (except in a fetus or neonate). Outpatient opioid withdrawal can be effectively managed in motivated patients, but most (especially intravenous and high-dose users) will require admission to an inpatient unit where there is no access to drugs and withdrawal can be managed appropriately with medication. Stimulant drugs such as cocaine and methamphetamine do not produce a withdrawal syndrome requiring detoxification with medication. Some high-dose stimulant users complain of depression, irritability, and insomnia that may last for several days or weeks after their last use, but many others experience no post-drug discomfort at all.

How can you determine when medical detoxification is required? If the patient has been abstinent for the preceding 2–3 weeks, there is generally no reason to be concerned about acute withdrawal. With opioids, you need only ask the patient whether she experiences withdrawal symptoms and wants medication to prevent or alleviate those symptoms. The most common symptoms of opioid withdrawal are stomach cramps, diarrhea, chills, restlessness, tearing eyes, runny nose, and insomnia. These symptoms are usually not health threatening, but they do cause considerable discomfort and sometimes make it intolerable for the patient to sustain the motivation to complete the withdrawal process. In general, the severity of withdrawal is directly related to the patient's level of opioid dependence, as measured by the total dose necessary to prevent the appearance of withdrawal symptoms. Patients with high levels of opioid dependence who have failed repeatedly to complete detoxification on an outpatient basis may find inpatient detoxification more helpful.

With alcohol and other central nervous system depressants, however, it can be more difficult to determine whether the patient is physically addicted and whether there is a strong likelihood of medical complications if consumption is markedly reduced or stopped too quickly. There is a great deal of individual variability in the severity of withdrawal symptoms with alcohol and sedatives. For example, some people who have several drinks every day experience clinically significant withdrawal symptoms upon stopping abruptly, whereas others who consume exactly the same amount of alcohol experience no withdrawal problems at all. Furthermore, it often happens that the patient does not know whether he is addicted, either because there have been no recent periods of abstinence in which consumption has ceased long enough to allow withdrawal symptoms to emerge or because the patient has not recognized the early signs of withdrawal as such and so has inadvertently ignored them. The clinician should ask pointed questions about any recent periods of abstinence that have extended for 2 or more consecutive days and what, if any, physical symptoms the patient experienced during those periods. For example, you should ask, "When was the last time you consumed no alcohol and no other sedative drugs for at least 2 days in a row? Did you feel sick or notice any physical changes during that time? Did you experience any vomiting, sweating, nausea, tremors, or insomnia? If so, were these symptoms relieved by drinking alcohol or taking sedative drugs? Have you ever experienced withdrawal symptoms or any other physical problems during previous attempts to stop drinking?" It is essential to keep in mind that with the longer-acting benzodiazepines (e.g., Valium, Librium) serious withdrawal reactions can be considerably delayed. Life-threatening seizures can occur as late as 7–10 days after cessation of use and without prior warning. The final determination of whether an alcohol- or sedative-dependent patient requires medically managed withdrawal should be made by a physician who is familiar with medical detoxification procedures.

Psychosocial Consequences

It is important to determine whether and to what extent the patient's substance use is associated with problems concerning work, family, finances, and legal matters. For example, to what extent is there a pattern of absenteeism or lateness, poor productivity, argumentativeness, or apathy at work, related to alcohol and drug use? Are there frequent arguments with a parent, mate, or significant others? Has a significant relationship broken up as a result of the patient's alcohol or drug use? Is there a current threat of this happening? Is there a pattern of social isolation and withdrawal? Are there financial or legal problems due to substance use? Whether and to what extent does the patient perceive the substance use to be adversely affecting her life?

In addition to substance-related vocational, financial, and interpersonal problems, the impact of substance use on the person's values, priorities, expectations, goal attainment, self-esteem, leisure activities, and overall quality of life should also be explored. Helping patients to think about how their aspirations and goals have been delayed, diverted, or perhaps even relinquished during the course of their substance use can be both informative and therapeutic.

SEXUAL CONSEQUENCES

It is important to ask about the sexual consequences of alcohol or drug use because many patients will not volunteer this information spontaneously.

Sexual problems associated with substance use generally fall into two categories: (1) sexual dysfunction and (2) hypersexuality or sexual compulsivity.

Sexual Dysfunction. Sexual dysfunction caused by alcohol or drug use is evidenced by reduced sex drive and/or impaired sexual performance. Impaired performance is manifest as erectile and/or orgasmic dysfunction. Whereas short-term and/or low-dose use of certain psychoactive substances (e.g., alcohol, stimulants, marijuana) often enhances sexual performance, chronic and/or high-dose use often impairs or eliminates sexual functioning. Complaints about lack of sex drive and inability to achieve erection or orgasm are common among substance-abusing patients. Fortunately, these problems usually remit on their own after cessation of use but can linger for several weeks or months, depending on the chronicity and amount of prior use.

Hypersexuality and High-Risk Behaviors. Considering that alcohol and other depressant drugs often reduce inhibitions while simultaneously increasing a person's willingness to act on impulse, it is no surprise that use of these substances alone or in combination with one another is sometimes associated with indiscriminate or risky sexual behaviors in both men and women. Drug-induced hypersexuality, characterized by extraordinarily powerful increases in sexual desire, sexual fantasies, and sexual acting-out behaviors, is a problem uniquely associated with the use of stimulant drugs (cocaine and methamphetamine), particularly in male users. Studies indicate that as many as 50% of male patients receiving treatment for stimulant dependence report that their drug use is strongly linked with various types of sexual acting-out behaviors. Although this stimulant–sex connection can be found to some extent in women, it occurs in fewer than 20–30% of female stimulant users. The reasons for this gender difference are unknown, but likely involve both biological and sociocultural factors.

Stimulant-induced hypersexuality in male users often involves compulsive masturbation and marathon encounters with prostitutes or other unknown sexual partners during prolonged drug binges. Some patients report that cocaine or methamphetamine use stimulates intense sexual fantasies, often involving "taboo" sexual behaviors such as cross-dressing, sadomasochism, and exhibitionism. In addition, some male heterosexual stimulant users report engaging in sex with transvestites (men dressed as women) while under the influence of cocaine and/or methamphetamine. These homosexual encounters often generate feelings of embarrassment, humiliation, and extreme anxiety, sometimes coupled with suicidal ideation. These individuals are typically repulsed by their behavior after each homosexual encounter. Many experience profound dysphoria as a result of seeing this behavior as sexually perverted and calling into question their sexual identity—although most have no history of homosexual behaviors or fantasies when not under the influence of stimulant drugs or before ever getting involved with these drugs.

The clinical importance of conducting a detailed assessment for stimulant-related hypersexuality cannot be overemphasized, considering how often this problem remains hidden despite being a major precipitant of relapse. Many of these patients become trapped in a repeating cycle of reciprocal relapse in which sexually compulsive behaviors lead inevitably to drug use and drug use leads inevitably to sexually compulsive behaviors. Once the sex–drug link is established, it becomes extremely powerful and thus difficult to break as it is repeatedly reinforced. Failure to address stimulant-related hypersexuality, when present, is associated with repeated relapse and treatment failure.

Unless you ask specifically about drug-related sexual behaviors, most patients will not report this information to you. They are often embarrassed and afraid that you will see them as sexually perverted. Many patients harbor the unverbalized hope that they can give up the drugs without giving up their sexual escapades. In addition to reciprocal relapse patterns, a potentially ominous consequence of stimulant-induced hypersexuality is increased risk of contracting and/or spreading serious sexually transmitted diseases such as HIV, hepatitis C, and genital herpes, among others. Safe sex is rarely practiced while a person is under the influence of cocaine or methamphetamine. Moreover, drug-induced hypersexuality leads to the indiscriminate choice of sex partners (whose health status is unknown), coupled with a markedly higher frequency of sexual contacts overall. Another consequence of drug-induced hypersexuality is that "regular" sex (i.e., without drugs) becomes boring and unsatisfying. This creates further incentive for the individual to seek the types of high-intensity sexual experiences attainable only under the influence of the drugs. As might be expected, loss of interest in having sex without drugs can cause serious marital or other relationship problems.

Developmental History Focusing on Substance-Related Issues

Another aspect of assessment is exploring the usual developmental stages in a person's life with special attention to issues that may be associated with or affected by substance use. Among the issues to explore are early traumas and neglect; insufficient or unattuned parenting; substance abuse by parents and/or significant others, including siblings, caretakers, and peers; peer group changes, dynamics, conflicts, and pressures to use drugs; sexuality, sexual identity, and sexual conflicts; separation–individuation struggles; development of coping skills; relationship history; intellectual, educational, and vocational development; learning disabilities; history of psychiatric problems, including mood disorders, attention deficit disorders, and antisocial or aggressive behavior. The developmental history should be interwoven with an assessment of the progression from earliest use of alcohol and drugs to the present pattern of use. Ideally, the patient's developmental history should provide a clearer picture of the internal struggles and significant life events that may have set the stage for emergence of an SUD and/or contributed to its escalation over time.

Other Addictive and Compulsive Behaviors

Addictive disorders often occur in clusters. Accordingly, the assessment should determine to what extent there may be coexisting problems with other addictive/compulsive behaviors such as compulsive gambling, compulsive sexuality, compulsive spending, and compulsive eating or noneating. Some people engage in two or more addictive behaviors simultaneously, whereas others may switch sequentially from one addictive behavior to another. The reciprocal relapse pattern mentioned earlier involving stimulant drugs and sex can occur with any addictive/compulsive behaviors that have been paired with each other. For example, compulsive gambling is often associated with alcohol consumption and sometimes with the use of cocaine. Compulsive spending is often associated with the use of stimulant drugs. Moreover, because cocaine and amphetamine are both appetite suppressants, people with eating disorders such as bulimia, anorexia, or compulsive overeating are frequently attracted to these drugs, not only for their psychoactive effects, but also for the help they provide in reducing hunger and food consumption. It is essential to identify these coexisting addictive/compulsive behaviors because they will otherwise remain unaddressed and thus increase the likelihood of relapse. Clinically useful assessment instruments have been developed to identify pathological gambling (Blume & Lesieur, 1987) and eating disorders (Fairburn & Brownell, 2001).

Prior Treatment and Self-Help Experience

In assessing patients with a history of prior treatment for substance abuse, inquiring about the particulars of these treatment episodes can be very informative. In addition to discovering when, where, and what type of treatment was received, it is important to know whether the course of treatment was completed as prescribed or terminated prematurely; whether the treatment was perceived as helpful and, if so, what aspects of the treatment were most helpful; what aspects were least helpful; for how long did patients remain substance-free after treatment; what helped them to remain abstinent; and what contributed to subsequent relapse.

In addition to seeking information about prior treatment episodes, similar information should be elicited about any past or present involvement in 12-step and other self-help programs. It is useful to know, for example, whether patients have ever attended self-help meetings, for how long they attended, and how deeply or meaningfully they were involved in a program. For patients who have attended 12-step meetings it is useful to know if they had a sponsor, worked the steps, read AA literature, did volunteer service, led or spoke at meetings. And for a patient who discontinued his involvement in self-help, what led him to drop out?

For patients who have never attended 12-step meetings or did so only for short periods of time or superficially, it is important to find out why. Many people object to AA and other 12-step programs for a variety of reasons. Some find the spiritual aspect of these programs, with frequent references to God or a "Higher Power" objectionable. Others feel uncomfortable in public meetings, do not relate to the content and philosophy of the program, or fail to identify and connect with others in attendance. It is important to explore the patient's feelings and objections about self-help meetings without taking the position that these objections represent resistance or denial. It is useful to know about the patient's attitude and prior experience with self-help programs so that they can be taken into account when later discussing treatment strategies and goals.

Family History of Substance Abuse

It is important to know whether and to what extent there is a history of alcohol or drug problems in the patient's family, including parents, grandparents, aunts and uncles, and siblings. In addition to the possibility of a genetic predisposition to addiction, social learning factors also warrant consideration when family members have a history of abusing alcohol and drugs. A positive family history for substance abuse is important because (1) the patient should be regarded as being at increased risk for developing alcohol or drug problems as compared with individuals with no family history of SUDs and (2) contact with family members who continue to abuse alcohol and drugs may hamper a patient's efforts to change. When taking a family history, it is important to ask for a description of family members' alcohol and drug use patterns rather than ask the patient to offer a diagnosis. For example, it is better to say, "Tell me about your parents'/siblings'/grandparents' use of alcohol and other drugs" rather than "Was anyone in your family an alcohol or drug abuser?" It is also important to ask whether any family members received treatment for substance abuse, ever attended AA, or suffered from substance-related medical problems such as liver disease.

Role of Family Members in the Patient's Current Use

In addition to obtaining a family history, it is essential to assess the current roles that family members may play in unintentionally perpetuating the patient's substance abuse. It is often said that chemical dependency is a "family disease," not only because there may be a familial biological (genetic) component to the problem, but also because the behavior of significant others toward the active substance abuser can provoke, maintain, or otherwise unwittingly "enable" an individual's continuing substance use. It is important to know, for example, whether any family members (1) currently use alcohol and drugs together with the patient, (2) financially support the patient's substance use indirectly by paying her living expenses while the patient spends most of her money on drugs, (3) inadvertently sabotage attempts by the patient to stop using, or (4) compensate for the patient's dysfunctional or irresponsible behavior by shielding her from actually experiencing negative consequences resulting from substance use. Whatever the circumstances, it is often helpful to interview the patient's spouse, parent(s), or significant others. But this should be done, of course, only with the patient's consent.

Meeting with family members can also help in assessing to what extent any of these individuals are available to support and encourage the patient's efforts to change. It also provides an opportunity to orient and educate family members about the treatment process, including how they can be involved in a positive way (assuming the patient agrees) and how they can maintain appropriate boundaries with the patient in the face of continuing substance use or other problematic behaviors. Often family members are eager to help in any way they can and clamor for guidance from the therapist about how best to deal with the substance abuser. However, some family members (especially spouses) are initially too angry and resentful to be supportive of the patient at the beginning of treatment before it is clear whether he is truly motivated to change and actually follows through on stated intentions.

Interviewing family members offers another perspective on the patient's substance use as seen through a different set of eyes. It may also help family members to realize that their involvement in the recovery process is essential and that changes in their own behavior may be needed to help facilitate changes in the patient's behavior. In some cases, failure to interview family members runs the risk of having therapeutic efforts inadvertently or even purposefully sabotaged by those for whom changes in the patient's behavior may be threatening and unwelcome. Any contact you have with significant others must take place only with the primary patient's full knowledge and consent. Often it is advisable to interview significant others with the patient present in order to avoid potential problems resulting from distorted communication about what took place during the interview and the patient's fears that private contact with others has shifted your loyalty in their direction. In this regard, if concerned family members or others call you, unsolicited, to offer information about the patient's substance use (usually fearing that the patient has not given you the full story), it is essential to inform the caller at the outset that you will share whatever is said during the conversation with your patient and that under no circumstances will you keep secrets from your patient, as this could severely damage your therapeutic relationship with the patient. If, after being informed of this fact, the caller decides not to offer the information he or she had hoped to convey to you, so be it. You must still inform your patient at the next visit that the person attempted to contact you and what transpired in the conversation.

OFFERING FEEDBACK AND ASSESSING READINESS FOR CHANGE

Once the assessment is completed, your next tasks are to (1) offer helpful feedback, (2) elicit the patient's response to your feedback, and (3) assess the patient's readiness for change in preparation for negotiating an initial treatment plan. Your feedback should present the most salient aspects of assessment results in a clear, concise, straightforward manner, followed by your request for the patient's response. Feedback should be presented using a motivational interviewing style devoid of confrontational or coercive tactics. The purpose of feedback is not to club the patient over the head with her resistance or to confront denial, but to highlight problematic aspects of her substance use, particularly its connection with any adverse consequences in important life areas.

With a patient who did not come seeking your help for an alcohol or drug problem, it is especially important to draw connections, wherever they may exist, between the person's substance use and the other problems that prompted him to seek your help in the first place. Motivation for change is enhanced when a person recognizes significant discrepancies between where he is now and where he wants to be (Miller & Rollnick, 2002). Thus, feedback that helps patients see that they are not where they want to be and that substance use is a major cause of this discrepancy can help to open their thinking about the possibility of making changes. You should not try to pressure or persuade the patient to accept your view of the situation, agree with your diagnosis, or commit to a particular course of action. Similarly, your feedback should not be aimed at proving anything or convincing patients that their perception of their own behavior is grossly distorted or an outgrowth of their "denial." An overbearing, controlling approach will only diminish a person's receptiveness to your feedback and stimulate defensiveness. Success in giving feedback is evidenced when it elicits the person's own concerns and he actively solicits your view and recommendations.

The process of offering feedback and assessing change readiness consists of the four steps in the following list. Assessing change readiness is the last step in the process because, according to the stages-of-change (SOC) model, the way a person responds to clinical feedback about a problem behavior provides strong clues about the person's motivation and readiness to change that behavior.

Although the exact sequence and degree of emphasis placed on each of these steps may vary with the individuals involved, this outline can serve as a general guide:

1. Summarize assessment results.
2. Present and explain the diagnosis.
3. State your clinical concerns.
4. Assess the patient's readiness for change.

Summarizing Assessment Results

Feedback should begin with a summary statement that highlights the most important aspects of the assessment results. When presenting the summary statement, you should adhere closely to the facts, leaving out interpretations, conclusions, and advice. At the end of the statement you should solicit the patient's view of what you have presented. Here is an example:

"Well, Jerry, let me summarize what I think I've heard from you thus far, and then I'd like to hear your reactions. You said that you came here because your supervisor threatened to fire you if you didn't take care of your 'drinking problem' as he saw it. He seemed to be reacting to your most recent failure to show up for work after a weekend of drinking and several similar absences over the past few months. You report that you drink, on average, two or three times per week, and most heavily on weekends. You don't always drink to the point of getting 'drunk,' but you have noticed that on weekends your drinking has led to some problems, including getting into arguments in bars, getting into a car accident when you were driving under the influence, and failing to show up for work on at least several Monday mornings. You stated that your wife gets angry when you come home smelling of alcohol, but otherwise your drinking has not led to major problems in your marriage. You emphasized that despite a recent string of absences you are a good worker and feel that your company views you as a valuable employee. You have also made clear that you are not sure that your drinking is enough of a problem to warrant being in treatment and that you would prefer to try to stop drinking on your own. However, you were quick to add that you have tried to stop on your own many times in the past, but were unable to refrain from drinking for more than 2 or 3 weeks at a time before going back to it again. So, what do you make of all this? Would you like to correct or add to anything I've just said? I'm interested in hearing your view of the situation."

Presenting and Explaining the Diagnosis

Part of giving feedback is to present patients with the formal diagnosis of their alcohol or drug problem. This involves not only making patients aware of the diagnosis, but perhaps even more important, explaining to them how you arrived at the diagnosis based on specific assessment results, and educating them about the defining features of relevant diagnostic categories. Historically, therapists either have refrained from presenting a diagnosis or have adopted a confrontational stance if the patient rejects or argues against the diagnosis. Neither approach is very useful. Failure to present a diagnosis often stems from the therapist's concern about offending the patient and provoking a negative response. Not giving a patient a clear statement about the nature and severity of her problem conveys the wrong message, that the problem is not serious enough to warrant clinical attention.

Presenting the diagnosis in a motivational interviewing style and explaining specifically how you arrived at that diagnosis can help to enhance the patient's willingness to consider change. This is a delicate process, requiring that you convey the severity of the problem and related consequences in a manner that does not overwhelm the patient or stimulate his defenses. Your prior observations of the patient's verbal and nonverbal reactions to your summary statement and other feedback can be used to decide when and how to present the diagnosis, based on your sense of the patient's readiness to receive this information. In some cases, for example, you may decide to wait until the next session to present the diagnosis in order to give the patient time to digest the feedback you have already given. In other cases, you may sense that the patient is ready to receive this information without further delay.

You should explain to patients what the diagnosis means and what implications it may have for how to proceed. It is important that you explain, for example, the definitions of "safe" versus "at-risk" drinking limits and the defining features of substance abuse versus substance dependence (as discussed previously in Chapter 2). This information not only provides a conceptual framework within which patients can better understand the nature and severity of their problems, but it gives added credibility to your diagnosis by referencing accepted norms. Clinicians often underestimate the extent to which at-risk or even heavy drinkers have difficulty in recognizing that their alcohol consumption falls well outside accepted definitions of safe drinking limits and population norms. Similarly, most patients are not familiar with the distinctions between substance abuse versus dependence. It can be helpful to present a written checklist of the criteria for relevant diagnostic categories and to use this information as the basis for discussing how you arrived at a particular diagnosis. For example, you might explain that although abuse and dependence are both characterized by a pattern of continued use despite adverse consequences and/or in situations where use is hazardous, dependence is often distinguished (according to DSM-IV) by additional criteria such as obsessive thinking about using, cravings and/or urges to use, giving inordinate priority to using to the point where it overshadows other aspects of a person's life, frequently using more than one intends to use, and by failure in previous attempts to stop. Where indicated, it is important to inform patients that physical addiction to a substance (i.e., the appearance of a withdrawal syndrome when use is discontinued) is neither necessary nor sufficient to warrant a diagnosis of dependence (i.e., addiction).

After presenting patients with this information, it is useful to ask how *they* view their substance use within the context of these diagnostic categories. For example: "Based on what we have been discussing about the various categories of use, how would you characterize your alcohol and drug use?" Ideally, this encourages the patient to examine various aspects of her substance use with an eye toward determining to what extent it falls within one category or another. The following are additional suggestions for presenting the diagnosis in a motivational style:

1. State that alcohol and drug problems are *not* indicators of character weakness, personality problems, immorality, or lack of willpower.

2. Avoid lengthy discussions with patients about why they use alcohol and drugs, especially speculation about the contribution of psychological, personality, relationship, or job problems to the development of an alcohol or drug problem.

3. Affirm, where appropriate, that having a substance abuse problem is not the patient's fault, inasmuch as no one uses alcohol or other drugs with the intention of developing a problem. You can explain, for example, that as a result of repeated alcohol and drug use, people unknowingly cross an invisible line from controlled use to abuse, and in some cases, to dependency—a process driven largely by changes in brain neurotransmitters induced by the repeated drug use itself.

4. Mention, where indicated, that a family history of alcohol or drug problems can predispose people to developing similar problems of their own by lowering the invisible threshold in the brain for setting off an addictive response.

5. Affirm that although they are not responsible for developing the problems, people with alcohol and drug problems are solely and personally responsible for the negative consequences of their behavior and for making the necessary changes to avoid intensifying existing problems or creating new ones.

6. Remain tolerant of the range of patient reactions your feedback elicits, including surprise, embarrassment, anger, and denial. You should also be prepared to respond appropriately when feedback evokes emotional reactions of sadness, fear, and hopelessness.

7. Resist provocation and avoid getting dragged into power struggles with patients over who is right or heated debates about how much alcohol or drug use is too much. Remember, the patient is not an adversary to be defeated. It is essential that you stay in the role of clinical expert who has important knowledge about the nature of alcohol and drug problems and how to deal with them safely and effectively.

Here is an example of presenting the diagnosis:

"David, at this point in our discussion I want to share with you my diagnosis of your alcohol and drug problem and how I arrived at that diagnosis based on information you gave me during the assessment. I think it is important for you to know how I am looking at the problem and what concerns this raises in my mind about the impact of your drinking on your health and general well-being. In my view, your current alcohol use qualifies for a diagnosis of alcohol *dependence* because it clearly meets the standard criteria that are required to give someone that diagnosis. Based on what you told me during the assessment interview, the following statements appear to characterize your drinking pattern. First, you often drink more than you intend to drink on a given occasion and frequently end up much more intoxicated than you had planned or expected to be. Second, you have tried several times to stop drinking on your own, and although you have been able to not drink for weeks or even months at a time, you have ended up returning to drinking despite your best intentions to remain alcohol free. Third, you have given up social and recreational activities because of your drinking, such as visiting with certain friends and family members, playing softball, and participating in leisure activities with your wife and children. And fourth, you have continued to drink despite the problems it has caused you on the job and in your marriage. To qualify for a diagnosis of alcohol dependence, which is more serious than a diagnosis of alcohol abuse, a person has to meet three out of seven criteria. Your drinking pattern meets at least four of these criteria. That's the bad news. The good news is that your problem is entirely treatable and your chances of success are really very good, especially because you have a lot going for you and a lot to lose by continuing to drink. You also have the good fortune of having a boss and a wife who you said are very supportive. And I am quite willing to help you deal with problem, if that's what you decide to do. I know that this isn't what you expected, and it looks like this is hard for you to hear. What are you thinking and feeling at this point?"

Some key points in this example are worth noting: (1) The statement makes deliberate reference to the fact that the diagnosis is based on information obtained during the assessment and not on preconceived ideas or assumptions; (2) to counterbalance the blow of presenting the diagnosis in rather stark factual terms, the problem is described as highly treatable, the patient's chances of success in overcoming the problem are described as very good, and the clinician clearly offers to help; and (3) the patient's feelings about hearing this information are solicited and acknowledged empathetically and nonjudgmentally.

Stating Your Clinical Concerns

After presenting the summary statement and the diagnosis, you should state your clinical concerns concisely, unequivocally, and in lay terms that can be easily understood. Be specific about the problematic aspects of the patient's substance use, including past, present, and potential consequences/ risks associated with the use. Recognize that the feedback you present may trigger opposition or elicit feelings of shame, embarrassment, and even hostility. Rather than approach or label patients as being resistant, unmotivated, or "in denial," focus instead on whatever connections you can draw between the patient's substance use and other psychosocial and/or physical health problems identified during the assessment. When stating your concerns, you should avoid labeling patients as "alcoholics" or "addicts" because these terms are stigmatizing and often provoke defensiveness. It is equally important to solicit the patient's view as to whether or not he sees the alcohol and drug use as a "problem." Rather than say something like, "Based on the assessment, it is clear to me that you are alcoholic and likely to lose both your marriage and your job if you continue drinking," it would be better to say, "I'm concerned that your drinking is causing problems with your job and your wife and that these problems could become more serious if your drinking continues. What's your view of the situation?" Limit your statements to concerns clearly supported by factual information gathered during the assessment. Each statement should be coupled with one or more open-ended questions asking for additional information and/or the patient's view of what you have just said. For example:

- "You complain of persistent insomnia and depression. I'm concerned that your drinking is either causing these problems or at the very least making them worse. What is your view of this?"
- "You mentioned that cocaine use has caused you to have financial problems and 'roller coaster' moods over the past year. I'm concerned about the emotional distress these problems appear to be causing you. How do you view your drug use, and to what extent does it concern you?"
- "You mentioned that you've been taking prescription (narcotic) painkillers to relieve headaches several days a week over the past year. I'm concerned that you may be dependent on these medica-

tions or at risk for developing dependence if you continue this pattern of use. I'd like to hear your thoughts on this."

- "You've said that you've been smoking marijuana for many years. I'm concerned that this may be contributing to the problems of depression and lack of motivation that brought you here today. What do you think?

Assessing the Patient's Readiness for Change

A number of factors appear to reflect change readiness. These include (1) the specific reasons that the person is seeking consultation at this particular point in time, including external pressure from family members, employers, and other outside forces; (2) the extent to which the person acknowledges negative consequences of substance use and perceives it to be a problem; (3) the individual's stated intentions to change in the near future; (4) the person's perception of her ability to make the desired changes and what obstacles might stand in the way; and (5) what if any changes she is willing to consider making at this point in time. Miller and Rollnick (2002) caution therapists not to base their judgments about patient motivation on variables such as the extent of the patient's agreement with the therapist, acceptance of the diagnosis, expressed desire for help, apparent distress about substance-related consequences, and compliance with the therapist's advice. Most of these variables are actually of little value in predicting the readiness for change. The actual task of eliciting the patient's response, and in the process assessing change readiness, is relatively straightforward. (Several instruments have been developed for this purpose, but they are not suitable in a busy office practice.) You can begin the assessment simply by asking open-ended questions such as:

- "What is *your* view of your alcohol and drug use?"
- "To what extent do *you* feel that it is a problem?"
- "What if anything do *you* think you should do about it?"
- "How confident are *you* about your ability to make the changes you see as desirable?"

Carefully listening to a patient's responses to these questions is likely to reveal the person's current stage of readiness for change. The following are examples of patient statements that typify the different stages of change:

- *Precontemplation*—"I just don't see my alcohol and drug use as a problem. I don't know why everyone is making such a fuss about it."
- *Contemplation*—"Maybe I have a problem, but I'm not so sure that I need to do anything about it right now."

- *Preparation*—"I know that I have a problem and I need help in deciding what to do about it. What are my options?"
- *Action*—"I stopped using alcohol and drugs on my own about 2 weeks ago, but I feel I need professional help to keep moving forward. How can you help me?"
- *Maintenance*—"I've been clean and sober now for over 6 months, but I feel that I need to do something more to prevent relapse and protect my recovery over the long term."

As part of assessing readiness for change, you should ask patients what, if anything, they are willing to do. A constructive way to initiate this discussion is to summarize what has been said thus far and to restate any concerns or intentions to change that the patient has expressed along the way. For example:

"Jack, You've told me that you have become increasingly concerned about your cocaine use over the past year although you remain unsure about whether or not it is really a problem and whether you need to do something about it. You also stated that previously, when you had stopped using cocaine for several months, you felt a lot better about yourself and your marital relationship improved—in particular, arguments with your wife and your depressed moods—the main reasons you are here today— were not nearly as severe back then as they are now that you have returned to using cocaine regularly again. Taking all of this into account, where might you want to go from here in terms of doing something about your cocaine use?"

It is also helpful to elicit fears the patient may have about the prospect of changing—for example:

"You say that you may want to consider stopping your use of prescription narcotics, but what concerns or fears do you have about how you will cope with the stresses in your life without taking pills?"

If the interview has uncovered a serious alcohol and drug problem, express your concerns straightforwardly, but without being unduly confrontational or trying to pressure for change—for example:

"I recognize that you didn't come here seeking or expecting help for an alcohol and drug problem, and I certainly can't and do not want to try to force you to do anything about it. However, I can help you take a closer look at how your substance use is negatively affecting your life and help you decide what, if anything, you might want to do about it. I recognize that it was not comfortable or easy for you to discuss your alcohol and drug use in such detail here today. Based on what I've heard from you, I think it might be a good idea for us to take a closer look at your use the next time we meet. I'm concerned that if we do not give it the attention it deserves, it will be much harder for us to deal effectively with the problems you came here to resolve. How does that sound to you?"

Solution-Oriented Techniques

Another way to both assess and enhance readiness for change is based on the solution-focused approach formulated by Berg and Miller (1992). These authors define five types of interview questions that are designed to assess and, ideally, influence how patients perceive their problems with alcohol and drugs. The goal of these questions is to stimulate thinking about possible solutions.

QUESTIONS THAT HIGHLIGHT PRESESSION CHANGE

Many patients make significant changes in their substance use in the days and weeks before coming for the first interview. Patients who do so need to be complimented and encouraged for their self-initiated efforts instead of being told that they should not be trying to treat themselves or underestimate their need for outside help. Rather than labeling such positive presession changes in negative terms as "reluctance to ask for help," "failure to admit powerlessness," or "unwillingness to give up control"—a tactic not uncommon in traditional (confrontational) treatment approaches—Berg and Miller (1992) suggest using patient-initiated change as a building block for working toward future goals. For example, a patient may come to the interview saying something like, "Since making this appointment several days ago I've cut my cocaine use in half, so I was wondering whether I should cancel the appointment because maybe I can do this on my own." According to Berg and Miller (1992), a useful response might be something like, "That's really great that you've somehow managed to cut down substantially since making the phone call. Tell me how you did it and what motivated you to get a head start on this? Whatever you did appears to have worked so far, and maybe we can work together to build on what you are already doing on your own."

EXCEPTION-FINDING QUESTIONS

Exceptions to the problem can always be found, inasmuch as inevitably there are spontaneous or preplanned instances when the person is not using alcohol and drugs. Berg and Miller (1992) emphasize the importance of looking for these exceptions and capitalizing on these non-occurrences of the problem to enhance the patient's feelings of self-efficacy and self-esteem. For example, a patient may describe a particular day or weekend when he managed to drink significantly less or abstain completely. The therapist can respond affirmatively, saying something along the lines of, "I'm impressed. How did you do that? Tell me step-by-step how you made this happen? This can be very useful to our going forward. If you did it on this one occasion, surely you have the ability to do it again."

THE MIRACLE QUESTION

Asking the so-called miracle question may be the most important technique of all, according to Berg and Miller (1992), for orienting patients toward solutions. Their example of the miracle question is as follows:

> "I want to ask you a slightly different question now. You will have to use your imagination for this one. Suppose you go home and go to bed tonight after today's session. While you are sleeping a miracle happens and the problem that brought you here is solved, just like that (snapping a finger). Because you were sleeping, you didn't know that this miracle happened. What do you suppose will be the first small thing that will indicate to you tomorrow morning that there has been a miracle overnight and the problem that brought you here is solved?" (p. 78)

In response to this question, patients are prompted to envision an alternate state of being for themselves in which they are no longer hampered by their alcohol and drug use. This can be an empowering and freeing experience that helps to instill optimism and hope about achieving positive change. According to Berg and Miller (1992), the miracle visualization is most useful to the patient when described in realistic, detailed, measurable terms. Useful follow-up questions include "When you wake up, how will you know that the problem is solved? What will you notice that is different? What will other people notice about you that is different? Describe specifically how you think you will feel."

SCALING QUESTIONS

Asking scaling questions is a technique for assessing the patient's view of the seriousness of the problem and monitoring future progress in working toward resolution. For example, the therapist might ask, "On a scale of 1 to 10, how bad were things when your alcohol and drug use was at its peak a few months ago, and where would you say the problem is today?" Similarly, "What rating would you give for how unhappy you feel now as compared with a year ago when things were going better in your life?" This technique can also be used, of course, to obtain ratings of the patient's perception of her progress at various points down the road.

COPING QUESTIONS

Coping questions are used to instill even the slightest bit of hope in a discouraging clinical situation with patients who feel pessimistic, hopeless, and that nothing will help. Patients are asked how they are able to muster the strength to "barely cope" with such a serious problem and "manage to get through each day." The aim of these questions is to help patients see that they do have some coping skills, no matter how rudimentary, that help them survive from day to day. It is a way of counteracting the mindset that everything is futile and positive change is impossible. Examples of coping questions include "Given the horrible things you have been through, it's amazing that you're still standing. What do you do to get through each day? How do you prevent things from getting even worse?"

Identifying Ambivalence: The Decisional Balance Analysis

Another important strategy to help patients identify their ambivalence and motivation about changing their substance use behavior is an analysis of the personal costs versus benefits of substance use—a technique known as the decisional balance analysis (Miller & Rollnick, 2002). This technique is based on the premise that people who develop strong attachments to substances often have a great deal of ambivalence about giving them up. Even when use is causing significant harm, many people are concerned about their ability to cope with life stressors without being able to chemically alter their moods with alcohol and drugs. Many therapists view this ambivalence as evidence of patient resistance and denial. However, it is more clinically useful to recognize that people often use psychoactive substances initially as an attempt to cope with difficult or unpleasant situations and to enhance certain aspects of their functioning. Substances may help them to relax, go to sleep, feel more energetic, feel more comfortable in social situations, overcome performance anxiety, be more creative, be more talkative, be less sexually inhibited, and so on. Over time, as an individual comes to rely more and more heavily on substance use for certain effects, it often becomes increasingly difficult, and in some cases extremely anxiety provoking, to consider what it would be like to function without using substances—a major source of ambivalence about stopping. Accordingly, it is important for therapists to acknowledge not only the benefits individuals may derive from substance use, but also their fears about stopping. There are pros and cons of stopping drug use just as there are both pros and cons of continuing use.

The decisional balance analysis can help patients acknowledge this conflict and see how it may be affecting their willingness to change their behavior. Miller and Rollnick (2002) emphasize that the decisional balance analysis is not merely a passive assessment of current motivation to change. Rather, it is a clinical intervention likely to *influence* motivation. A simple balance sheet can be prepared for a patient by drawing a vertical line down the middle of a blank sheet of paper and a horizontal line across the middle of the page, thus creating a grid with four cells. The two columns are labeled "pros" and "cons" and the two rows are labeled "continuing use" and "stopping or drastically cutting down." It is important to recognize that the decisional balance strategy is not simply a matter of listing the number of pros versus cons or tallying scores for deciding whether or not to change. Some patients, for example, provide many negatives (cons) associated with their substance use, counterbalanced by only one or perhaps two very important positives. For example, a multitude of negative consequences resulting from cocaine or methamphetamine use may be outweighed by the perceived positive benefits of increased sexuality, energy, or work productivity. Understandably, you should expect patients who perceive their substance use as enhancing rather than impairing important aspects of their functioning to be reluctant about giving it up even in the face of rather severe consequences.

To begin the decisional balance analysis, you can ask:

- "You said that you want to stop using alcohol and drugs. What are the benefits or positive things you might gain from quitting?"
- "You've been using alcohol and drugs for a very long time and they've become a routine feature of your day-to-day life. Can you imagine what the drawbacks or downside of quitting might be?"
- "What are some of the good things about your alcohol and drug use that you still like?"
- "What are some of the not-so-good things about your alcohol and drug use?"

Some patients may not be able at first to list both the pros and cons of their substance use or may be hesitant to do so. This is especially true if they are actively experiencing negative consequences resulting from their use, have made a firm decision in their minds to stop using, or have been mandated to appear for the assessment. In such cases, you should be prepared to take a more active role in initiating and perhaps even doing the lion's share of the work in filling out the decisional balance worksheet. In addition to exposing ambivalence, the decisional balance analysis helps to build trust and rapport with the patient and facilitates development of a cooperative therapeutic relationship.

FINAL COMMENT

In this chapter we have described the various components of a comprehensive assessment of substance use and a clinical approach to the assessment relying heavily on motivational interviewing techniques. As stated earlier, assessment is much more than a fact-gathering procedure. It is the first and often the most critical phase of the treatment process. If utilized properly, it presents a window of opportunity to engage patients in a therapeutic relationship that reduces their defensiveness and enhances their willingness to change. The goal of assessment is to determine the nature and extent of an individual's substance use behavior within the broader multidimensional context of his current life.

Offering therapeutic feedback based on assessment results is a critical step in determining appropriate treatment strategies. In order to maximize the clinical value of feedback to your patients, you should adhere as closely as possible to motivational interviewing techniques. The purpose of feedback is not to club patients over the head with their resistance or denial, but to highlight connections between the substance use and adverse consequences that are meaningful to the *individual*. A patient's reaction to feedback provides strong clues about her stage of readiness for change and the types of treatment interventions that are most likely to be effective. Solution-focused techniques offer additional tools to help identify and enhance your patient's readiness and motivation for change.

CHAPTER 8

Individualized Goal Setting and Treatment Planning

Meeting Patients "Where They Are"

Individualized treatment planning is an essential feature of the integrative approach. Unlike standard approaches, in which treatment plans are often predetermined for patients who enter addiction treatment programs, in the integrated model treatment plans are developed collaboratively to meet patients "where they are," based on information gathered during the assessment. This process recognizes that patients' presenting needs and problems vary substantially from one person to the next, as do their strengths, available resources, personal goals, and motivation/readiness for change. The more precisely the treatment plan takes into account these individual differences, the greater the patient's personal investment in making the desired changes and the greater the likelihood that treatment goals will actually be achieved. It is important that patients view whatever goals are established as being realistic, stepwise, and achievable. Motivation for change, sense of self-efficacy, and retention in treatment are all enhanced significantly when patients experience early success in achieving their initial treatment goals. Conversely, failure to achieve initial treatment goals often leads to discouragement, a sense of hopelessness, and early dropout from treatment.

The process of developing an individually tailored treatment plan requires that the therapist and patient work collaboratively to identify and prioritize a list of specific treatment goals and then define strategies and approximate time frames for achieving those goals. It is important for both the patient and the therapist to acknowledge that the initial treatment plan must be flexible and subject to change, based on what actually transpires as treatment proceeds. The treatment plan is best viewed as a temporary draft or road map for change that *can* and most likely *will* be modified during the course of treatment. It is likely, for example, that certain needs and problems will emerge during treatment that had not been present or anticipated during the pretreatment assessment. Moreover, treatment priorities and goals may change as some problems are resolved and others become evident.

In this chapter we describe a variety of important factors that influence and shape the development of an individualized treatment plan. Toward the end of the chapter we describe in detail how to match specific treatment goals and interventions with the individual patients' stage of readiness for change in order to find the best fit and meet them "where they are."

RISK FACTORS REQUIRING IMMEDIATE ATTENTION

Urgency and risk factors identified in the pretreatment assessment must be taken into account in developing an initial treatment plan. These factors include the need for medical detoxification and other types of serious medical and psychiatric concerns often requiring immediate clinical attention.

• *Is the patient an imminent danger to self and/or others?* This includes not only substance-related suicidality, homicidality, and psychosis, but other high-risk behaviors such as driving while intoxicated, having unprotected sex with strangers, and acting violently toward self and/or others. Of similar concern is a pattern of continuing to use alcohol or drugs despite recent life-threatening overdoses, especially if resuscitation and/or other heroic emergency medical interventions were needed to prevent the patient from dying. The risks of suicide, accidental injury to self or others due to impaired judgment or motor coordination (including vehicular accidents), and physical injury to self or others due to substance-induced aggressive behavior are extraordinarily high among this patient population and must not be overlooked in assessing risk.

• *Is the patient at risk of suffering serious medical consequences if substance use either continues or stops too abruptly?* Important considerations here are whether there are already signs of potentially serious organ damage (e.g., liver problems) that can only be made worse by further substance use and/or the patient is at risk of experiencing serious withdrawal complications (e.g., delirium tremens, seizures) if use of alcohol and/or other depressants is stopped too abruptly.

• *Is the patient in imminent danger of serious and potentially irreversible psychosocial consequences if substance use continues?* Such consequences may include loss of job or professional licensure, breakup of a marriage or other valued relationship, loss of child custody and/or visitation rights, and loss of personal freedom (i.e., incarceration).

When the patient's physical health and safety are at risk, encouraging the patient to accept an immediate referral for physician consultation or hospitalization is the most prudent course of action. It is important to recognize that containing risk must always be given priority over addressing the patient's substance abuse problem, whether or not the risk is a direct result of alcohol and drug use. Patients in need of medical detoxification and/or treatment for serious substance-related health problems should be referred to an addiction medicine physician or facility where the needed services can be obtained. This should be done before negotiating or initiating any psychosocial interventions to address the patient's substance disorder. In cases where the patient is at risk of suffering serious psychosocial, but not medical, consequences from continued substance abuse, it is important to express straightforwardly your serious concerns about the very real dangers of continued use and, where indicated, suggest the possibility of immediate inpatient care.

What if patients in any of these risky situations refuse to accept your directive or recommendation? Depending on the severity of the risk, you have a limited number of options about how to proceed. In the most serious and urgent cases (e.g., patients who are suicidal or homicidal), you have both a clinical and legal obligation to intervene. If such a patient refuses immediate hospitalization, you are obliged to enlist the help of local police and emergency medical services to ensure that the patient is placed in a protective environment and receives the needed clinical services. In less urgent cases that are not life-threatening, you can ask for the patient's permission to contact available family members and enlist their help in encouraging the patient to take immediate action. You must guard against becoming cynical and unduly frustrated in dealing with severely addicted and troubled patients who are not yet ready to let you (or perhaps anyone else) help them.

ANTICIPATED LENGTH OF TREATMENT

Just as some patients come to treatment with certain preconceived goals, they often harbor certain expectations about the length of treatment. Many patients expect treatment to be briefer than the therapist may think is optimal. Rather than challenge the patient's view, which may only increase the potential for early dropout, it is best to negotiate a treatment plan that focuses initially on short-term goals and then renegotiate the plan as these goals are accomplished or changed. Unlike most traditional treatment programs that usually require patients to commit in advance to a predetermined length of treatment, office-based practitioners are in a better position to individually tailor the length and other aspects of treatment to address patients' individual and changing needs.

PREFERRED TREATMENT MODALITY AND SETTING

In addition to having preconceived ideas about treatment length and goals, some patients arrive with definite ideas about the modality and type of treatment they desire. Some will be strongly against or in favor of structured inpatient or outpatient substance abuse treatment programs and 12-step meetings. Others will have no strong preferences or preconceived ideas about the type of treatment they are willing to consider and instead will look to you for advice and guidance. Many, if not most, patients who seek help from an office-based practitioner come hoping that individual therapy alone will suffice to address their substance abuse problem. Recognizing that some patients will inevitably require levels of care that go beyond what any office practitioner can provide, it is important to familiarize yourself with the various types of substance abuse treatment resources available in your practice community and elsewhere, including inpatient detoxification and rehabilitation programs, intensive outpatient and day (partial hospitalization) programs, dual diagnosis programs, halfway and sober living houses, addiction psychologists and other mental health clinicians specializing in substance abuse treatment, and physicians specializing in addiction psychiatry and/or addiction medicine.

PRIORITIZING TREATMENT GOALS

It is important that therapists not underestimate the possible impact of substance use on the patient's clinical presentation and functioning and proceed with the therapy assuming that substance use is only a symptom of an underlying disorder. It is equally important not to focus exclusively on the patient's substance use while ignoring other problems that the patient considers pressing and important. Current substance use and related consequences are often matters of primary concern, and initial treatment goals must reflect this priority. But sometimes addressing other issues is higher on the patient's priority list, issues such as a relationship crisis, negative moods, and intrusive thoughts related to early trauma and abuse. Considering that alcohol and drug problems are almost always associated with dysfunction in other life areas (e.g., marital, family, legal, health, psychiatric, vocational), these areas should be given sufficient priority in the initial treatment plan even though stopping or reducing the substance use is likely to alleviate some of the more acute problems. For example, reaching an initial goal of not using alcohol for 2 consecutive weeks is likely to help alleviate the problem of lateness and absenteeism at work that has been caused directly by the patient's drinking.

It is likely that a variety of patient problems and needs will have been uncovered in the pretreatment assessment that must be addressed in order to forge a working alliance with the patient and foster treatment retention. Denning (2000) emphasizes the importance of formulating a needs hierarchy with substance-abusing patients, and Morgan (2001) offers several strategies for striking a balance between addressing SUDs and giving sufficient attention to problems that are of greater concern to the patient. These strategies include (1) heightening patients' awareness of connections, wherever they exist, between their substance use and other problems that are matters of concern to them, and how these problems may be alleviated by stopping or markedly reducing their substance use; (2) striking an agreement with patients to devote a portion of each session to addressing these other problems and a portion to focusing specifically on their substance use; and (3) when the therapist encounters difficulty in redirecting the patient's focus from other problems to substance abuse issues, raising this issue for discussion as a possible sign that the person is highly ambivalent about changing his substance use behavior.

ABSTINENCE OR MODERATION GOALS?

It is essential to keep in mind that no matter what your theoretical orientation or clinical biases may be, only the patient has the power to choose the treatment goals, regardless of what you think may be best. Some patients already have certain goals in mind when they appear for treatment, such as reducing rather than completely stopping their alcohol or drug use. Others have vague notions about possible treatment goals and are looking for some guidance, and still others assume that total abstinence is the only legitimate or acceptable goal. It is essential for therapists to recognize that treatment goals must be negotiated, agreed upon mutually, and not predetermined or imposed unilaterally. The decision of whether and how to change is always the patient's choice to make. Even when it seems clear to you, based on the pretreatment assessment, that total abstinence offers the safest and most clinically appropriate treatment goal and that continued use at any level will only increase the likelihood that your patient will suffer serious consequences, it is the patient, not you, who has the ultimate say about whether and to what extent the substance use behavior should be changed. Certainly, you should not hesitate to express your concerns clearly, straightforwardly, and respectfully, but ultimately your task is to find a starting point for making positive changes that the patient feels is acceptable. The overall strategy here is to negotiate, not mandate, treatment goals in a spirit of meeting patients "where they are," rather than insist that they be where you and others would like them to be. Doing so provides patients with a greater sense of ownership and personal responsibility for whatever treatment goals emerge from this negotiation. As mentioned previously, this approach to treatment planning contrasts sharply with traditional approaches in which goals are often predetermined and patients are expected to accept them without challenge—a strategy that frequently evokes power struggles, patient resistance, and early dropout from treatment.

In the integrative approach, abstinence is seen as the preferred treatment goal for patients who have a history of serious problems with alcohol and drugs. Patients with less serious problems may also derive significant benefits from trying abstinence at least temporarily. A useful strategy that can help to enhance patients' willingness to consider abstinence is to propose a short-term (e.g., 2- to 4-week) trial period or "experiment" with stopping all alcohol and drug use temporarily. You need not try to convince patients that alcohol and drug use is the primary cause of their distress, but you can suggest temporary abstinence as an assessment tool to determine more precisely whether and how the substance use figures into the overall clinical picture. Nor is it necessary to convince patients that they are "addicts" or "alcoholics" to justify the need for an experiment with abstinence. Engaging patients in a time-limited experiment with abstinence helps to avoid debates and power struggles around issues such as how much alcohol or drug use is "too much," whether the substance use really is a "problem," and whether abstinence should be a temporary or permanent goal. Once patients stop using alcohol and drugs completely, the extent to which prior substance use had been adversely affecting their psychological status and functioning often becomes much more apparent to them and others (including the therapist). Even patients who do not meet the criteria for substance dependence often report substantial improvements in energy, sleep, concentration, mood, and judgment when they stop using substances. It is important to recognize that alcohol and drug use can impede therapeutic progress in resolving other psychological and life problems long before the use meets the diagnostic criteria for abuse or dependence. This is not surprising, considering that all psychoactive drugs profoundly alter neurochemical activity in the brain.

Many patients are uninformed and thus unclear about the potential benefits of trying abstinence, especially if they see quitting alcohol and drug use as capitulating to the wishes of others. You can describe to patients the personal advantages of trying an experiment with abstinence, as follows:

- "Abstinence is clearly the safest choice. There is no guaranteed 'safe' level of alcohol and drug use that will cause no harm. If you do not use alcohol and drugs, you eliminate the possibility of incurring any additional adverse consequences (e.g., legal problems, health risks, etc.) caused directly or indirectly by your alcohol and drug use."
- "Abstinence provides a unique opportunity to see things through a 'different set of eyes' and to acquire valuable information about the ways you think, feel, and behave in the absence of alcohol and drugs that is simply not attainable by other methods. It helps to reveal the nature and extent of your attachment to substances, including the degree to which you rely on chemically altering your mood to help you cope with stress and other negative emotions."
- "Abstinence can give you better access to your emotions and provide an opportunity to learn how to deal with them more effectively after the chemical blanket of alcohol and drug use is removed."
- "Abstinence gives you a chance to break old habits, experience a change, and build some confidence."
- "Abstinence helps you to identify more clearly the internal (emotional) and external (environmental) 'triggers' associated with your alcohol and drug use."
- "Abstinence can help to reduce conflicts with family members and significant others (e.g., spouse, parents, etc.) caused or exacerbated by your alcohol and drug use."
- "Abstinence provides an indication of how easy or difficult it is for you to stop using."
- "Abstinence exposes voids and unmet needs in your life that you may be filling up or distracting yourself from with alcohol and drugs."
- "Abstinence may enhance or restore the effectiveness of prescribed medications you are taking for other problems such as depression, anxiety, and the like."

Here is an example of how to present to a patient the idea of trying an "experiment" with abstinence:

"Jennifer, let me try to explain how you might benefit from attempting a trial period of abstinence. Not using any alcohol or drugs whatsoever during the trial period is likely to provide you with valuable information that is not attainable by other means. In particular, it may give you an opportunity to see how you think and feel on a day-to-day basis and how well you cope with problems without chemically altering your brain activity and mood. In other words, not using anything will give you a chance to experience things through a 'different set of eyes.' This will, I hope, allow you to better define the role that alcohol and drug use plays in your life, including how it may help and/or hurt you. For example, you may notice that you become more stress sensitive or perhaps more bored when you are not using any mood-altering chemicals whatsoever. Another benefit of total abstinence is that it can help you to identify specific 'triggers' that encourage and perpetuate your alcohol and drug use. These triggers include external factors such as certain people, places, objects, and situations associated with your prior use, as well as internal factors such as certain thoughts, feelings, and moods linked with your use. Giving abstinence a serious try may also give you an indication of just how easy or difficult it is for you to stop using. Last, but not least, refraining from all alcohol and drug use provides an opportunity to learn and practice new (nonchemical) coping skills for dealing with problems and uncomfortable feelings. Abstinence maximizes both the speed and effectiveness of your learning process. There are also reasons why you might want to consider abstaining at least temporarily from *all* mood-altering substances rather than stopping only your substance of choice. In addition to all the reasons I just mentioned regarding the potential benefits of abstinence, there are two more reasons why total abstinence from everything can be valuable. One is that using any mood-altering substance is often associated with impulsive behavior and decision making. Thus, when you are trying to refrain from using your substance of choice, using another substance can make it much harder to resist temptations and impulses to use. For example, while trying to stay away from cocaine many people find that having only one or two drinks of alcohol leads them right back to using cocaine. Another reason to consider total abstinence is the well-known phenomenon of drug substitution. While people are trying to stay away from their drug of choice, they sometimes switch to another drug that they may view as 'safer'—often because they have no prior history of problems linked directly to using that substance. Over time, however, many individuals begin to develop problems with the substance they had previously regarded as safe."

Despite the many potential benefits of abstinence and regardless of how severe a person's substance abuse problem might be, some individuals find a goal of abstinence (now matter how brief or temporary) undesirable or view it as unattainable. Accordingly, therapists should be prepared to negotiate alternative treatment goals. Insisting on abstinence as the only worthwhile or acceptable goal may serve only to increase patient resistance and the risk of dropout. Regardless of the therapist's goal preferences, patients will ultimately and inevitably decide what treatment goals are acceptable to them. This includes alcohol-dependent patients who reduce but do not stop their drinking even when treated in abstinence-based programs and patients who choose abstinence even after they have been treated in moderation-based programs. Clearly, patients' self-selection of treatment goals has an important influence on the motivation and commitment to change their substance use behavior.

Many patients refuse to consider complete abstinence but are willing to attempt to moderate their use or to change other aspects of their behavior in order to reduce harm. Keep in mind that the therapeutic alliance is your most powerful tool, and many people who have successfuly overcome a serious addiction took years to conclude that abstinence was the only reliable solution for them. You can begin wherever the patient shows willingness to make changes. You do not need to endorse the patient's view that moderation will suffice in order to maintain an atmosphere conducive to exploration. Indeed, you should offer clear recommendations while conveying respect for the patient's desire to take one step at a time: "Your greatest benefits would come from eliminating alcohol completely, but I can understand that you find that too big a leap and it doesn't make sense to you right now. How could you change your drinking habits in a way that seems manageable to you?" The key is giving the patient a framework for self-observation and an arena to explore the issue regularly. This approach has been described as "an experiment with abstinence" (Margolis & Zweben, 1998) or "sobriety sampling" (Miller & Page, 1991).

A variety of strategies can be used in moderation experiments. A powerful intervention is to ask the client to commit to complete abstinence for 1 month, and then to moderate use (e.g., 2 drinks, standard units of 1.5 ounces of alcohol, 12 ounces of beer, 5 ounces of wine) in the succeeding month. Alcohol dependent clients often have much more trouble with moderation than with abstinence. It is common for someone who insists on a moderation goal to conclude that the daily struggle to drink less is too difficult. Such individuals tire of the continuing preoccupation with attempting to control their drinking and eventually conclude that complete abstinence is the best course of action. Many are unable to moderate their use for any period of time, or can do so but find it a daily struggle. It is important to frame this difficulty as part of the learning experience, not a sign of weakness or failure. You can emphasize that it is quite normal for people to underestimate the hold their preferred substance has on them, and that it takes courage to acknowledge and address this issue.

Be careful to avoid suggesting that the ability to moderate drinking or drug use is proof that an addiction does not exist. The natural history of alcohol (Vaillant, 1995) and other drug use is that many people, with or without treatment, move in and out of abstinence and what appears to be periods of controlled use over a lifetime. This feature of the disorder allows patients to conclude that they are not "really" addicted. However, it is the absence of dependable control and the accumulation of adverse consequences that are the defining features of an SUD. You can remind the patient that one reason SUDs are described as "cunning, baffling, and powerful" is that periods of apparent control allow individuals to believe there is a magic formula that will permit them to consume safely, if only they can find and perfect it.

Inasmuch as most substance abuse problems are dose related, moderation strategies certainly reduce harm in the short run. However, once your patient has crossed the boundary into uncontrolled use, relapse vulnerability remains high. Good clinical judgment as well as liability considerations indicate that you should avoid suggesting that one goal is as good as another. Abstinence offers the widest margin of safety. It is important for patients to feel they have options, and important for you to describe some potential consequences of each option. A binge drinker who reduces the frequency and duration of her binges is improving her circumstances, but is still at risk of injuring someone in an automobile accident. The therapist who has suggested that harm reduction goals are adequate is potentially at legal risk if the patient injures someone while intoxicated and the therapist's notes indicate that the patient was advised that moderate drinking was a realistic goal.

As discussed earlier, controlled or moderate drinking is an appropriate and attainable goal for many individuals with *less severe* alcohol problems, particularly those who have never met the diagnostic criteria for alcohol dependence. The goal of moderation approaches is to help patients establish and maintain a pattern of *responsible* drinking, defined as drinking that provides positive effects (e.g., relaxation, enhanced sociability, etc.) without putting oneself or others at increased risk for suffering negative consequences (Rotgers, Kern, & Hoeltzel, 2002). Although individuals with severe alcohol problems are clearly not appropriate candidates for controlled drinking approaches, moderation strategies can still be effective as a starting point to engage these individuals and move them incrementally toward accepting abstinence as a goal. In fact, proponents of moderation approaches suggest that one of the best ways to get a head start on moderating drinking is to take a temporary vacation from alcohol. Understandably, clinicians who operate within the framework of disease model abstinence-based approaches have strong reservations about offering moderation goals to patients with significant alcohol problems. Their major concern is that condoning continued drinking at any level will only feed into these patients' denial and rationalization, worsen their problems, and lead inevitably to a downward progression resulting in more and more serious consequences and possibly death. The counterarguments are that such progression is not inevitable in all cases (as discussed in Chapter 2) and that engaging patients in working toward moderation goals holds much greater promise of generating positive outcomes than alienating patients with a rigid approach that turns them away.

There is even greater hesitation and concern among clinicians about offering moderation or harm reduction goals to patients using addictive drugs other than alcohol who are not interested in stopping their use of these substances entirely. Nonetheless, the most critical question here is, What types of treatment goals are these patients willing to pursue in regard to changing their use of specific substances? Some patients are willing to abstain, at least temporarily, from their drug of choice (i.e., the one causing them the most trouble), but do not want to give up other substances they feel capable of using in moderation. For example, patients using opioids or stimulant drugs are often unwilling to give up alcohol or marijuana, seeing these substances as much more benign, especially if prior use has caused them no significant problems. Within the harm reduction model, potential goals such as using less frequently and in smaller amounts, using fewer drugs and drug combinations, shifting from more to less hazardous drugs and routes of administration, and changing from more to less intensive and impulsive patterns of use, are all considered feasible goals in the service of reducing drug-related harm. It is important to keep in mind that within the harm reduction framework, any steps taken to reduce the harm or risks associated with substance use are seen as steps in the right direction.

Miller (1999) emphasizes that it is important to be clear that by offering moderation or harm reduction alternatives to total abstinence you are not *advocating* continued use of dangerous substances. Your overall goal is to help the patient move away from harmful substance use, including illegal drug use. In certain cases you may feel especially obliged to encourage abstinence, particularly if the patient's use is associated with clear and present dangers. This must be done in a persuasive but noncoercive manner, consistent with the overall tone of motivation interviewing techniques. ("It is entirely your choice to make, but I do want to honestly and straightforwardly express my serious concerns to you about the risks associated with your continued drug use and to say very clearly that I think that abstinence, even if only for a short while, would be the best way to go.") It is also important to remain clear about the fact that it is not up to you to "permit," "let," or "allow" your patients to use or not use substances. The choice is theirs and theirs alone to make, and you cannot make it for them, although you should certainly state your recommendations and express your concerns in a respectful, empathic, nonauthoritarian way in keeping with principles of motivational interviewing.

There are at least several important reasons to advise against nonabstinence goals for patients with serious alcohol and drug problems (Miller, 1999). These include legal and other risks involved in procuring, possessing, and using illicit substances; medical and psychiatric conditions exacerbated by use; strong external demands to abstain; pregnancy; hazardous interactions with prescribed medications; and a prior history of severe alcohol or drug problems. Interestingly, when given the option of choosing moderation, many patients who initially reject abstinence later choose it as a goal after finding themselves unable to limit their use reliably. This underscores the importance of offering choices rather than dictating treatment goals. Insisting rigidly at the outset that abstinence is the one and only acceptable treatment goal often engenders an oppositional dynamic that breeds power struggles between patient and therapist. The harder the therapist pressures for abstinence, the more the patient digs in his heels, arguing that abstinence is neither necessary nor desirable. Acknowledging to your patients that only they can choose the goal can help to enhance your credibility and encourage them to participate more actively in formulating a treatment plan.

THE PATIENT'S MOTIVATION
AND READINESS TO CHANGE

According to the stages-of-change model (Chapter 4), certain types of clinical interventions are likely to work best with patients in each of the five different stages of change. Conversely, interventions that are not properly matched or synchronized with the patient's stage of change are likely to heighten patient resistance, reduce treatment effectiveness, and cause premature dropout. Thus, developing a keen sensitivity to the patient's location on the continuum of readiness for change is one of the most important keys to developing a treatment plan that fosters patient engagement, retention, and successful outcomes. Table 8.1 outlines the types of clinical interventions that appear to be most appropriate for patients in each stage of change.

The overall strategy here is to "meet patients where they are" as a starting point to help them move forward in the process of change. Treatment–patient matching has been a topic of much discussion and debate in the literature on treating addiction. The following discussion draws heavily from the recent work of several authors (Connors, Donovan, & DiClemente, 2001; Miller & Rollnick, 1991; Miller, Zweben, & Rychtarik, 1994; Miller, 1999).

Strategies with Patients in the Precontemplation Stage

Patients in the precontemplation stage, by definition, do not realize that their substance use is a problem and thus see no reason to reduce or stop their use. The primary therapeutic task with these individuals is to raise their awareness of substance-related problems without raising their resistance to change. Traditional approaches to dealing with people "in denial" rely heavily on advice giving, confrontation, and warning of dire consequences. Such patients are often characterized as "unmotivated," "noncompliant," and/or "resistant to change," and confrontation is seen as the only way to break through their denial and persuade them to change. How-

TABLE 8.1. Appropriate Motivational Strategies for Each Stage of Chan

Precontemplation

The patient does not perceive substance use as a "problem" and is not yet considering change or is unwilling to change.

- Establish rapport, ask permission to discuss the topic of change.
- Acknowledge the patient for willingness to talk openly.
- Raise the patient's doubts or concerns about his substance-using patterns.
- Explore the sequence and meaning of events that brought him to see you or to seek previous treatments.
- Elicit the patient's perception of the "problem."
- Explore the pros and cons of substance use.
- Elicit, listen to, and acknowledge the aspects of substance use the patient enjoys.
- Examine discrepancies between the patient's and others' perception of the "problem."
- Offer factual information about the risks of substance use.
- Educate the patient about DSM-IV definitions of use, abuse, and dependence and NIAAA categories of low-risk, at-risk, and problem drinking.
- Express concern, keep the door open, continue the dialogue.

Contemplation

The patient acknowledges concerns about substance use and is considering the possibility of change, but is ambivalent, wavering, and uncertain.

- Normalize the patient's ambivalence about using and about reducing or stopping the use.
- Help the patient "tip the decisional balance" toward change.
- Elicit the patient's views about the pros and cons of change.
- Examine the patient's personal values in relation to change.
- Emphasize the patient's free choice, responsibility, and ability to change.
- Examine the patient's understanding of change and what it might involve.
- Discuss the idea of an "experiment" with abstinence or markedly reduced use as potentially informative and a helpful way to "get off the fence."

Preparation

The patient is committed to and planning to make changes in the immediate future, but is still considering what exactly to do.

- Clarify the patient's own goals, timetables, and strategies for change.
- Offer a menu of different treatment options.
- Offer guidance and suggestions.
- Explore what has worked or not worked in the past.

(cont.)

Note. Adapted from Miller (1999).

TABLE 8.1. (*cont.*)

- Negotiate a plan for change that includes smaller achievable goals for a successful plan.
- Explore treatment expectations and the patient's role.
- Identify and enlist available social supports.

<u>Action</u>

The patient is actively taking steps to change, but has not yet reached a stable state.

- Engage the patient in treatment and reinforce the importance of remaining in treatment until goals have been achieved.
- Support a realistic view of change through taking small steps.
- Acknowledge common difficulties in early stages of change and explore how to handle them.
- Educate the patient about cravings and how to deal with them safely.
- Help the patient identify high-risk situations through a functional analysis and develop appropriate coping strategies to avoid and overcome these.
- Assist the patient in finding new reinforcers of positive change.

<u>Maintenance</u>

The patient has achieved initial goals, such as abstinence, and is now working to maintain gains.

- Help the patient identify and sample non-drug sources of pleasure (i.e., new reinforcers).
- Support positive lifestyle changes.
- Affirm the patient's resolve and self-efficacy.
- Help the patient practice and use new coping strategies to avoid a return to substance use.
- Maintain supportive contact.

<u>Recurrence</u>

The patient has returned to previous substance-using behaviors and must now cope with the consequences and decide what to do.

- Help the patient reenter the change process, overcome self-blame and guilt, and recommit to specific treatment goals.
- Commend the patient for not dropping out and for willingness to reconsider change.
- Convey empathy, understanding, and positive regard.
- Explore the meaning and reality of the recurrence as a learning opportunity.
- Explore how to prevent it from happening again—"What will you do differently this time?"
- Maintain supportive contact.

ever, too often these types of heavy-handed tactics backfire. Confronting people in the precontemplation stage often evokes resistance and oppositional behavior. Arguing with patients in the precontemplation stage about the need for change or pressuring them to accept treatment when they have not yet even acknowledged that a problem exists is likely to rupture whatever rapport and therapeutic relationship you have been trying to establish up to that point. With patients in this stage you generally should avoid prescribing action-oriented strategies requiring specific or immediate changes in behavior. Expecting these individuals to accept without challenge your recommendation to reduce or eliminate their alcohol and drug use, go to an AA meeting, or seek help at a substance abuse treatment program is not only unrealistic, but a setup for failure. Instead, you must work hard to establish an open dialogue with these patients about their alcohol and drug use and look for ways to coax them forward toward making a commitment to change. Agreeing to disagree about the presence of a substance abuse problem is often the only workable starting point. The goal is to find ways to work *with,* rather than *against,* the patient's resistance and to enhance the patient's willingness to change.

Understanding transference and countertransference dynamics can be very helpful in minimizing power struggles and avoiding other destructive interactions that frequently drive these patients out of treatment (Imhof, 1995; Kaufman, 1994; Zweben, 1989). When working with patients in the process of acknowledging an alcohol or drug problem, you must closely monitor and contain your negative countertransference reactions, especially when patients flatly reject or argue against your well-intentioned recommendations. Moving these patients toward acknowledging the problem and accepting the need for treatment is not a simple task. Leading them on a path of closer examination of their involvement with psychoactive substances requires empathy, patience, and persistence. It also requires your willingness to accept small positive changes in patients' *thinking* that may be unaccompanied by immediate changes in *behavior* as initial steps in the right direction.

The following are suggested strategies for working with patients in the precontemplation stage:

1. Explore with the patient in detail the reasons why she has come to see you at this particular point in time. In other words, ask, *why now?* Individuals in the precontemplation stage are by definition not self-motivated for treatment, and thus there are almost always other (external) reasons why they are seeking professional help. The goal for many individuals is to satisfy a mandate (legal or otherwise) in order to avoid consequences or get out of trouble. Many are looking to placate a spouse who is threatening to leave, a parent who is threatening to cut off financial assistance, or an

employer who is threatening to suspend or terminate employment. Sometimes individuals in precontemplation are looking for confirmation by a professional that they do not have an alcohol and drug problem. Many openly admit that their only reason for seeking treatment is to satisfy an external demand. It is important to recognize that motivation for treatment is not synonymous with motivation for change. When considering how best to intervene with patients in this stage, it is especially important to follow the general guideline "start where the patient is rather than where you want him to be."

2. In an effort to raise the patient's consciousness about potential consequences, ask, "What would have to happen for you to decide that your alcohol and drug use has become a problem?" Help the patient assess the obvious and not-so-obvious potential risks of continuing to use.

3. Examine discrepancies between the patient's and others' perception of her substance use. Ask, "What have your spouse, other family members, and friends said about your alcohol and drug use? In what ways are their perceptions different from yours?"

4. Use the "Columbo approach" (Miller, 1999), a Socratic interviewing style portrayed humorously by actor Peter Falk in his TV role as Detective Columbo. When interviewing a suspected criminal, Columbo had a good sense of what actually had occurred, but acted naive, curious, and confused while strategically posing questions in an attempt to get suspects to explain apparent inconsistencies in their alibis and, in the course of doing so, unwittingly expose their own culpability. Similarly, the "Columbo clinician" can enlist the patient's help in explaining discrepancies and how seemingly contradictory pieces of information might fit together. When this type of intervention works well, it encourages the patient (rather than the therapist) to explain apparent discrepancies and how they can be reconciled. For example, "I'm really not clear at all why others think that your alcohol and drug use is a problem. Why do you think your family members appear to be so concerned about your use?" Or, "Maybe I'm not entirely correct. I suppose it's possible that your substance use is not nearly as serious as my impressions have indicated up to this point. I wonder where I may have gone wrong."

5. Suggest bringing in a spouse or significant other to a session (only with the patient's permission). It can be very illuminating for both you and the patient to hear the viewpoint of others regarding the patient's substance use behavior and related consequences, including those the patient may not have mentioned previously.

6. Educate patients (and family members) about alcohol and other drug abuse, including but not limited to the definitions of substance abuse and dependence and NIAAA categories of low-risk and at-risk drinking. Provide educational pamphlets and other take-home materials that you keep on hand in your office, together with a list of helpful books and

websites (see Appendix 4). Consider giving patients brief reading or workbook assignments that can serve as the basis for discussion in subsequent sessions. Educate patients about some of the subtle, insidious effects of substance use on values, priorities, self-esteem, coping abilities, mood, and personal growth. Taking an educative, nonconfrontational stance avoids the problems of stimulating defensiveness and getting into power struggles—the primary pitfalls of working with patients in the precontemplation stage.

7. Although suggesting an "experiment with abstinence" is not likely to meet with a positive response from individuals in the precontemplation stage, discussing the idea of a temporary reduction in the amount and/or frequency of alcohol and drug use can sometimes spark their curiosity.

8. Express your interest in keeping the door open, and resist the temptation to pressure for change. At all costs, do not antagonize or alienate the patient. Don't give up prematurely and don't get frustrated in thinking that you are just wasting your time: subliminal or hidden change still may be occurring! If all of these efforts fail, your fallback position is to simply agree to disagree with your patient and to ask his permission to continue the dialogue about substance use and related issues.

Strategies with Patients in the Contemplation Stage

The primary goal with patients in the contemplation stage is to increase their awareness of problems caused by their substance use and heighten their ambivalence about continuing their current pattern of use so as to tip the balance in favor of change. Toward this end, you should present patients with objective feedback about their substance-related problems and help them evaluate realistically the consequences and risks associated with continuing their alcohol and drug use. The decisional balance exercise described in Chapter 7 is especially helpful, inasmuch as being embroiled in ambivalence is a defining characteristic of patients in the contemplation stage. Similarly, asking the "miracle question" (also described in Chapter 7) can help to define more clearly what the potential benefits of reducing or stopping substance use might be.

A word of caution: You must be careful not to focus exclusively on the negative consequences of substance use. It is important for you to normalize the patient's ambivalence about addressing her substance use by acknowledging that whenever people consider the possibility of moving away from or completely letting go of something to which they have become strongly attached, they are likely to feel ambivalent or conflicted about making changes of this type—whether that something is alcohol or drugs or anything else. Another technique for exposing ambivalence is to help patients see that they are of "two minds" about their substance use. Part of them wants to give it up, but another part of them does not—or at the very least is unsure about giving it up. To help expose this ambivalence, ask the following question: "Speak to me from the side of you that still feels positively about your alcohol and drug use and wants to continue using despite the problems it may have caused you." Accordingly, it is important explore, without challenge, whatever positive effects or benefits patients feel their alcohol and drug use provides. An open, unbiased discussion of positive drug effects instills trust, encourages more honest disclosure, and enhances your credibility with these patients. You should ask patients to describe the "good" and "not so good" things about their substance use and describe the same for any prior periods of abstinence or markedly reduced use. For example: "Although your marijuana use may be contributing to your problems with depression and insomnia, I wonder what positive effects you get from it and how it has helped you in the past." You should also ask about positive and negative aspects of the patient's past experiences with abstinence. For example, "What was it like for you the last time you stopped smoking marijuana with regard to both the positives and the negatives?" It is important to ask about the patient's expectations of problems, difficulties, and obstacles involved in considering the possibility of stopping or reducing use. Some patients recoil from thinking too seriously about trying to stop, fearing that they are likely to fail and feel humiliated. They may be willing to change but do not feel confident about their ability to do so successfully.

A potential trap for therapists working with patients in the contemplation stage is to jump too far ahead and press for change when these patients are just beginning to acknowledge the problems associated with their substance use. This is likely to activate the wrong side of the patient's ambivalence. If you push too hard for change, the patient is likely to retreat into a defensive posture and rationalize the use. It is important to educate patients in this stage about some of the subtle, insidious, and not-so-obvious effects of substance use on values, priorities, aspirations, coping abilities, mood, relationships, self-esteem, and personal growth. Another strategy is to offer to schedule a family interview that includes that patient and significant others, not only to obtain information from collaterals, but also to enlist their help in encouraging (not coercing) the patient to address her substance use. Here too, the goal should not be to try to press for change, but to establish and maintain a therapeutic relationship that can serve as a vehicle for enhancing the patient's motivation to change.

Patients who do not meet the criteria for alcohol abuse or dependence, but are nevertheless drinking above low-risk consumption levels and/or are at increased risk for developing alcohol problems (as defined by the NIAAA criteria described previously in Chapter 2), should be encouraged to cut down substantially on their alcohol consumption or consider a trial period of abstinence. (Offering this advice assumes that you have already determined that the patient is *not* physically dependent on alcohol and does *not* require medical detoxification.) For example, you might ask the patient if he is willing to try an "experiment" with abstinence for a period of 2–4 weeks. This can be an effective way to help patients "get off the fence" about the prospect of taking action. The proposed length of the experiment can be whatever time period the patient finds acceptable and feels confident that he can reasonably manage. If the patient is not receptive to considering a trial period of abstinence, you should ask, "What do you think you would be willing and able to do at this point? Would you consider cutting your use in half for the next week or so?" The patient handout entitled "10 Tips for Cutting Down on Your Drinking" (Appendix 2) offers specific suggestions for reducing alcohol consumption. Additional resource material to facilitate patients' efforts to reduce or control their drinking is available in other publications that describe moderation techniques in much greater detail (Rotgers et al., 2002; Miller & Muñoz, 2005; Sanchez-Craig, 1993; Sobell & Sobell, 1993).

Strategies with Patients in the Preparation Stage

Patients in the preparation stage are, by definition, receptive to discussing treatment options and to being actively involved in developing a treatment plan that they are ready to implement in the very near future. What works with patients in the preparation stage? Patients in this stage can be actively engaged in discussions about the potential benefits and drawbacks of particular treatment options and what types of change strategies they may want to utilize. The key to success with individuals in the preparation stage is to offer a menu of options and negotiate, but not impose, treatment goals and methods. Patients in this stage often are willing to actively explore various treatment options, to comply with follow-up appointments, and to accept referrals for outside consultations and/or treatment, where indicated. In order to reinforce patients' self-change efforts and their sense of optimism that change is indeed possible, you must be sure to acknowledge and compliment them for making a decision to seek help and for whatever positive changes they have already made on their own, no matter how small these changes may be. For example: "It's a really good sign that you've been able to follow through on your decision and reduce your cocaine use over the last month from 4 days to 2 days per week. Let's talk about possible treatment options that may help you realize your stated goal of taking the next step toward stopping completely."

A critically important task with patients in the preparation stage is to help them explore and then choose a type of treatment that feels right to them. Even if you think that, ideally, the patient would be better off with a different or more intensive level of care than she is willing to accept at this point in time, you can still support the patient's choice as a positive step in the right direction and also express your concerns. In helping patients decide what type of treatment may be best for them, other important considerations include (1) whether the patient is physiologically dependent on any substances (e.g., alcohol, sedatives–hypnotics, opioids) requiring medical detoxification as an inpatient or outpatient and (2) what contributed to the success/failure of previous attempts to achieve/maintain abstinence, including what methods were tried, what led to relapse after periods of abstinence, and what could be done to improve the current chances of success.

Strategies with Patients in the Action Stage

Patients in the action stage have not only committed themselves to a specific plan, but often have already begun to act on this plan by making specific changes in their substance use behavior. They are committed to working toward specific goals (whether abstinence, moderation, or harm reduction) and generally welcome your assistance in helping them define and realize these goals. Your role with these patients may be to provide the primary or only treatment for their alcohol or drug problem (as discussed in greater detail in subsequent chapters of this book) or to provide supportive therapy in conjunction with treatment delivered by other caregivers.

A "Change Plan Worksheet" (Miller, 1999) can help to concretize the action plan:

- *"The changes I want to make are. . . . "* In what ways or areas does the patient want to make a change? Be specific. It is also wise to include goals that are *positive* (wanting to begin, increase, improve, do more of something), and not focus only on negative goals (to stop, avoid, or decrease behaviors).
- *"The most important reasons why I want to make these changes are. . . . "* What are the likely consequences of action and inaction? Which motivations for change seem most impelling to the patient?
- *"The steps I plan to take in changing are. . . . "* How does the patient plan to achieve his goals? How could the desired change be accomplished? Within the general plan and strategies described, what are some specific, concrete first steps the patient can take? When, where, and how will these steps be taken?
- *"The ways other people can help me are. . . . "* In what ways could other people (including significant others, if present) help the patient in taking these steps toward change? How will the patient arrange for such support?
- *"I will know that my plan is working if. . . . "* What does the patient hope will happen as a result of this change plan? What benefits could be expected from this change?

- *"Some things that could interfere with my plan are. . . . "* Help the patient to anticipate situations or changes that could undermine the plan. What could go wrong? How could the patient stick with the plan despite these problems or setbacks?

Strategies with Patients in the Maintenance Stage

Patients in the maintenance stage have already made changes in their substance use behavior and now want help in maintaining these positive changes indefinitely. The primary focus of treatment in this stage is to prevent relapse to the former pattern of substance use and, where appropriate, foster other personal gains as well. Many individuals in the maintenance stage seek help from psychotherapists, hoping to address certain lingering problems that have not been resolved automatically and have either persisted or grown worse in the absence of alcohol and drug use. Strategies for patients in this stage include a variety of cognitive-behavioral therapy techniques designed to help prevent relapse (Chapter 10) as well as other psychotherapeutic interventions designed to address a range of psychological issues in ongoing and later-stage recovery (Chapter 11).

AVAILABILITY AND INVOLVEMENT OF SIGNIFICANT OTHERS

An important consideration in developing a treatment plan and deciding how to proceed with treatment is the availability of significant others and the nature of their investment and involvement in the patient's substance abuse problem and recovery. For example, spouses, parents, adult children, close friends, and others may be available and quite eager to participate in treatment sessions and/or lend support to the patient's efforts to change. Some will need guidance in how best to help their loved one, and in some cases how best to address their own issues. If neither the patient nor significant others see her substance use as a problem, you should provide education and address any tendencies to minimize the problem. It is also possible that significant others have long recognized the problem and are angry, frustrated, discouraged, exhausted, and perhaps traumatized by their experiences in trying to get their loved one to address the problem seriously. In these cases, it is important to offer family members a plan that provides adequate support and an opportunity to work on their own issues. Significant others can be asked how their loved one's substance use affects *their* emotional state, relationship satisfaction, sexuality, financial status, social life, and relationships with others within and outside the family. As part of the groundwork, family members should be asked how they have tried to handle problems and what has worked or not worked. You should consider suggesting their attendance at several Al-Anon and Nar-Anon meetings for peer support from others in similar situations and to help them come to grips with the impact of the patient's addiction on their own well-being. Significant others often need a place to learn about addiction and recovery, express and process their own feelings, and develop healthy ways of coping with their relationship to the primary patient. Although the self-help groups educate significant others over time, it is beneficial to provide them with relatively systematic coverage of issues such as alcohol and drug effects in intoxication and withdrawal, long-term effects, health hazards (particularly related to HIV, hepatitis C, or other transmissible diseases), and common forms of damage to relationships. Such education should describe the process of addiction and how to view the problem as a treatable disorder to help reduce family members' sense of shame and stigma and orient them toward taking constructive action. It should also describe the stages-of-change model and the stages and tasks of recovery, indicating realistic expectations for progress and providing guidelines for appropriate participation. Educational sessions should also address relevant psychiatric disorders and how the symptoms and treatments interact. This is a good time to identify any resistance family members may have to psychotropic medication, clarify misconceptions, and identify potential problems. Family members should be educated about patterns of reciprocal relapse, a process by which a relapse in one area will likely lead to a relapse in another. Discontinuing psychotropic medication is a common precursor of relapse to alcohol and drug use and may be promoted by significant others who want their loved one to be "normal," or who are troubled by some of the medication side effects. Although the patient may function adequately off medication for a while, once anxiety, depression, and other symptoms return, the progression to relapse can be rapid.

In early stages, it may be preferable to postpone confronting the dysfunction of other family members, as this often results in their feeling blamed and they may refuse to participate further. The concept that each family member has his or her own personal issues to address is something that family members often appreciate better once work is underway. Family members are much more quickly engaged if you can provide specific help in an area of pressing need. For example, parents may be struggling with how much financial assistance to provide their adult child who is professing readiness for treatment. They may be frantic about how to interrupt the flow of drug users visiting their daughter who is living in their in-law apartment adjacent to their house. Once you supply practical assistance or relief from a key source of distress, the therapeutic alliance is greatly strengthened and family members are more receptive when you introduce charged issues.

It is very important for you to give a perspective on the time frame needed to build a solid recovery. Family members need to hear from an outsider that an extensive time investment is needed in the early stages. For example, family members frequently resent the time commitment needed to attend self-help meetings regularly, particularly because these often occur during dinner hour for working patients who cannot go at other times. They can be angry and distressed because of the neglect by the addicted family member over the years and anxiously hope for "normal" participation in family-related activities. Some express bitter disappointment; first they lost the person to alcohol and other drug use, and then they lose to recovery-related activities. You can offer a realistic view of the time investment needed for everyone to achieve a satisfying stability in the long run.

As early as possible, you should establish guidelines about the presence of alcohol or other intoxicants in the home. This issue often generates considerable feelings, and you can often identify other family members who likely have a problem by the strength of their objections to removing intoxicants from the home. Although alcohol is legal and readily obtainable, deterrents to impulsive use can make a big difference. For patients struggling with abstinence in early recovery, buying time often allows them to call on their newly acquired skills and build success experiences when they encounter dangers. You can also emphasize that everyone needs a safe place and ask, "If that is not your home, where is it?" It also increases empathy in family members if they accompany the alcohol- or drug-addicted person on the journey by also abstaining from alcohol and other drugs. Many eventually conclude that this is a profoundly symbolic form of support that is not obvious at first glance. Family members who use alcohol or drugs but do not meet the diagnostic criteria for substance dependence will likely notice the loss when they abstain, and they gain a new appreciation of the extent to which alcohol use is embedded in our culture as essential to the good life. In addition, if they abstain, the patient is protected from the behavioral cues and smells of someone else who is drinking or using other drugs. These cues can be triggers even if they are not consciously noticed by the identified patient. Do not get into a power struggle if family members reject this recommendation. It will have great value as a catalyst, even if compliance takes a long time to secure or is never achieved. A clinical stance that promotes exploration is more valuable than struggles over rules.

The balance of engagement and detachment is often an ongoing therapeutic theme. The 12-step-based treatment and self-help system have focused on the overinvolvement of family members and have emphasized the need for the alcohol and drug user to disengage and center on his own needs. Family members are often uneasy about this, as they are conflicted about abandoning their loved one in time of need. Indeed, the treatment outcome literature repeatedly confirms the importance of family and social support in producing positive outcomes. Our task is to shape helping behavior, not to pathologize it. Therapy sessions can explore desirable forms of assistance, examine problematic interactions, and encourage appropriate forms of nurturing.

Family therapy sessions can provide an arena to apply new concepts and knowledge and explore how to make changes. What can be accomplished is closely tied to the primary patient's stage of recovery. Family members need help to work on family issues while supporting the recovery process. For example, it is typical for the primary patient to stop drinking and/or using for several months, to appear to be much better, and for spouses or partners to expect dramatic improvements in the relationship or vigorous atonement for past misdeeds. Significant others want their anger and frustrations to be "heard," often at a time or in a form that your patient cannot tolerate. They need to be reassured that these feelings are understandable but must be expressed selectively and are often best worked on in a separate therapeutic relationship with someone familiar with addiction. It may be most appropriate for significant others to develop a variety of outlets for their negative feelings until the primary patient reaches a stage where these feelings can be constructively addressed.

As the recovery process evolves, the power balance in intimate relationships inevitably shifts. Typically, the addicted person has abdicated important responsibilities while drinking and using, and family members have filled in the gaps. The identified patient, feeling disempowered and resentful, may seek to reclaim adult status in the family. The spouse may be reluctant to relinquish the checkbook; the teens may resent diminished freedoms. Once crises no longer center on drinking and drug use, other family members can more easily be held accountable for their contribution to stress and unhappiness. The change process can be tempestuous, even when everyone believes it is going in positive directions. The intervention of a skilled family therapist experienced in treating couples affected by addiction can go a long way toward helping the family negotiate these transitions adaptively without severe disruption to the relationships.

It is desirable for the office-based practitioner to form affiliations with other professionals who can collaborate effectively in these situations. The more knowledgeable these colleagues are about treating addiction, the more productive the collaboration is likely to be. The therapist of the primary patient may be able to manage couple/family issues if they are relatively circumscribed, but these can quickly become complicated and adversely affect the practitioner's therapeutic relationship with the primary patient. Thus, referral to a trusted colleague who can provide the needed couple and/or family therapy is an important option.

Clearly, family members who have alcohol and drug problems themselves pose an ongoing threat to the patient's attempt to establish and sustain abstinence. You should make every effort, within reason, to encourage them to get help and, at the very least, not to drink or use in the presence of your patient. This can be a thorny issue that may require you to meet with the substance-abusing family members at least several times, but you must avoid becoming the primary therapist for these individuals in order to maintain the integrity of your therapeutic relationship with the primary patient.

FINAL COMMENT

When determining how best to intervene, the patient's own choice of treatment goals and stage of readiness for change are among the most important factors to consider. Different types of clinical interventions are likely to work best with patients in different stages of change. Conversely, interventions that are not properly matched to the patient's stage of change are likely to heighten resistance and reduce treatment effectiveness. Therapists who are able to meet patients where they are on the continuum of change are more likely to engender patient engagement, retention, and good treatment outcomes. Some patients will require treatment services and levels of care that go beyond those that any office-based practitioner can reasonably provide. Accordingly, it is important for you to be familiar with the various types of substance abuse treatment services available to your patients.

CHAPTER 9

Taking Action

This chapter describes specific action stage strategies designed to help patients make positive changes in their substance use behavior. We begin with a brief discussion of moderation and harm reduction techniques for individuals whose initial goal is to reduce rather than stop their substance use and its negative consequences. We follow with a more in-depth discussion of cessation techniques for those individuals who choose abstinence as their initial goal and are committed to discontinuing the use of all psychoactive substances, at least as a starting point. Although cessation techniques are intended primarily for patients who are attempting to stop using all psychoactive substances, these techniques are also applicable to patients working toward the more limited goal of stopping only their primary substance, that is, the one causing them the most trouble.

The cessation techniques described in this chapter emanate not only from our own clinical experience, but also from an extensive literature on the treatment of SUDs that has developed over the past three decades describing a wide range of empirically validated abstinence-based approaches (Carroll, 1998; Gorski & Miller, 1986; Marlatt, 1985; Mercer & Woody, 1999; Rawson, 1999; Washton, 1989; Washton, 1995). Clinical protocols and patient workbooks based on these approaches are available in a variety of publications (Gorski, 1988; Kadden et al., 1995; Rawson, Obert, McCann, Smith, & Scheffy, 1989; Washton, 1990a, 1990b, 1990c; Zackon, McAuliffe, & Ch'ien, 1993).

MODERATION AND HARM REDUCTION TECHNIQUES

Because we are much more familiar and experienced with abstinence-based approaches, our discussion here of moderation and harm reduction techniques is relatively brief and general. These clinical strategies are described in much greater detail elsewhere (Rotgers et al., 2002; Miller & Munoz, 2005; Sanchez-Craig, 1993; Sobell & Sobell, 1993).

An essential feature of controlled drinking strategies for reducing alcohol consumption is to help patients establish and maintain clearly defined drinking limits. Most controlled drinking approaches strongly advise patients to begin with a period of total abstinence of 30 days or longer before attempting moderation, while recognizing that many individuals are simply not willing to start with a trial period of abstinence. At whatever point an individual attempts to reduce rather than stop drinking, evidence suggests that setting specific limits rather than having a general intention to "cut down" is a key element of successful moderation. For patients whose alcohol consumption is significantly above the NIAAA limits for low-risk drinking, described previously in Chapter 2, a reasonable starting point may be to reduce consumption to levels at or significantly below these limits. Successful moderation requires that drinking should be reduced to a level that is neither causing new problems nor exacerbating preexisting ones. In preparation for establishing specific drinking goals, it is important to educate patients that a standard "drink" consists of either a 12-ounce bottle of regular beer (5% alcohol), 5 ounces of wine (12% alcohol), or 1.5 ounces of 80-proof distilled spirits (40% alcohol), all of which contain equivalent amounts of alcohol.

Another moderation technique is to establish certain rules for drinking, such as no drinking in bars or clubs, no drinking within at least 2–3 hours before bedtime (i.e., no "nightcaps"), no drinking on consecutive days, and no drinking when feeling emotionally upset (e.g., depressed, angry, lonely, etc.). Other drinking control techniques include (1) keeping accurate track of both the amount and number of drinks consumed per hour during any episode of drinking; (2) switching to beverages containing a lower concentration of alcohol, such as mixed drinks, lower-alcohol beer, and table wine, instead of straight liquor, fortified wines, or malt liquor, without increasing the overall consumption of the less-concentrated beverages to compensate for the difference; (3) deliberately spacing drinks and sipping more slowly to keep the blood alcohol concentration within predefined limits and, especially, slowing down the first drink or two to set the pace for moderation and avoid inducing rapid intoxication, in which the decision to moderate dissolves almost immediately in the alcohol; (4) eating both before and while drinking to keep the rise in blood alcohol concentration in check; (5) drinking water or soda in between alcoholic beverages to dilute the effects of the alcohol; and (6) avoiding drinking together with others who drink heavily. When patients are unable to adhere to their own rules to reduce or reliably keep their drinking within defined limits, the need for a trial period of abstinence becomes more apparent and the cessation techniques described in the next section may be seen as more helpful than continued attempts at moderation.

For patients attempting to reduce their use of drugs (other than alcohol) and the negative consequences associated with this use, a variety of harm reduction techniques have been described in detail by other authors (Denning 2000; Denning, Little, & Glickman, 2004). These techniques include (1) changing the amount of drug used, (2) changing the numbers and types of drugs used together, (3) changing the frequency of use, (4) changing the route of administration, (5) changing the situation or setting in which the drug use occurs, (6) making drug substitutions, (7) taking overdose prevention measures, and (8) tapering toward abstinence or quitting altogether. Understandably, many clinicians are hesitant to offer these alternatives to patients whose drug use is clearly out of control, but proponents of harm reduction techniques claim that many of these individuals can and do successfully reduce their drug use and its negative consequences. Here, too, a patient's failure to adhere reliably to her own rules about drug use and avoid drug-related harm can help to support there therapist's request for a trial period of total abstinence as a more clinically viable alternative.

CESSATION TECHNIQUES

The therapist's toolbox for helping patients establish abstinence includes a combination of cognitive-behavioral, motivational, supportive, directive, and psychoeducational techniques, all aimed at cessation of alcohol and drug use. Patients require direction and support because in the early stages of coming to grips with an alcohol or drug problem, most have not yet acquired the skills needed to break their pattern of habitual substance use. A basic structure and daily routine is needed to interrupt and replace the repetitive ritual of seeking, using, and recuperating from alcohol or drug use. They need a simple plan to follow on a day-to-day basis—a framework and set of basic guidelines for avoiding alcohol and drug use. Healthy rituals and positive habits must replace destructive ones. The therapist must be both directive and supportive: educating, encouraging, instructing, and advising patients through their initial triumphs and setbacks. A firm but flexible and accepting take-charge posture is called for here; neither a passive analytic stance nor a harshly confrontational or controlling one will work very well. Your role is that of teacher, providing information about addiction and recovery; coach, giving guidance about concrete behavior change strategies that are helpful; and therapist, addressing emotional obstacles to giving up alcohol and drug use.

Once your patient has made a commitment to stop using, it is important for you to provide encouragement and guidance. Those who have been using alcohol and drugs for a very long time especially need your reassurance that the difficulties of the early abstinence period are temporary and that making good use of a recovery support network can help greatly to weather the storm. Many are anxious about the loss of their substances, and some are convinced that life will be intolerable without them. You need to convey a realistic expectation that nothing will work as instantly as alcohol and drugs to obliterate negative feelings, but that other strategies and activities will help, especially as new behaviors and coping skills are acquired and established. If you have reason to think your patient has a co-occurring mental health problem, such as an anxiety or mood disorder, you can prepare him for the possibility that symptoms may initially get worse during the early phases of abstinence, but ultimately it will be possible to intervene more effectively when the confounding effects of alcohol and drug use are eliminated. For example, low energy, depression, and irritability are common complaints in the first few weeks of abstinence whether or not the patient has been physically dependent on any substances. The therapist can instill hope, giving information about how long before certain symptoms will subside and reassuring patients that some benefits of abstinence will become apparent relatively quickly. The individual's prior alcohol and drug use pattern itself often determines how long symptoms will last, but giving patients a range (in days or weeks) provides an element of predictability that can help to counteract the fear that their current unhappiness and discomfort will be endless. You should also watch for positive behaviors and call them to the patients' attention, especially because they may not recognize what they are doing that is working.

STARTING WITH SHORT-TERM GOALS

It is important to start the treatment with a clear statement of mutually agreed upon short-term goals that patients feel are realistic and accomplishable. For example, achieving 1 week (7 consecutive days) of complete abstinence is often a good starting point. This initial short-term goal helps to focus the patient's attention on the day-to-day task of achieving abstinence instead of the seemingly impossible task of not using for months, years, or ever again. Early success in achieving a short-term abstinence goal helps to build positive momentum and a foundation for continued progress. It bolsters feelings of self-efficacy, counteracts defeatist attitudes, and helps to build the therapeutic relationship. For binge users, the initial short-term goal should be a period of abstinence that is at least twice the usual time period between binges. For example, if cocaine binges occur roughly once every 2 weeks, then the first goal would be to remain abstinent for a period of at least 4 weeks. In the course of working toward that goal, the patient is likely to experience increased cravings and urges for cocaine at the 2-week point and will need extra support and more frequent contact to avoid resumption of the binge cycle.

MAINTAINING FREQUENT CONTACT

The importance of maintaining frequent contact with patients in early phase of establishing abstinence cannot be overemphasized. During the first week or two, see your patients as frequently as possible for brief (e.g., 30-minute) individual sessions and maintain telephone or e-mail contact with them between sessions. Frequent contact provides structure, support, accountability, encouragement, and positive reinforcement. During each contact you should review what has transpired since the last contact and offer advice and encouragement for bridging the gap until the next contact.

CLINICAL USE OF URINE DRUG TESTING

Urine testing is an extraordinarily valuable clinical tool that can serve as a key element in providing the much needed structure, support, and behavioral accountability for patients attempting to establish abstinence, especially in the early stages when their commitment to change is often tenuous. Understandably, most nonmedical therapists have no experience with urine testing, are unaccustomed to obtaining urine samples from patients, and may fear that patients will react negatively to it. Adding to these therapists' hesitations is the fact that urine testing is often viewed as a medical procedure that lies outside the scope of what mental health therapists can or should know how to do.

It is important to work past these hesitations and concerns, because urine testing can be very helpful to patients who want to stop using, but are aware of their own ambivalence about doing so and how this can unintentionally sabotage their efforts. Most patients respond positively to the idea of being tested, seeing it as a safety net and additional check against their unpredictable and often uncontainable impulses to use. Agreeing to urine testing is part of openly acknowledging their ambivalence about stopping and recognizing their need to have an external check on their impulses to use. Countless patients over the years have told us how comforted they feel in knowing that urine testing would be a routine component of their treatment, especially those who previously hid their alcohol and drug use from unsuspecting therapists. In this regard, patients who are trying to stop using, despite their ambivalence about giving up alcohol and drugs, tend to devalue and feel unsafe with therapists whom they are able to deceive reliably—a situation that often leads patients to either drop out of treatment or remain unproductively in therapy for long periods of time without ever addressing their substance use. It essential for you to inform patients at the outset of treatment that the purpose of urine testing is not to challenge their honesty or catch them in a lie, but rather to enhance their efforts to achieve their chosen goal to stop using, assuming that they have chosen this goal. Urine testing should be used only with the patient's consent and full cooperation. It should not be used to create a "cat and mouse" dynamic between therapist and patient—a situation that is clearly not helpful.

In addition to enhancing truthfulness and limit setting, urine testing provides an objective marker of clinical progress and positive reinforcement for remaining abstinent. It is quite common for patients to feel a sense of accomplishment when they are able to demonstrate objectively via urine testing that they are remaining drug free. It also helps to keep the focus on the behavioral task of establishing and maintaining abstinence, evidenced most concretely by producing clean urine. Family members also feel comforted when their loved one is being urine tested regularly. It helps to quell their anxiety about whether or not she is using again and relieves them of the onerous task of being hypervigilant for any signs of substance use. Keep in mind that even experienced addiction treatment specialists, including those in recovery themselves, often cannot detect subtle signs of a patient's alcohol and drug use.

When utilizing urine testing as a clinical tool, it is essential that you discuss with patients what will happen if they test positive for drugs on one or more occasions. Most assume that you will terminate them from treatment for test results unless you say otherwise. It is essential to emphasize that positive test results or self-reported instances of use will not be dealt with punitively. Your goal is to help them identify what led up to the use and how to prevent it from happening again. Some patients learn from relapses and demonstrate a willingness to adjust their behavior in order to reduce the likelihood of further drug use. Others remain highly ambivalent about giving up their substance use and are reluctant to make the changes necessary to support abstinence. If a patient's inability to establish and maintain abstinence reveals that he does not want or simply is not ready to take that step, despite having made an initial commitment to do so, it is important address this issue and make the necessary adjustments in treatment goals and/or methods. This may involve scheduling more frequent visits, encouraging the patient to become more involved in a self-help program, and possibly involving significant others who can lend support. In some cases, it may mean switching, at least temporarily, from abstinence to reduced use or harm reduction as a treatment goal.

There is an important caveat to keep in mind about the drug screening you do in your office: it must be used only for clinical purposes and never to impose external consequences on your patients. For example, if an external agent (e.g., employer, judicial system, regulatory agency) wants to use the results of these tests in order to impose certain consequences (e.g., job termination, incarceration, loss of professional license) on your patient, you should categorically refuse to make the test results available to them. This is not to say that such consequences are always unjustified, but as a treating clinician you should not be party to such an arrangement. You cannot be both therapist and executioner at the same time. If external agencies want to impose consequences based on a patient's drug screening results, they should arrange for testing of the patient that is not connected with the treatment you provide.

Urine testing should be discussed at the very beginning of treatment when negotiating an initial treatment plan with patients who have elected abstinence as a treatment goal. It should be presented as a therapeutic tool and not as a police tactic. If you present drug screening as a normal part of an abstinence-oriented treatment process, rather than as a confrontation of the patient's denial and motivation, most patients are able to see the benefits in being tested and accept it quite readily. However, if you come across as apologetic, hesitant, or mistrustful of patients, they may balk at the idea. If you approach drug screening in a matter-of-fact manner as a standard procedure for your patients who are striving for abstinence, you are more likely to enlist their cooperation. It can be helpful to have a written policy about urine testing for new patients, stating the purpose of the testing, how it will be conducted, the cost, and its potential therapeutic benefits.

A number of logistical considerations are involved in implementing urine testing in an office-based practice. Using on-site urine testing kits has many advantages and offers the most viable option. These kits provide instant results and incorporate certain safeguards against falsification. Whereas laboratory-based drug testing requires physician authorization (prescription), on-site urine testing kits are readily accessible to nonmedical clinicians. On-site, as compared with laboratory-based, testing has the added advantage of providing immediate results while the patient is still in your office. Most laboratories do not provide results for several days or more after the sample is received. The easiest way to find suppliers of on-site drug testing kits is by doing an Internet search for "drug testing kits" or "urine drug tests." This usually generates an extensive list of relevant websites and suppliers. Available kits vary widely in terms of accuracy and price, as well as the number and types of drugs that the test can detect. Some suppliers give the purchaser the option of customizing the testing kit in terms of the number and types of drugs included in the test panel. Most kits contain a standard panel of five drug classes known as the "NIDA-5," a standard test panel defined by the National Institute on Drug Abuse (NIDA) that tests for amphetamines, cocaine, benzodiazepines, opioids, phencyclidine (PCP), and cannabinoids (THC). As of this writing, NIDA-5 test kits range in price from $10 to $20 each. It is best to limit your choice to kits that are self-contained so that you do not have to handle the urine specimen. Self-contained kits come with reagent strips already attached to the inside of the specimen jar or to the underside of the specimen cap. Once the patient voids the urine sample into the jar and tightens the cap, the reagent strips become immersed in the urine and results appear within a few minutes, typically in the form of certain color changes on the reagent strips. Also look for kits that contain a temperature strip and other indicators of sample adulteration. These are important because they provide at least some degree of assurance that the sample is valid without having to directly observe the patient voiding urine into the sample cup—a task that most patients and therapists would find unacceptable and is forbidden in cases where patient and therapist are not the same gender.

Urine testing should be done twice weekly (Mondays and Thursdays are ideal) wherever possible so as not to exceed the sensitivity levels of most tests, especially for rapidly metabolized drugs such as cocaine. When regular testing is not practical, testing on a random unannounced basis may be a viable option. You should be aware of the limitations of urine testing. No test is 100% accurate or foolproof. Despite its potential limitations, however, urine testing remains one of the most reliable ways to detect recent drug use. All urine tests have established cutoff levels for detecting each type of drug. This means that both false positive as well as false negative results are possible with any test. For example, false positives for amphetamines can be produced by certain diet supplements and over-the-counter medications. Ingesting poppy seeds can produce false positives for opioids. False negatives can result when the drug concentration in the urine falls below the limits of detection. Urine screening will detect most drugs used within the past 2 or 3 days, but this varies greatly according to the type and amount of drug that is used as well as physiological differences between individuals in rates of drug metabolism. In general, short-acting rapidly metabolized drugs such as cocaine, amphetamines, heroin, and certain benzodiazepines (e.g., alprazolam—Xanax) can be detected with reasonable accuracy within only 48–72 hours or so after last use. Marijuana, however, is metabolized very slowly and may be detectable for as long as 1–6 weeks after last use, depending on the frequency and chronicity of use. Alcohol leaves the body very quickly, and thus urine screening for alcohol generally is not very effective. Instead, breathalyzers and saliva test strips are often used to detect recent alcohol use or legal intoxication, but here too the limits of reliable detection rarely extend beyond a few hours after the last drink.

False negatives can also result from deliberate attempts to nullify the accuracy of a test, including (1) drinking large quantities of fluids for several hours before giving the urine sample or by adding tap water to the specimen jar in an effort to dilute the concentration of drugs in the urine to levels below the sensitivity limits of the test; (2) drinking certain types of acidic beverages that alter urinary pH in ways that invalidate the test; (3) ingesting certain types of herbal, over-the-counter, or other urine adulteration products available on the Internet and elsewhere that can produce negative urine test results despite recent drug use; and (4) submitting a specimen of previously voided urine presumed to be free of drugs or submitting someone else's urine that is expected to yield negative test results. Fortunately, there are a number of ways to detect falsification of urine samples, although none of these methods is entirely foolproof. Temperature strips indicating whether the urine sample is at or near normal body temperature can detect dilution of the sample with tap water or attempts to submit previously voided urine. Otherwise, direct observation of urination is needed to prevent this problem—a procedure that is impractical and unacceptable (and perhaps countertherapeutic) for therapists and patients alike. Dilution resulting from preemptive ingestion of a large volume of fluids can be detected by measuring the specific gravity of the urine. Attempts to acidify the urine can be detected by measuring urinary pH.

MANAGING WITHDRAWAL

Assisting the patient to become abstinent requires working collaboratively with physicians when medical detoxification is indicated. Medical management is advisable, and in some cases essential, to safely manage the withdrawal syndrome associated with certain types of drugs. Withdrawal from alcohol or other depressants (sedative–hypnotic drugs) such as barbiturates, or anxiolytics such as benzodiazepines (Valium, Ativan, etc.), can be extremely dangerous if not managed properly with medication. Although many patients can and do withdraw from alcohol safely without medical assistance, we recommend that you consult with an addiction medicine physician who can make that determination. Medication certainly makes alcohol withdrawal more comfortable, and it may be essential to avoid seizures and other life-threatening complications. Withdrawal from opioids (narcotics) may be uncomfortable, but does not in itself pose life-threatening dangers. Opioid withdrawal can be highly unpleasant and stressful, and the patient can be made considerably more comfortable with appropriate medication. When withdrawal symptoms are not properly managed, patients are far more likely to seek relief by medicating themselves. It is important to keep in mind that other than medical considerations, there is no long-term benefit to managing withdrawal unless clinicians take the opportunity to engage the patient in ongoing treatment. Nontraditional and expensive detoxification methods (e.g., ultra-rapid opioid detoxification under general anesthesia) may pose more danger than benefit and have not been demonstrated to be superior to more commonly used methods that are safer and less costly. In the relatively uncommon situation of a patient who is severely debilitated owing to other medical conditions, such as severe heart or liver disease, medically managed opioid withdrawal may be imperative. In this case, it is not the drug withdrawal itself, but the coexisting medical conditions that pose a threat to the patient's health and well-being.

Therapists should identify addiction medicine physicians in their communities who can provide screening, monitoring, and medical management of withdrawal, when needed. Physicians board certified in addiction medicine can be located through the American Society of Addiction Medicine (ASAM; www.asam.org).

The therapist's role during the withdrawal process is to provide patients with encouragement, structure, and support. You can do a great deal to enhance patients' compliance with prescribed medication regimens, their ability to cope with withdrawal discomfort, and their resolve to stay the course. To be maximally effective in supporting patients through withdrawal, you should be familiar with the characteristic withdrawal syndromes associated with the different types of drugs and with the medications most commonly used to manage these syndromes. Psychosocial interventions during detoxification should be kept simple, aimed at preparing the patient for the next set of treatment activities and directing them to appropriate services.

ESTABLISHING STRUCTURE AND EXTERNAL CONTROLS

Structure is an essential element in establishing abstinence. Unplanned and unstructured time breeds both boredom and fantasies about using to relieve the boredom and fill up the time. At the most basic level, structuring time involves working out a schedule that serves to avert and contain impulses to drink and use. People in early recovery typically have problems in organizing their time, even if they are otherwise good at doing so. This time structure should include treatment activities, self-help meetings, exercise sessions, school, work, community activities, and anything else that may be helpful in restoring healthy functioning. It provides a contrast to the more unproductive or chaotic lifestyle associated with active addiction. The concept of "one day at a time" provides a manageable unit that patients generally perceive as more achievable.

Especially during the first few days of abstinence, you should help patients construct a written 24-hour time plan for each day. Doing so is particularly important when 2 or more days will elapse before the next session, as well as just prior to weekends and holidays. The plan should specify not only the activities that will occupy the person's time during each block of hours, but also where these activities will take place and with whom. Specifying these details is important because patients often do not recognize the dangers inherent in certain types of situations (see the section "Managing Triggers") that have the potential to lead them quite easily back to alcohol and drug use. Sometimes these details reveal a pattern of workaholism or simply taking on too much without sufficient time set aside for rest and recreation. If appropriate measures are not taken to interrupt this pattern, it too can set the stage for returning to alcohol and drug use, as many people with addiction histories often turn to mood-altering substances as a way to relieve stress instantaneously and "nurture" themselves.

Certain external controls can be put in place temporarily, with the patient's cooperation, as stopgaps or barriers to alcohol and drug use. These strategies usually require the participation of significant others. For example, limiting the person's access to cash can be an effective short-term deterrent to impulsive use. This may involve relinquishing ATM cards, credit cards, and check books and perhaps temporarily turning over complete control of financial affairs to a trusted family member or friend. Because payday can be a powerful relapse trigger, a person's handing over her paycheck immediately to a significant other or depositing it directly in her bank account can be a helpful short-term strategy. In general, and wherever possible, patients struggling to establish abstinence should avoid having direct access to substantial amounts of cash.

DEVELOPING A RECOVERY SUPPORT SYSTEM

The challenging task of giving up alcohol and drugs, especially after substance use has become a routine part of life, often requires a great deal of support and encouragement from others to accomplish successfully. Trying to do it alone can be emotionally and physically exhausting and often diminishes the chances of success. Accordingly, it is important not only to encourage your patients to make use of self-help programs (see Chapter 13), which provide the most focused and widely available support system for people dealing with alcohol and drug problems, but also that you help them identify those among their family members, friends, and concerned others whom they might enlist to be part of their recovery support system. Certainly, any among these people who are in recovery will intuitively understand the patient's plight and be eager to help. Family members and concerned others who are not familiar with recovery and may not know how to help but sincerely want to, may benefit from the education and guidance you can provide. This is best accomplished in joint meetings involving your patient together with whomever he has chosen to be potential members of the support network. Concerned others need to know the basic do's and don'ts of helping someone to get clean and sober (Rogers & McMillan, 1989; Washton, 1989; Washton & Boundy, 1989). For example, perhaps the most important role that concerned others can play in fostering the patient's efforts to stop using alcohol and drugs is to be empathetic, supportive, and available when the patient feels a need to make contact, to avoid being alone, or to talk through urges, cravings, or other disquieting thoughts and feelings to someone with a sympathetic ear. However, concerned others must be helped to relinquish any fantasies or hopes that they can stop the patient from using again, especially if she is intent on using. The only help from concerned others that works is help that is requested and welcomed by the patient. It is also essential to educate concerned others about the importance of refraining from enabling and provoking behaviors that unintentionally increase rather than decrease the likelihood of further use (Washton, 1989).

MANAGING TRIGGERS

The process of becoming addicted to psychoactive substances creates the ability for a wide variety of conditioned stimuli or "triggers" to set off drug cravings and drug-seeking behavior. Most of these triggers involve people, places, things, circumstances, and emotional states associated with prior alcohol and drug use. For example, the mere sight of drug dealers, other users, drug paraphernalia, cash, photographs or video images of drug-using situations, or a liquor store, bar, or nightclub can elicit strong physiological reactions, including cravings and urges to use alcohol and drugs. A particular part of town, a particular street, or a particular building where the addicted person previously obtained and/or used drugs can elicit overwhelming urges to use again. The sight of a highway exit sign leading to the location where drugs were purchased can send an addicted person's car on "automatic pilot" back to that spot.

Negative affect states such as feeling depressed, bored, stressed, emotionally exhausted, anxious, angry, or frustrated also can be powerful triggers for alcohol and drug use, largely because these substances have worked so well in the past to remove negative feelings and moods instantaneously. Alcohol and drugs are so tempting in the face of negative feeling states because they replace the empty void of boredom with instant euphoria and relieve feelings of anxiety and helplessness (Kaufman, 1994).

Positive feelings can also jeopardize efforts to remain abstinent. Wanting to celebrate an accomplishment or another joyous occasion and feeling like taking a well-deserved break from the rigors of daily life are often overlooked as triggers for substance use. In addition, certain memories, anniversaries, holidays, sensations, and experiences can be triggers for alcohol and drug use. For example, cravings can be set off by certain songs on the radio associated with prior drug use. A birthday, a significant anniversary (e.g., the death of a loved one or the breakup of a relationship), or a holiday associated with "partying" can all set off the desire to use. For patients whose prior drug use was associated with sex, feeling sexually aroused can lead to overwhelming urges and cravings to use again. This is particularly true for patients whose use of stimulant drugs (cocaine or methamphetamine) is powerfully linked with sex (Rawson, Washton, Domier, & Reiber, 2002; Rawson & Washton, 1998; Washton, 1989)

Other relapse triggers include having a lot of cash on hand, engaging in other addictive behaviors such as gambling, the use of drugs other than the person's drug of choice, and hearing "war stories" that glorify the "good times" on drugs. Physical illness, pain, and fatigue can also serve as triggers for drug use, particularly for individuals who preferred the activating and pain relieving effects of certain types of drugs (e.g., stimulants, opioids). In short, unless appropriate preventive measures are taken, no matter how motivated individuals may be to remain abstinent in the early stages, premature exposure to powerful conditioned cues and other high-risk situations can pull them rapidly back into using.

The Inventory of "Triggers" for Alcohol and Drug Use (Appendix 3) can help patients identify potential hazards to establishing and maintaining abstinence. However, it is not enough to merely identify these hazards, although it is a crucial first step. To establish and maintain abstinence, patients need your help in developing a specific action plan to avoid relapse-risky situations whenever possible and to cope effectively with those that are truly unavoidable or appear suddenly without warning. It is essential to review with patients both actual and potential triggering situations that might occur and what can be done to avoid or cope with them. Advance planning and rehearsal are the keys to dealing with risky situations successfully. Individuals who want to stop using must do anything and everything possible (within reason) to avoid triggers, risky situations, reminders, and sources of access to drugs.

Avoidance strategies include removing alcohol from the home, staying out of bars, getting rid of drugs and paraphernalia, avoiding contact with drinking and drug-using friends, and breaking off contact with dealers (Washton, 1989, 1990a, 1990b, 1990c). When contact with high-risk situations is inevitable, such as at weddings or other celebrations, you can work with your patient to identify strategies to reduce the risks. You can use a "risk meter" to help the patient communicate his subjective level of risk on a scale of 1 to 10, and ask for ways to bring the risk level down. Your patient can generate the strategies, with you adding suggestions if he runs out of ideas.

> Marie was newly sober and dreaded the upcoming family wedding. She rated it at a risk level of 8. When asked how she might reduce the risk, she indicated she could speak to her relatives and ask that nonalcoholic alternatives be available. She would also ask her husband, a close cousin of the groom, to run interference if the social pressure to drink became intense. This brought her risk level down to 5. Asked to lower it still more, she and her husband agreed that if the situation became too difficult, she would signal and they would leave as unobtrusively as possible.

You can also role-play alcohol and drug refusal skills in a therapy session. Although discussing strategies is helpful, role plays give the opportunity to master a situation through rehearsal and then polish the strategy. For example, many patients adopt an apologetic tone when refusing a glass of wine or feel compelled to give elaborate explanations. In the role of coach, you can help your patient practice a neutral tone and experiment with simple statements such as "No thank you." These role plays may surface larger issues, such as needing to conform in order to belong or fearing the displeasure of others. Although early recovery is not the time to probe deeply into anxiety-provoking areas, you can flag these issues and frame the situation as an opportunity to experiment with new behavior patterns, monitoring how this feels. You can ask your patient to enact her preferred way of dealing with the situation as a person who is calm and confident. "Act as if you were the person you aspire to be" is a venerable drug treatment concept, referring to the fact that there is benefit in practicing new behaviors until they become comfortable and internalized.

It is a mistake to assume that your patient does not need explicit focus on these skill areas just because he is highly intelligent and perhaps high functioning in a professional situation. In the case of substance use, the correlation between intelligence and common sense can be tenuous, if not imperceptible, in early recovery, and you can assist the patient to make a plan to address challenging situations. High-functioning patients may dismiss these discussions as mundane and then succumb to the hazards of an ordinary situation:

> Dr. S. had agreed to a trial period of abstinence after colleagues expressed concern about his midday drinking and made it clear they were considering reporting him to the medical board. He and his wife hosted a lavish dinner party, and several guests brought bottles of fine wine. He was chagrined when offered a glass and could think of no

way to refuse that did not involve confessing he might be alcoholic and was now trying to stop drinking.

This type of dilemma can be anticipated and preferably addressed prior to the occurrence of a high-risk situation. Proactive behavioral planning reduces "accidental" use and gives your patient confidence about achieving success.

DEALING WITH CRAVINGS AND URGES

Patients attempting to establish abstinence should be educated about cravings and how to deal with them in order to prevent an impulsive return to alcohol and drug use. Although cravings are usually triggered by conditioned cues such as those discussed earlier, sometimes they seem to occur spontaneously or "out of the blue" with no apparent provocation. Cravings can be brought on by events and circumstances that are not always obvious, including subtle changes in mood, having unstructured time, feeling fatigued or sexually aroused, daydreaming about the "good times" on alcohol and drugs, or anticipating future situations in which drugs might be available. Regardless of what stimulates cravings, patients must be prepared to deal with them whenever and wherever they might occur.

Facts about Cravings

Conveying to patients the following points about cravings can be helpful (Washton, 1989, 1990a; Washton & Stone-Washton, 1990; Zackon et al., 1993):

1. Cravings are a natural outgrowth and predictable result of chronic substance use that are thought to be caused by drug-induced changes in brain activity. Cravings are not a sign of poor motivation or that treatment is ineffective. Cravings often continue to occur, albeit less frequently, long after the drug use has stopped.

2. Cravings, no matter how strong, do not have to lead to drug use. It is a grave mistake to think that the intensity of cravings always builds to a point where drug use becomes inevitable. Cravings are like waves: they build to a peak, stay there for a short time, and then drop off. Patients should be encouraged to "surf the craving" or "ride it out" until it passes. Detaching from the craving and looking at it from the vantage point of an outside observer can also help to deflate its power.

3. Cravings tend to be strongest and occur most frequently during the first few days and weeks after stopping the drug use. Thus, it is essential to

address the issue of cravings immediately, as soon as your patient begins the task of establishing abstinence.

4. Cravings tend to diminish in frequency and intensity over time, but only while a person remains abstinent. Cravings lose some of their power through the process of extinction each time they are not followed (reinforced) by drug use. Any instance of cravings followed by drug use will rekindle cravings. Thus, complete abstinence from all psychoactive substances is the most reliable way to facilitate the extinction of cravings. Deliberate exposure to drug triggers in the hope of speeding up the extinction process is a dangerous tactic that is likely to provoke strong cravings and initiate further drug use.

Tips for Handling Cravings

Offering patients the following tips for handling cravings can also be helpful (Washton, 1990a; Washton & Stone-Washton, 1990; Zackon et al., 1993):

1. *Think beyond the high, play the tape to the end.* Cravings are almost always associated with thoughts about the euphoric effects of drugs to the exclusion of the negative effects, such as those that brought the person into treatment—a phenomenon known as "euphoric recall" or "idealizing the high." In order to counteract euphoric recall and short-circuit cravings, patients should be encouraged to think beyond the high, recall the negative aftereffects of drug use, and "play the tape" to the end as a reality check about the adverse consequences of use and the fact that they are no longer to able to experience the "good" effects of the drugs without also experiencing the bad effects.

2. *Leave the situation and engage in alternative activities.* Sometimes the only way for a person to stop cravings is to physically leave whatever situation she is in at the time and do something else, even if that situation does not appear at first to be the cause of the cravings. Alternative safe activities may include talking a walk, engaging in physical exercise, or visiting a trusted relative or friend.

3. *Use thought-stopping techniques.* It is important for your patient to stop the craving when it first occurs, to prevent it from building into an overpowering compulsion. Effective thought stopping often involves changing visual cues and focusing attention outward, not inward. Thus, leaving the room, performing exercise, or turning on music (not associated with alcohol or drug use) while changing activities are examples of such techniques.

4. *Reach out for help.* The patient can contact someone in his support system as soon as possible when cravings first start to appear. This is one of the best ways to contain cravings and prevent them from initiating drug-seeking behavior. Talking out cravings with a supportive person on

the telephone, face-to-face, or by e-mail is almost always helpful. The worst strategy for dealing with cravings is to ignore them or minimize their power.

5. *Detach from the cravings and delay any intention or decision to use.* Another way to short-circuit cravings is to pull back and try to look at them from the vantage point of an outside observer. This strategy can be coupled with postponing any intention to use for 5–10 minutes at a time or until the cravings have peaked and then receded. Remind your patients that cravings are always temporary and usually pass within 20–30 minutes or less. Relaxation exercises and other stress reduction techniques may also be helpful.

ADDRESSING THE USE OF OTHER SUBSTANCES

Patients' reluctance to at least temporarily give up substances other than those that have caused them the most serious problems can, in some cases, severely hamper their efforts to establish abstinence from their substances of choice. Secondary drugs of abuse are frequently involved in a relapse to a person's primary substance or may evolve into problems themselves. Being under the influence of any intoxicant can impair a person's ability to resist the temptation to use her primary drug, and in some cases can directly trigger cravings for the primary drug. For example, because cocaine users often drink alcohol before, during, and after episodes of cocaine use, alcohol becomes a trigger that can elicit cravings for cocaine, even long after they have stopped using cocaine. For many patients, giving up alcohol is one of the most important keys to giving up cocaine. Labeling a patient as "alcoholic" in order to justify recommending abstinence from alcohol is virtually guaranteed to elicit resistance. It is simply not real to the patient. Instead, you can talk about alcohol-induced changes in the brain that increase vulnerability to relapse to stimulants. Thus, you can inform the patient that your recommendation is pragmatic; all intoxicants must be eliminated to maximize chances of success. There is certainly nothing magical about this piece of education and recommendation; patients will almost certainly test it out for themselves. However, informing your patients about the potential hazards of secondary substance use provides the foundation for dealing with resistance when it appears down the road.

The following is a list of 10 reasons (adapted from Washton, 1990b) why total abstinence from all substances is the safest strategy.

1. Using other drugs can stimulate your desire and cravings to use your drug of choice.

2. Using other drugs can act as a "permission giver" by reducing your ability to resist temptation and impulses to use your drug of choice.

3. Using other drugs can lead to irresponsible and inappropriate behaviors.

4. Using other drugs can become more appealing in the absence of your primary drug and can develop into a substitute addiction.

5. Using other drugs can thwart the development of non-drug-coping and problem-solving skills.

6. Using other drugs can prevent learning how to have fun and enjoy life without resorting to chemical mood alteration.

7. Using other drugs often keeps you in contact with people, places, and high-risk situations that trigger cravings for your primary drug.

8. Using other drugs can impair your judgment and decision-making skills.

9. Using other drugs can cause health and behavior problems of their own.

10. Using other drugs can prevent you from forming relationships with potentially supportive people who are committed to abstinence.

PROVIDING PSYCHOEDUCATION

Providing information about addiction and recovery is an important part of therapeutic work. Explaining the nature of the addiction process, particularly how alcohol and other drugs affect the brain, gives a framework to help your patient get beyond confusion, shame, and guilt and accept the behavioral changes needed to become abstinent. It also offers hope to family members and provides a rationale for their efforts to provide more constructive assistance. It is important to avoid giving long monologues, but to introduce information in brief segments, keeping in mind that repetition is important in early recovery. You can encourage your patient to read, access materials on informative websites, and view films in addition to hearing the information you provide during the sessions. As with any therapeutic intervention, timing is important, and you should be sure you are focusing on the most relevant issues as you proceed. Sometimes therapists become so involved in providing information on how to quit using that they fail to recognize the patient's ambivalence about giving up alcohol and drugs.

Psychoeducation should also include information about any relevant co-occurring psychiatric disorders. This includes the nature of the disorder, its usual course, and prognosis with proper treatment. You should review influential factors, such as the importance of genetic heritage, traumatic and other stressors, and benign or unfavorable environments affecting outcome. Patients with stabilized psychiatric conditions should be assisted in recognizing the early warning signs of a recurrence and knowing how to maximize their recovery potential. It is particularly important to address misconceptions about and resistances to psychotropic medication. Patients in early or later recovery may have a keen sensitivity to the idea of using a pill to feel better, and they may have difficulty separating this from their use of alcohol and drugs to change their feeling states. They often think that it is more noble to avoid the use of medications, as they feel it detracts from their achievements. These and other resistances may have to be explored over a considerable period of time. Good teamwork with the prescribing physician is essential, which includes coaching the patient about how to work well with her physician. The patient may need to be reminded that mounting evidence and clinical consensus indicates that appropriate treatment of co-occurring conditions improves the chances of recovery from addiction.

DEALING WITH POST-ACUTE WITHDRAWAL

Individuals who have used large amounts of alcohol and other drugs over long periods of time are especially prone to experiencing disruption in mood, affect, and memory that may linger for weeks or months after establishing abstinence. This phenomenon has been labeled the post-acute withdrawal syndrome, or PAWS (Gawin & Kleber, 1986; Gorski & Miller, 1986). The most common symptoms of PAWS are labile and depressed moods, anhedonia, irritability, short temper, low energy, sleep disturbances, short attention span, distractibility, and memory deficits. It is easy to see how PAWS can create serious diagnostic problems, inasmuch as these symptoms overlap with many psychiatric disorders. If symptoms are due to PAWS, psychotropic medication is not likely to provide much relief. It is important to educate patients about PAWS so that they do not become demoralized by continuing to feel bad despite working hard on abstaining from alcohol and drugs. Otherwise, they may be inclined to return to drug use out of a sense of extreme frustration and in the hope of alleviating the lingering symptoms. Returning to drug use, however, often makes the PAWS symptoms worse, not better.

ADDRESSING DRUG-RELATED SEXUAL BEHAVIORS

The use of cocaine and methamphetamine, in particular, and sometimes alcohol (Rawson et al., 2002; Washton, 1989), is associated with various types of sexual acting-out behaviors, as discussed previously in Chapter 3. If cravings for cocaine, for example, are triggered by sex, you should encourage patients trying to establish abstinence to avoid or interrupt sexual stimuli that trigger these cravings. For example, Scott regularly sought out anonymous sex partners in the midst of weekend cocaine binges. Sexual arousal became associated with his drug use, and "ordinary" sex paled in comparison. He learned that sexual stimuli inevitably elicited strong drug cravings, and in order to avoid using, he needed to interrupt his sexual fantasies promptly and categorically avoid both people and places associated with sex and drugs.

Some patients may need a temporary "cooling off" period (e.g., 30 days), during which they refrain entirely from sex in order to diminish the power of the sex–drug connection. Subsequently, you can help them differentiate between sexual behaviors that are compulsive and potentially life damaging and those that are healthy and self-affirming. For many if not most of these patients, recurrent fantasies about drug-related sexual escapades fade over time as they continue to remain abstinent from drugs. Those who experience persistent preoccupation and obsession with sex despite drug abstinence, particularly those with pre-drug histories of sexual compulsivity/addiction, often require targeted treatment interventions for these sexual issues as part of an overall recovery plan (Carnes, 1991; Earle & Crow, 1989).

DEALING WITH DRUG DREAMS

Nearly every addicted person who establishing abstinence will at some point have dreams about using. These dreams are usually quite vivid and often generate a great deal of anxiety and distress when they occur. People wake up from drug dreams uncertain at first about whether they actually used or not, and often they may remain unsettled about this for several hours into the day. In addition, they frequently feel that a dream is prophetic, an indication that returning to alcohol or drug use is imminent and unavoidable. It is important to allay such fears and offer constructive alternatives. You should inform patients that although drug dreams are not predictive of relapse, they often do contain valuable information about potential areas of vulnerability and hidden fears. Drug dreams frequently contain clues to vulnerabilities that can seriously undermine recovery efforts. Thus, it is important to help patients examine the content and symbolism in a dream that could help to reduce their risk, rather than leave them adrift in uncomfortable feelings. Drug dreams often are triggered by events outside or on the periphery of the patient's awareness, and it is important to "do the detective work" to identify such triggers clearly so that cognitive-behavioral strategies can be applied. This is an example of how focused, insight-oriented work is useful in formulating an effective behavioral strategy. Often, patients can readily identify internal and external triggers, given appropriate therapeutic inquiry. It can be useful to ask your patient in the early abstinence phase to examine a dream from the perspective of discovering a message about where his support system needs strengthening. This approach is different from an open-ended exploration of dreams and certainly does not address the richness of dream content. Dreams in the later stages of recovery may have much broader meanings and can be explored in greater depth (Flowers & Zweben, 1996, 1998).

ADDRESSING PSYCHODYNAMIC ISSUES ARISING IN EARLY TREATMENT

Although early treatment intervention focuses primarily on changing substance use behavior, psychodynamic issues inevitably arise and, where appropriate, they need to be addressed. Powerful transferences and countertransferences often are evoked during the early phase of treatment and require a high level of therapist awareness (Kaufman, 1994). It is important to attend to these phenomena not only to prevent patients from dropping out prematurely and re-engaging in self-destructive behaviors, but also to prevent therapists from engaging in unhelpful enabling and provoking behaviors. Among the most important issues are recognizing and addressing the patient's ongoing ambivalence about stopping or reducing her alcohol and drug use and the related issue of whether the therapist is more invested than the patient in the treatment outcome. Most patients disavow and unconsciously suppress their ambivalence about changing their substance use, often because of fear that anything short of an unwavering, ironclad commitment to maintaining abstinence will guarantee failure. This stance often causes them to minimize or ignore the power of their addiction and put themselves in harm's way unnecessarily. For example, they may not accept the need to diligently avoid triggers and high-risk situations, feeling that their willpower and strong determination to remain abstinent will get them through. Moreover, they may be hesitant to let the therapist know that they are feeling vulnerable to using again, wanting to be seen as model patients highly motivated to succeed.

In addition to disavowed or unrecognized ambivalence, many patients have strong transferential responses to the therapist (and other authority figures) leading to various "people pleasing" and other approval-seeking behaviors at great expense to themselves. Some patients drop out of treatment prematurely because they cannot tolerate the idea of disappointing the therapist. To proactively prevent this dynamic from playing out, the therapist must normalize the patient's ambivalence by stating from the outset that feeling unsure or being "of two minds" about giving up alcohol and drugs is not only expectable, but the norm. Often the most important step in dealing with ambivalence is acknowledging that it exists. Putting the patient's ambivalence "on the table" can be very helpful in preventing it from being acted out destructively. Related issues warranting attention are patients' fear of failure and the need to be perfect.

Therapists must also be on guard for the types of countertransference reactions frequently evoked during early phases of treatment. These include enabling behaviors, such as overlooking clear signs that a patient is highly ambivalent about changing his substance use and becoming frustrated with patients who do not follow recommendations, which may cause the therapist to label these patients as "unmotivated." This can lead to taking an unnecessarily confrontational, aggressive stance that alienates patients who are floundering and drives them out of treatment, thus fulfilling what is often an unconscious wish to be rid of patients who elicit feelings of impotence and ineffectiveness in the therapist. Because patients with alcohol and drug problems are often more ambivalent about change and often more prone to acting out this ambivalence than many other types of patients who seek help from mental health practitioners, you must be especially aware of your potential for acting out destructive countertransference reactions and, where indicated, seek peer support and/or professional supervision to help manage these dynamics therapeutically.

FINAL COMMENT

We have described in this chapter a variety of specific strategies to help patients change their substance use behavior, whether their goal is to reduce or completely stop using alcohol and other drugs. The clinician's role in this early treatment phase has been described as that of teacher, providing information about addiction and recovery; coach, giving guidance about specific strategies that are helpful; and psychotherapist, addressing emotional obstacles to changing behavior. This chapter also touched on several psychodynamic issues that arise during this phase, including transference and countertransference issues that need to be recognized and addressed. The next phase of treatment focuses on maintaining abstinence and counteracting the gravitational pull toward relapse, the topic of the next chapter.

CHAPTER 10

Preventing Relapse

"It's easy to stop smoking—I've done it hundreds of times." When Mark Twain made this humorous remark, he was referring to the problem of relapse as applied to his own nicotine addiction. In this one simple statement he described a major dilemma encountered by people trying to overcome addictions—specifically, that stopping an addiction in the short term is relatively easy and not nearly as difficult as keeping it stopped over the long term. In other words, quitting may be fairly easy, but staying quit tends to be a more formidable challenge. Many addicted individuals are able to stop for a few days, weeks, or months (sometimes even years), but many if not most fall back into using again despite their best intentions to quit for good. This experience is so common among addicted persons that it is safe to say that one of the most distinguishing features of an addiction—whether to drugs or something else—is the proclivity for relapse, especially during the weeks and months immediately following cessation of use.

This phenomenon was demonstrated quite dramatically in a study comparing relapse rates in cigarette smokers, alcoholics, and heroin addicts. Hunt, Barnett, and Branch (1971) found that relapse rates, based on the numbers of subjects who returned to using their substance of choice during successive weeks after quitting, were nearly identical to one another. This study suggests that the relapse dynamic cuts across different substances of abuse and may be a fundamental aspect of all addictive behaviors.

Marlatt and Gordon (1985) proposed a cognitive-behavioral theory of relapse and formulated a set of specific relapse prevention (RP) strategies and interventions designed specifically to prevent a resumption of addictive behaviors. High relapse rates have long been the nemesis of attempts to treat alcohol and drug dependencies. But prior to the appearance of Marlatt's work, relapse and its prevention had not been given much attention in addiction treatment programs. This can be attributed partly to clinicians' fears that even raising the topic of relapse with patients might communicate an expectation of failure and promote a self-fulfilling prophesy of failure by inadvertently giving patients "permission" to use alcohol and drugs again. However, as the RP model became more widely accepted and its efficacy was supported by empirical research (Rawson, Obert, McCann, & Marinelli-Casey, 1993), addiction treatment programs began to incorporate RP strategies more routinely into their work with patients. During the past two decades, RP strategies have been applied to many different types of chemical and behavioral addictions (Washton & Boundy, 1989) and different substances of abuse, including alcohol (Gorski & Miller, 1986; Monti, Kadden, Rohsenow, Cooney, & Abrams, 2002), cocaine and other stimulants (Rawson, 1999; Rawson, Obert, McCann, Smith, & Ling, 1990; Washton, 1988, 1989), opioids (Zackon, McAuliffe, & Ch'ien, 1993), and nicotine (Fiore et al., 2000).

Although in addiction treatment programs RP is often provided as a distinct component or phase of the program delivered in a group format, RP strategies are embedded in all good treatment of SUDs and are easily integrated into individual sessions provided in office-based practice. RP strategies rest on the premise that the factors that help to initiate abstinence from addictive behaviors are different from those needed to maintain abstinence. These techniques involve a combination of education, therapeutic confrontation, and skill development. Educating patients about the relapse process and helping them acquire problem-solving and affect management skills are essential components of the RP approach, as described more fully in this chapter.

In this phase of treatment, as in all other phases, one of the key elements in working with patients who have SUDs is the attitude and stance of the therapist toward these individuals. Therapists must be cognizant of their personal attitudes and beliefs about relapse and their countertransference reactions to patients who return to using alcohol and drugs despite the therapist's best efforts to help prevent this from happening (Imhof, 1995; Kaufman, 1994). Negative, judgmental, controlling attitudes by therapists are likely to fracture the therapeutic alliance and cause patients to drop out of treatment prematurely. The therapist must never downplay the potential dangers of relapses or ignore them, but it is essential to show empathy, concern, and a positive problem-solving attitude that reframes relapses as avoidable mistakes, not tragic failures. A genuine belief that patients can learn from these mistakes and move forward in their recovery must be communicated unequivocally.

UNDERSTANDING THE RELAPSE PROCESS

"Relapse," as the term is traditionally used in the addiction treatment field, refers to returning to substance use after a period of abstinence. More recently, however, relapse has come to be seen as a complex phenomenon involving much more than the act of using mood-altering chemicals again. Relapse is now seen as a process or dynamic that is set in motion by certain forces and as involving both overt and subtle shifts in patients' attitudes, behaviors, and choices that move them progressively closer to the point of using again. Thus, individuals can be in a backsliding or relapse mode, caught up in the process of heading for relapse, before they actually use alcohol and drugs again. In reviewing relapse experiences, many patients can identify specific clues or warning signs that preceded their return to alcohol and drug use. Typically, they were either totally unaware of these warning signs or paid little attention to them while heading for relapse. Thus, a significant aspect of relapse prevention strategies is helping patients to become aware of the earliest signs that they are in a relapse mode and learn how to take appropriate action to short-circuit this process before it culminates in a return to alcohol and drug use.

Although relapse can occur at any point after initial abstinence has been established, most relapses occur within the first 3–6 months. A wide range of variables contribute to the relapse process, and in most instances the actual causes of relapse are determined by a multitude of factors. Rarely does one factor alone precipitate a relapse to alcohol and drug use. Several categories of relapse precipitants have been defined by earlier investigators (Marlatt & Gordon, 1985), some of which were mentioned in the preceding chapter. These include (1) both positive and negative mood and affect states, (2) environmental cues or triggers associated with prior substance use, (3) inadequate coping and problem-solving skills, (4) sexual triggers, (5) unrealistic expectations and other "mind traps" or cognitive distortions, (6) lingering withdrawal including post-drug anhedonia and dysphoria, and (7) conscious and unconscious motivations to use mood-altering substances again including shame, guilt, and residues of earlier trauma and abuse.

Patients in early stages of the relapse process usually exhibit a variety of changes in thought, emotion, attitude, and behavior. At this point, the clinician can intervene to help short-circuit the relapse process before it leads to resumption of substance use. However, this depends on the ability of the clinician to recognize the warning signs coupled with the patient's ability to receive feedback and make the necessary preemptive changes. Sometimes the warning signs are subtle and therefore very difficult to recognize as such. Adding to the difficulty is the fact that different patients show different warning signs. Moreover, because behavior is at times unconsciously motivated, the client may actually be unaware of warning signs that are apparent to other people.

The Relapse Chain or Progression

The relapse process has been described as a progressive chain reaction or set of behaviors, attitudes, and events set in motion most often by negative feelings and/or stressors. This chain reaction can take many different forms, but may look something like this (Washton, 1989):

1. There is a buildup or onset of stress caused by negative events (e.g., relationship conflict, financial pressures, etc.).
2. The stress activates overnegative thoughts, moods, and feelings that lead the person to feel overwhelmed or emotionally numb.
3. Either overreaction or emotional numbing causes failure to take action, leading to continuation and eventual escalation of the problem.
4. The person gradually withdraws from his established recovery support system and daily routines.
5. There is a resurfacing or exacerbation of denial, as evidenced by increasingly skeptical and cynical attitudes toward treatment, self-help, and other commitments.
6. Feelings of futility about the ability to manage life comfortably without using alcohol or drugs, coupled with an increasing belief that relapse is inevitable, begins to overshadow whatever progress the person has been achieved up to this point.
7. Signs of impaired judgment and impulsiveness become evident as the individual makes poor decisions that result in even greater stress.
8. As the person's life becomes increasingly unmanageable, feelings of frustration, despair, and self-pity set in and trigger obsessive thoughts about using again.
9. Irresistible urges and cravings lead to drug-seeking and drug-using behavior. The relapse chain is complete.

Mistaken Beliefs about Relapse

Several mistaken ideas and beliefs about relapse are common and should be addressed (Washton, 1989; Washton & Stone-Washton, 1990). They are as follows:

1. *Relapse starts when the person starts using drugs again.* As stated earlier, the relapse process is activated long before the person actually starts using again. Using is the end point, not the beginning of the relapse.

2. *Relapses are unavoidable, unpredictable, and often appear "out of the blue" without warning.* The fact is that relapses are avoidable and rarely if ever occur without warning signs, if the person knows what to look for and attends to the warning signs.

3. *Relapse is synonymous with treatment failure.* Although relapses do suggest that some aspects of the patient's treatment plan may need to be changed, they are best construed as "bumps in the road" or temporary setbacks. Patients sometimes overreact to relapses and in the process make it harder for themselves to get back on track.

4. *Relapse erases all progress achieved up to that point.* Relapse does not mean that all progress achieved up to that point is lost, and it does not have to destroy a person's recovery plan. Because many patients are frustrated and discouraged by the prospect of having to start all over again from square one and as a result may decide to drop out of treatment rather than face this frustrating situation, they need help in acknowledging the progress they were making before the relapse occurred and in seeing how they can use whatever information can be gleaned from the relapse to move forward from that point.

Slips versus Relapses

According to Marlatt and Gordon (1985), one of the most important aspects of the RP approach is to distinguish between a lapse or "slip" and a full-blown relapse. The purpose of drawing this distinction is not to make the idea of using again acceptable or to tacitly condone the use as long as it is not taken too far, but rather to make clear that emergency action can be taken to "put on the brakes" and short-circuit any instance of alcohol and drug use before it "skids out of control" and escalates into a full-blown relapse with all of the attendant dangers. Whether or not a slip leads to relapse depends on how the person reacts to it. Unlike relapses, which tend to have a negative impact on a person's motivation and commitment to regain abstinence, slips, if handled properly, can be valuable learning experiences that decrease the likelihood of a person's using again. Slips should never be recommended or condoned, but the fact is that they often do occur, especially during the early and middle phases of treatment, when patients are still struggling with ambivalence and have not yet acquired sufficient coping skills as substitutes for self-medicating with alcohol and drugs. Although less destructive than relapses, slips also carry significant risks. For example, they can rekindle intense cravings; renew doubts that the addiction truly exists; lead to irresponsible and inappropriate behaviors; adversely affect a person's health, relationships, and financial well-being; re-establish a person's contact with dealers and other users; impair judgment; and postpone learning of non-drug coping skills (Washton, 1989).

A slip is defined as a single (isolated) instance of substance use after a period of abstinence. Slips are usually incidental, impulsive, and unplanned. They commonly result from unexpected exposure to a high-risk situation that overwhelms a person's ability to resist temptation. That is not to say that the individual has no personal responsibility for the slip's occurring. Often there are unconscious and unrecognized desires to use alcohol and drugs, but patients are not adequately aware of their ambivalence (vulnerability) inside and do not take sufficient behavioral measures to guard against acting on their impulses. Slips may also result from a deliberate attempt to "test control" in order to see whether reduced or controlled use may indeed be possible. By definition, a slip is a momentary setback in the effort to remain abstinent that can be contained so that it does not destroy or derail continued progress. It can be viewed productively as a mistake, an opportunity for learning, and as a signal for more careful planning to avoid future slips. A slip can be seen as the behavioral manifestation of a person's ongoing ambivalence about giving up chemical mood alteration. How a slip is responded to by the clinician and/or group will have a significant impact on whether the patient responds constructively or destructively. Harsh confrontation is likely to exacerbate the individual's sense of failure and guilt about having "messed up" again and to increase the chances that the slip will escalate into a full-blown relapse. How patients react to a slip can be very revealing of their level of motivation and readiness to make the changes required to support abstinence. It is a good sign when patients are remorseful about using again, disappointed in themselves for letting it happen, and receptive to advice and suggestions from others about how to prevent it from happening again. It is not a good sign, however, when they express defiance rather than remorse about using, minimize the importance or significance of the event, and are generally unreceptive to feedback.

A relapse can be seen as the result of a slip that has gotten out of control. Instead of being isolated instances of use, relapses are characterized by a return to the former (pretreatment) pattern of use and a re-emergence of addictive patterns of thinking and behavior. Relapses, unlike slips, are associated with a regressive attitude shift that erodes or nullifies a person's desire to regain abstinence and often leads to dropout from treatment. Relapses can be very dangerous and, in some cases, fatal. The major difference between slips and relapses does not rest on the quantity of drugs used, but on the intent and the outcome. If the person who returns to using fails to re-establish abstinence and get back on track immediately after an episode of use, continues to use, rejects offers of help, and/or drops out of treatment, it is a relapse. Relapses that are allowed to get out of control almost always involve serious backsliding, erosion of progress, and regression to an earlier stage of change.

In considering the issue of when relapse prevention strategies should be introduced into the therapeutic work, it is important to distinguish between a failure to establish abstinence in the first place and a return to alcohol and drug use after achieving various benchmarks of stability and clinical progress, as described earlier in this chapter. The former may reflect the patient's ambivalence about an abstinence commitment and reluctance to take the steps necessary to remain abstinent for more than a few days at a time. In such cases, instances of alcohol and drug use should not be seen as relapses, but perhaps more accurately as a continuation of the former pretreatment pattern of use interspersed with brief forays into abstinence. Drawing this distinction is important for a number of reasons. First, labeling these forays as relapses is a misnomer that fosters an unrealistic assessment of what stage of change the patient is currently in and thus what types of interventions are likely to be effective in moving the patient ahead in the process. Whereas relapse prevention strategies are appropriate only for patients in the maintenance stage, patients whose behavior is indicative of inadequate commitment to sustaining abstinence are more likely to be in the action stage, or perhaps in an even earlier stage. Sometimes the motivation and readiness of patients to do the work required in the maintenance stage does not become evident until they actually try. A second reason for making this distinction is that introducing relapse prevention (maintenance) strategies prematurely, before patients are ready to make use of them, can actually encourage rather than prevent relapse. For example, presenting these unstable, marginally motivated patients with a long list of potential relapse precipitants and warnings signs is likely to be misinterpreted by them as justification to use alcohol and drugs again. Instead of using this information proactively to avoid returning to alcohol and drug use, they are likely to see it as evidence that relapse is inevitable and/or expected. Discussion of relapse prevention strategies followed by repeated failure to apply them is a clear indication that the patient's motivation and readiness for change, not her behavior, is the most critical issue to address. A third reason is that the notion of relapse involving a series of events that culminate eventually in alcohol or drug use is simply not applicable to patients who truly are not in the maintenance stage. Returning to substance use for these patients is not the end product of a complex relapse progression, as described earlier, but rather a near instantaneous event, inasmuch as the person has yet to achieve stable abstinence in the first place.

RELAPSE PREVENTION STRATEGIES

Relapse prevention strategies incorporate a variety of cognitive-behavioral, psychoeducational, and supportive techniques. The major thrust of RP strategies is to teach patients specific cognitive, behavioral, and problem-solving skills and to heighten their awareness of potential relapse precipitants, warnings signs, and "mind traps" to reduce the likelihood that they will return to using alcohol and drugs again and to improve the overall quality of their lives.

Educating Patients about Relapse and Its Prevention

Education is an important relapse prevention tool. Patients need to be educated about certain attitudes, thinking, and behavior patterns that are characteristic of addiction and often contribute to relapse. The primary purpose of doing this is to help them anticipate the "traps" most commonly faced by people trying to maintain abstinence and learn how to deal with these traps in order to avoid returning to alcohol and drug use. You should provide patients with education about relapse as soon as possible after initial abstinence has been reasonably well established. Even if they are not strongly motivated to maintain abstinence and do not acknowledge the true severity of their addiction, education on relapse can still be helpful. Educational interventions tend to be nonthreatening ways to counteract denial and motivate patients to change. You can provide these interventions systematically in topic-oriented sessions or spontaneously in individual therapy sessions as specific issues emerge. You can also give patients a list of suggested readings or specific homework assignments in RP workbooks designed specifically for this purpose (Daley, 2000; Washton, 1990a, 1990b, 1990c; Zackon et al., 1993). It is important, however, not to make relapse education a purely intellectual or didactic experience. Information about relapse should be made as personally relevant as possible by helping patients apply this information pointedly to their current life problems, circumstances, and experiences.

Relapse Precipitants and Warning Signs

One of the most important RP strategies is to help patients identify and become increasingly aware of circumstances most likely to initiate or herald an impending relapse. Through discussions during individual therapy sessions as well as homework (workbook) assignments, you can help patients define the specific conditions that are most strongly associated with their prior use and/or most likely to set the stage for resumption of their alcohol and drug use. Relapse precipitants and warning signs have been divided into several categories (Daley & Lis, 1995; Marlatt & Gordon, 1985; Rawson et al., 1993; Washton, 1988), including:

1. *High-risk situations:* certain times of the day or night; people, places, and things previously associated with substance use; idle, unstructured time; access to cash; parties; bars; anniversaries; celebrations.
2. *Behavioral warning signs:* interpersonal conflict; failure to cope adequately with life problems and stressors; engaging in other addictive and compulsive behaviors; impulsive decision making and poor judgment; returning to secondary drug use.
3. *Affective warning signs:* negative moods; emotional lability; anger, frustration, hopelessness, and irritability; identity and role confusion; positive moods and excitement; desire to celebrate; sexual arousal.
4. *Cognitive warning signs:* euphoric recall and selective forgetting; repetitive drug using dreams; relapse justification; rationalizations to let up on disciplines and reduce or discontinue recovery-supportive activities.
5. *Physiological warning signs:* unremitting PAWS; resurfacing of intense cravings and urges; physical illness; chronic pain.

One way to help your patients anticipate and deal with relapse triggers and warning signs is to ask them to describe in detail a likely relapse scenario. This technique can help to make the possibility or threat of relapse more real for patients and encourage them to become more mindful of forces that may propel them toward using again. Their descriptions of a relapse scenario should include exactly what type of situation might put them into a relapse mode, where and with whom, what thoughts and feelings might be evoked, and what options might be available for avoiding alcohol and drug use. If there have been previous relapses, help the patient conduct a detailed retrospective analysis ("microanalysis") of early warning signs and other precipitants that led up to the relapses. Previous periods of abstinence ending in relapse provide valuable information about how relapses happened and, more important, how to prevent them from happening again.

Another intervention is to ask patients routinely at each visit if they have had any close calls since the last session and if they have experienced any cravings, fantasies, or dreams about using. If patients report any of these, it is important to discuss in detail specifically what events, circumstances, and feelings may have led up to these occurrences. Careful detailed inquiry can help to focus needed attention not only on environmental, but also on psychological and interpersonal issues. Conflict in intimate and work relationships and significant personal losses are common relapse precipitants. Helping patients to be mindful of their increased relapse potential around certain holidays, birthdays, anniversaries, and celebrations of various kinds and to learn how to manage whatever feelings are elicited by these events are essential components of the ongoing therapeutic work.

Substance-Specific Relapse Factors

Although the basic principles and strategies of relapse prevention apply equally well to all substances of abuse, it is important to take into consideration some of the unique features of different substances when developing specific relapse prevention plans. Knowledge of key differences between drugs can help therapists attend to certain details that might otherwise seem insignificant and be overlooked. For example, with regard to alcohol, key relapse factors include its social acceptance and legality, widespread availability, low cost as compared with the cost of illicit drugs, and social pressures to drink. Thus, effective relapse prevention strategies for alcohol-dependent patients must include teaching them how to comfortably and politely refuse offers to drink and how to cope with abundant opportunities in which, whether requested or not, alcohol is going to be quite literally put in their faces. For users of stimulants such as cocaine and methamphetamine, the awesome power of urges and cravings triggered by conditioned cues and the strong connection between drug use and sex are common relapse factors. Accordingly, effective relapse prevention strategies must attend pointedly to identifying and managing drug triggers, learning how to cope with cravings, and addressing the connection with sexual arousal and behaviors. For users of opioids such as heroin and prescription narcotics, relapse factors often include physical discomfort or pain (which in some cases can be due to protracted withdrawal), low energy, and intense anger or rage. Relapse prevention strategies include dealing with protracted withdrawal, appropriate use of opioid antagonists such as naltrexone, stress reduction and anger management techniques, and alerting physicians responsible for providing medical care to these patients about the dangers of prescribing opioids unnecessarily to them and the need to have significant others retain possession of prescription opioids and dispense them according to doctors' orders if and when these medications are truly needed to alleviate intolerable pain. There are countless examples of individuals who have relapsed to opioids after receiving narcotics to alleviate intolerable suffering related to surgery, kidney stones, gall bladder attacks, back and nerve pain, dental pain, broken bones, and other traumatic illnesses and injuries. For benzodiazepine users, relapse factors include generalized and/or panic anxiety and chronic insomnia. Sometimes these are rebound symptoms due primarily to protracted withdrawal. As with users of opioids, physicians can inadvertently contribute to relapse by prescribing sedative medications unnecessarily to these patients or without implementing appropriate precautions to prevent abuse. Relapse prevention strategies include cognitive and behavioral techniques for coping with insomnia, using physical exercise to reduce stress and anxiety, and teaching progressive relaxation, medication, and thought-stopping techniques.

Dealing with Slips and Relapses: Avoiding the Abstinence Violation Effect

Patients must be prepared to deal with the reality of slips and relapses if and when they occur. As mentioned earlier, one of the most important strategies is to teach patients how to prevent a slip from developing into a full-blown relapse. Cognitive reframing of a slip from a tragedy into a learning opportunity and making an effort to "put on the brakes" helps to reduce the shame, guilt, and exasperation often experienced by patients when they start using again.

The abstinence violation effect, or AVE (Marlatt & Gordon, 1985), is one of the cognitive distortions or "mind traps" elicited by a slip. Essentially, the AVE is an overreaction, a strong defeatist response to a slip. Using again contradicts the person's identity as an abstainer and instantly transforms him back to the identity of an active user—thus the term "abstinence violation effect." The person often attributes the slip to personal weakness, instead of viewing it as an avoidable mistake. When immersed in this cognitive distortion with its attendant self-loathing, frustration, and self-blame, the individual is more likely to give up on abstinence and the slip is more likely to escalate into a full-blown relapse. Clearly, an important component of relapse prevention is warning (educating) clients about the AVE and, more important, helping them to plan strategies to prevent this reaction from escalating to the point where it completely derails their recovery.

It can be very beneficial to outline for patients responses to slips that can help prevent them from turning into relapses, as compared with responses that are unhelpful (Washton, 1990b). For example, people who slip without relapsing are likely to (1) take the slip seriously and regret that it happened, yet do not become demoralized but learn whatever they can from it; (2) discuss it openly and honestly with members of their recovery support system; (3) carefully examine the circumstances to determine what aspects of their attitudes, lifestyles, behaviors, and moods may have contributed to the slip; (4) re-establish routines, structure, support, and positive activities to prevent further slips; and (5) redouble their commitment to maintaining abstinence and working a good recovery program. In contrast, those who let slips turn into destructive relapses are likely to (1) feel shamed, humiliated, and demoralized by the slip; (2) become secretive, withdrawn, and uncommunicative; (3) blame others and external circumstances for the slip and fail to take adequate personal responsibility for it; (4) feel pessimistic about stopping and justified in continuing to use; and (5) reestablish contact with drinkers, users, and dealers.

Another important strategy is to debrief patients after a slip or relapse. As mentioned earlier with regard to relapses that may have occurred prior to the current treatment episode, conducting a "microanalysis" (Daley & Lis, 1995) or relapse debriefing can provide valuable information that can be used to help prevent relapses from happening again.

Heightening Awareness of "Seemingly Irrelevant Decisions"

The phenomenon of making seemingly irrelevant decisions is an example of how forces beyond an individual's conscious awareness can insidiously lead her back to using again. Individuals headed for relapse sometimes unknowingly make a series of self-defeating choices, including "accidentally" exposing themselves to high-risk situations that are likely to cause relapse. Through a series of subtle self-sabotaging acts and seemingly irrelevant decisions (Marlatt & Gordon, 1985) they end up in situations that virtually guarantee exposure to drug-related cues that overwhelm their impulse control. For example, a person who has been abstinent for several months might "unintentionally" find himself driving down a certain street, ignoring the fact that this is the very street where his former drug dealer lives. Similarly, patients may accept an invitation to a party, overlooking the fact that people who drink excessively and use drugs will be there and that the temptation to join in will probably be overwhelming.

Dealing with Fantasies of Returning to "Controlled" Use

Success in establishing abstinence can bring a return of ambivalence, a feeling that life has improved so greatly that controlled use might be possible now. Stimulant users, in particular, are likely to experience euphoric recall, in which memories of adverse consequences seem to evaporate along with the lessons of their painful struggles to rebuild their lives. It is as if a cloud comes over them and they are preoccupied with re-experiencing the intense pleasure of the early stages of their stimulant use. This particular phenomenon is manifested in different forms with other types of alcohol and drug users. It does not appear to be as distinct, yet there is often a longing for the "fun" of the hard drinking days, particularly in those who have not developed alternative recreational activities in recovery. Those with untreated depression are particularly vulnerable, as their dysphoria makes recovery seem gray to them. Those who have made substantial progress may be particularly vulnerable to the seductive idea that their accomplishments have now put them in a position to control their use. Participation in a recovery group or in self-help meetings can be an important influence to offset relapse drift, as others can almost certainly describe traveling down that path. There are times, however, when no intervention seems effective, and the therapist must maintain a firm therapeutic alliance so that the patient will not drop out of treatment if a relapse occurs.

The desire to test control is most likely to occur when patients have been abstinent for several weeks or months, feel stronger, more in control of their lives, and are no longer acutely or noticeably feeling the "sting" of drug-related consequences. Consider the words of one patient:

"I thought I'd prove my therapist, my wife, and everyone else wrong, so I went out and tested myself with cocaine again. I tried a little experiment just to see if I could handle doing it again without getting crazy and out of control. I figured that if I passed the test, maybe, just maybe, I could go back to doing it just once in a while again. I thought to myself, what an accomplishment that would be! After all, my life was back in order, I still had my job, I was making good money, and my wife was still with me. Well, I failed the test miserably and ended up on a 4-day binge of cocaine and alcohol. There I was, right back in the coke scene, disappearing on a binge and running after prostitutes again. Looking back, I realize how foolish and self-destructive I was to think that I could pull it off, but at the time it all seemed within reach to me. If nothing else, it showed me that my addiction and my potential for relapse were there all along, even though I had not used in several months and on the surface everything else seemed okay. I wish I didn't have to learn the hard way and go through the horror all over again. Now, when I get those nutty thoughts about trying to be a 'controlled' user, I reach out immediately to people in my support system for a reality check."

Ongoing Resistance to Abstaining from Secondary Drugs of Abuse

As stated in the preceding chapter, one of the most difficult clinical challenges is the issue of abstinence from secondary drugs of abuse. Patients are typically vigilant about desires for their primary drug of abuse, but many minimize the importance of their lesser preferences. Research data and clinical experience support the view that the widest margin of safety is obtained when the patient maintains abstinence from all intoxicants. Many, however, view their other drug use as insignificant. It is common for stimulant or opioid users to protest that they never had a problem with alcohol prior to their use of these drugs. However, they are often unaware of their escalating alcohol consumption during the periods of drug use; some even suffer serious alcohol withdrawal once they enter inpatient treatment for drug dependence. They would like to believe they can return to normal social drinking once they have had an extended period of abstinence from drugs. This supposition carries great risk. In addition, there is the problem of drug substitution. Alcohol problems usually develop more slowly than problems with other substances, but it is common to find former users of illicit drugs entering treatment for alcohol dependence, often years after their last use of other drugs.

Part of the difficulty in helping patients fully acknowledge the risk is that the major relapse may take place weeks or months after the use of the secondary drugs. Most stimulant users readily acknowledge that if they have a few glasses of wine, and someone offers cocaine, there is little chance they will be able to refuse and leave the situation immediately. It is much harder for patients to integrate the idea that the glass of wine or beer today bears on the relapse 6 weeks from now, though clinicians observe this repeatedly. This is an extension of the principle that drug use consequences that are removed in time are less influential than those that are relatively immediate. We can hypothesize several levels of contribution. On the biological level, the use of any drug stimulates the craving center in the brain, which in turn stimulates the hunger for the primary drug of abuse. On the psychological level, patients long for the rewards they get from intoxicants and convince themselves that there is little danger, because, "after all, I don't even like alcohol that much." Again, a recovery group or self-help meetings can provide valuable feedback to the patient entertaining these rationales, but the drift may be inexorable and even those who have been through several relapse episodes precipitated this way may persist in such behavior. It is nonetheless desirable to explore a range of psychological possibilities: rebellion for having been good for so long; longing to get high to counteract sustained negative moods; feelings of "I deserve this" for working so hard in recovery; a resurfacing of traumatic material; a desire to be "normal." The therapist can become exceedingly frustrated at this point, and it is necessary to work to maintain a healthy balance of engagement and detachment. Patients are very sensitive to their therapists' disapproval, and it is certainly important to avoid power struggles, but excessive detachment can leave the patient feeling that he is without a lifeline.

Dealing with the "Pink Cloud" and Feelings of Being "Cured"

The initial positive effects of stopping alcohol and drug use can be striking—at least for a while, until the stress and problems of everyday life reappear full force and burst the patient's bubble or "pink cloud" and end the "honeymoon" phase of early recovery. Although some patients do not experience such effects, but feel distinctly worse, not better, after stopping alcohol and drug use, many if not most will show some evidence of being on the pink cloud. Related to the pink cloud phenomenon are illusions of being "cured" of the addiction or that it no longer exists (and maybe did not exist in the first place) after several weeks or months of abstinence, especially if remaining abstinent has not been very difficult and has been devoid of crises,

The danger of being in this state is that it fosters overconfidence and a belief that the problem is solved and not likely to return. Having given up alcohol and drugs, the true source of all their problems, so it seems, patients often feel that they can now go on happily with their lives by simply remaining determined to not use again. Patients in this frame of mind are extraordinarily prone to overreacting to almost any negative event that threatens to throw them off their cloud, no matter how large or small that problem may be. Accordingly, they are at high risk for relapsing in response to feeling disappointed and resentful when problems arise.

Patients on a pink cloud pose a dilemma for the treating clinician. On one hand, it is important to applaud the patients' progress and compliment them for making positive changes. On the other hand, it is equally important to not foster unrealistic hopes and expectations that may set patients up for being blindsided by serious setbacks. The best approach is to compliment patients for making progress and also call their attention to the importance of remaining vigilant about dangers that may lie ahead. Reminding patients of their vulnerability to relapse and describing scenarios that others have experienced as a result of not being sufficiently aware and proactive, can be both instructive and motivating.

Creating a Balanced and Satisfying Lifestyle

Achieving a balanced, satisfying lifestyle is an essential part of reducing the potential for relapse. Often, using alcohol and drugs has occupied a significant part of a person's time and caused her to give up other healthy pursuits to the point where stopping the use leaves a large void that can be filled too easily by using again. Many individuals have become so accustomed to instantly modifying their moods and mental states with psychoactive substances that the idea of having to plan, expend effort, and engage in physical activity for enjoyment and stress relief may be daunting at first. In addition, some patients are severe workaholics whose daily lifestyles are severely out of balance. Often, using alcohol and drugs is the only form of gratification they have allowed themselves on a regular basis. Thus, once stable abstinence has been achieved, it is essential to encourage and guide the development of new leisure and recreational activities that serve intrinsically to reinforce a recovering lifestyle devoid of alcohol and drug use. The primary goal is to learn how to have fun and reap the rewards and pleasures of life without relying on alcohol and drugs. Pleasurable activities should be integrated with work and family responsibilities on a regular basis. The particular types of activities should be based on the patient's needs, interests, and preferences and ideally should include activities that can be pursued alone as well as those that involve the participation of others.

In regard to individuals who previously were in the process of establishing a balanced lifestyle, the discontinuation of regular exercise, self-help meeting attendance, or other self-care activities without thought or discussion should be a warning signal for the therapist. Other warning signs include neglect of stress management techniques, such as avoiding being hungry, angry, lonely, or tired (HALT). The therapeutic structure offers the advantage of a context in which to notice shifts in routine activities and discuss their implications. How did you decide to cut back your exercise regimen? How did you drift into thinking you could manage on less sleep for extended periods of time? This allows the patient to increase awareness and make appropriate behavioral corrections. It is always easier to interrupt relapse drift in the early stages than when the risk factors have accumulated.

Keeping Ugly Reminders in View

To counteract the tendency of patients in early recovery to experience euphoric recall (i.e., idealizing or romanticizing the previous good times on alcohol and drugs and selectively forgetting the bad times), they should be encouraged to maintain vivid and, where possible, visible reminders of the negative consequences caused by their previous alcohol and drug use. For example, one patient was encouraged not to immediately repair the fender of a new car that she had smashed into a fire hydrant while under the influence of alcohol. Similarly, another patient pinned a rent eviction notice on the wall of his home office to remind himself of the horrible financial situation he was in as a result of being addicted to cocaine.

Maintaining Drug and Alcohol Monitoring

Although not specifically considered an RP technique, urine testing (as described in Chapter 9) can be an effective tool for reinforcing abstinence. The unique benefits of this tool are discussed at length in the preceding chapter, but suffice it to say that continuing the monitoring through at least the first three months or so of recovery, or until the patient leaves treatment, is advisable. In fact, patients who have been on drug and alcohol monitoring for a while often feel reluctant and apprehensive about discontinuing it, realizing the significant role it has played in helping them control impulses to use at earlier points in treatment.

Filling Social and Recreational Gaps

Patients typically underestimate how much time they have devoted to using alcohol and drugs and how profoundly it has affected their social relationships. For those who use alcohol or marijuana, the changes are slow and can be almost imperceptible. Gradually, the person focuses attention on social groups that drink at the same level and disengages from other relationships. Forming a relationship with a partner who does not drink, or drinks responsibly, can reverse this trend in people who have not progressed to severe dependence or who are without risk factors such as a genetic predisposition. Those who develop serious problems have typically selected their social networks in ways that camouflage their drinking patterns and allow these patterns to appear normal. Indeed, what passes for normal drinking in many social groups is in fact well above the limits of what is considered nonproblematic or responsible drinking. Alcohol problems can take a long time to show themselves clearly, particularly in men. Women have a more telescoped course, but can also appear functional for lengthy periods.

Marijuana is associated with problems that are difficult to pinpoint until the user stops for a period of time. After 3 or more months of abstinence, marijuana users report a longer attention span, less forgetfulness, less fatigue, and fewer low-level symptoms of depression. They are then in a much better position to reconstitute their social networks and focus on improving their quality of life in other ways. This is especially true for those whose marijuana use has promoted social isolation.

The slow and gradual onset of problems results in lengthy participation in a social network in which drinking or drug use seems necessary in order to belong. Patients may need to grieve not only the loss of their substances of abuse, but also the social networks surrounding them. They will need to construct new social networks in order to be successful. Understandably, many resist this and may have several relapse episodes before concluding that they cannot continue to socialize with heavy drinkers or users and be successful in changing their behavior. Drugs like cocaine and methamphetamine are associated with a rapid downhill course, which often means patients have more low-risk social possibilities once they have become abstinent. They may not have to regenerate a social network that has been shaped by decades of drinking or marijuana use, but can resume at least some of their familiar contacts.

Coping with Social Pressures to Use

Many patients work in environments where there is strong social pressure for co-workers to drink together or where drug use is common. Patients may participate in order to belong or to achieve performance goals they have set for themselves. Regular drug and alcohol use almost always results in reduced performance; the drug effects change over time and the "downtime" typically increases. For example, the woman who depends on wine to help her feel comfortable in meeting strangers for a business lunch may fail to appreciate the subtle decrease in ability to focus and think clearly that develops over time. Stimulants tend to promote a person's narcissistic overvaluing of the quality of the work produced; they rarely improve judgment about work products. Medical professionals with relatively easy access may begin using prescription drugs out of curiosity, but then quickly become dependent and unable to ask for help while their performance deteriorates.

It is important to assess the many factors promoting drug use in the workplace and in social situations and to formulate action plans accordingly. Are the difficulties so daunting that the patient must consider changing her friends, job, or career? What protective factors can be introduced to allow your patient to remain in a job she may value highly? For example, naltrexone, a narcotic antagonist discussed in Chapter 4, allows many medical professionals to continue working in clinical settings, despite the availability of opioids in these locations. Disulfiram (Antabuse) may help someone in the restaurant business continue to work there despite the endemic presence of alcohol. However, medications can be only one part of a recovery effort; there must be psychosocial changes as well. Changing from an evening to a daytime shift may reduce vulnerability by placing the patient in a situation with more supervision and eliminating some of the conditioned triggers like fatigue and the presence of drug-using co-workers. Developing rituals to prepare for creative activity may allow your patient to get past the conviction that drugs are necessary to open the mental doors to meaningful work. Learning that in the absence of drugs, the quality of one's work is likely to be just as adequate as it was with the help of drugs, or even better, can take time. Interacting with others who have found and developed their creative voices without reliance on intoxicants is invaluable for reassuring your patient that this is an achievable goal.

Learning New Ways to Cope with Feelings

In early recovery, impulse control is a primary issue. Once abstinence is stable, you can address more subtle issues of experiencing and expressing emotions. If possible, it is useful to determine, on the basis of his history, your patient's strengths and deficits in this area prior to the onset of his alcohol and other drug use. Substance use distorts behavior, but it is important to know whether you are promoting a return to earlier, healthier coping patterns or helping your patient develop new skills. For example, many patients who are drinking and using become accustomed to expressing their anger freely, whether intoxicated or not. They may come to rely on intimidation rather than communication. Patients who never had good controls need much more attention to skill building than those who can reclaim skills they once exercised.

Substance users become accustomed to rapid change in feeling states and relatively instant relief from discomfort, and thus need to learn to approach their feelings in a different way. Acquiring the ability to tolerate arousal of difficult emotions, or the experience of any emotion for more than a few moments, can be a challenging task for your patient and may need to be an explicit focus of your work. Some emotions may be taboo, others acceptable. Anger may be expressed quite easily, but sadness or vulnerability is less tolerable and thus less likely to be expressed. Teaching your patient to simply maintain an ongoing awareness of changing feeling states without feeling compelled to alter them is an important task.

It is also important for you to help the patient determine when feelings reflect symptoms of mood or anxiety disorders and medication should be considered. Overwhelming anxiety or sustained periods of low mood increase vulnerability to relapse and interfere with learning new skills, developing new relationships, and building confidence in new ways of coping. Although some therapists prefer to have a sustained period of psychosocial intervention before considering medication, this can promote demoralization over lack of progress or allow a major depressive episode to get underway before medication is initiated. Depression is more easily treated if medication is initiated at the onset of an episode, so it is important that the therapist avoid the practice of referring patients for medication consults only when all else has failed.

Timing is best decided in collaboration with your patient. The patient must understand that learning to experience and express feelings appropriately is a part of recovery, but extended distress is not necessarily useful. Does depression interfere with mobilizing to attend self-help meetings? Does anxiety promote social isolation or fearfulness about trying new ways of handling relationships? Medication is not always useful, but patients can be asked to consult a psychiatrist whether they are prepared to begin medication or not. An addiction psychiatrist is particularly likely to offer a productive discussion on the potential benefits or contraindications. Patients may agree to a medication trial or may want time to digest the new information and consider a change in approach. You should explore and address any resistances to psychotropic medication, because you, as a therapist, spend more time with your patients than physicians and other treating professionals and are more likely to have relevant information about a patient's history. Patients with family members who have severe psychiatric disorders may view medication as a sign of "being crazy." Use of medication to feel better is a charged issue for people in recovery, especially if they have abused prescription drugs. This must be sensitively handled, and it may take time to work though. Fortunately or unfortunately, it takes time for many psychotropic medications to begin working, so that such medications gradually become distinguishable from drugs of abuse. This can be framed as part of the larger issue of learning to invest time and effort in the service of later improvements, rather than expecting instant results. The issue of control may also be important. Considering that substance use is often an important if not primary activity that gives your patient an illusion of control, it is common to resist sharing this control with a physician. Patients often stash supplies of antianxiety and other medications just so they won't be at the mercy of a physician if they reach a period of desperation. It is important to discuss and monitor your patient's willingness to build a good team relationship with the prescribing physician, one in which the parameters of patient decisions about dose changes and frequency are explicit and it is clear when the physician should be included in deviations from the agreed-upon plan.

Moving Beyond All-or-None Thinking

It is important to keep in mind that a rigid yes-or-no thinking style is quite adaptive in early recovery. No drinking or drug use, no exceptions, gives the widest margin of safety. This often extends to rigid rejection of certain social gatherings, determination to maintain specific schedules around 12-step attendance, and devotion to particular exercise regimens. Any disturbance of the protective routine is threatening. As recovery progresses, it is important for your patient to increase ambiguity tolerance and be able to handle complex considerations.

Some patients are inherently rigid in their character structure and may do best if left unchallenged. Others need encouragement to expand their perspectives and test out more flexible coping strategies. For example, a 30-year-old methamphetamine user who regularly engaged in sexual adventures while using the drug understood that sexual arousal was a powerful trigger and rigidly avoided sexual encounters and other forms of intimacy in his first year of recovery. Sexual arousal was frightening because of the associated cravings for methamphetamine, and he felt insecure about any attempts to connect with a woman. Although his rigid posture helped him achieve a year clean and sober, it was clear this coping strategy had decided limits as a permanent solution. His therapist encouraged him to form friendships with women with whom he did not have intense sexual chemistry. He also began to air his fears that sex would be awkward without using the drugs he had relied on since he became sexually active as a teenager. Sharing experiences with members of his small recovery group, as well as in his self-help meetings, reassured him that he was on a well-traveled path that many have navigated successfully.

Managing Anger

Because anger is one of the most common and compelling relapse precipitants, anger management techniques are an essential component of RP strategies. Anger management skills focus on helping your patient identify signs of anger, particularly in the early stages, and find appropriate and constructive modes of expression. Some people have to get furious in order to set a limit, and have to learn to monitor their own signals of discomfort so they can assert themselves before their anger builds up. Patients also learn to discern whether they are overreacting or displacing anger from one situation to another. They learn to recognize when their anger is a cover for fear and anxiety. In many situations, it is important for your patient to identify someone who is not part of the problem whom he can use as a sounding board. In early recovery, it may be important to be able to reach someone immediately. Members of the patient's self-help group, particularly sponsors, are good candidates. Substance abuse treatment settings often use cognitive-behavioral techniques in groups focused on anger management. These can be adapted to individual sessions if your private practice is not conducive to offering group treatment (Reilly & Shropshire, 2002).

In the beginning stages it is desirable for your patient to dilute her dependencies rather than concentrate them on the therapist, partner, or spouse. Many patients cannot tolerate intense feelings of vulnerability and dependency concentrated on one individual, and either abruptly withdraw or display storms of ambivalence. The self-help system is ideal to provide a support system that is diffuse enough to be well tolerated.

Patients in anger management also identify strategies for cooling off. Physical exercise is excellent, as it helps dissipate arousal. "Time outs" also define a cooling-off period for patients, who become increasingly able to use this structure with frequent practice. Patients are encouraged to wait before responding, organize their thoughts, and consider their options. They are encouraged to avoid solutions that have created problems in the past.

Accepting the Identity of a Recovering Person

The patient who accepts the identity of a person in recovery has a matter-of-fact acceptance that it is not possible to use intoxicants safely and it is necessary to develop a comfortable and satisfying life without them. Critics of AA have assumed that the identity of a recovering person is inevitably negative and argue that it is disparaging and prolongs low self-esteem. The identity of recovering person need not perpetuate a poor self-image. Those well along in a solid recovery process have worked through much of their shame and guilt, while taking responsibility for their behavior, and can acknowledge the importance of abstinence without harsh self-criticism. They also understand that they must remain mindful of potential relapse hazards, such as increased stress, interpersonal conflict or loss, and high-risk social situations. Their behavior reflects the changes in self-image, for example, disengaging from social networks in which drinking is glamorized or viewed as essential to having a good time.

Feelings of deprivation often reflect areas in which further therapeutic work is needed, such as management of feelings or development of new social networks. For example, patients who have not developed new friendships or attractive recreational activities often miss the lack of camaraderie and excitement they associate with drinking and drug use. Prolonged negative feelings may also reflect untreated psychiatric conditions such as depression. Although they may not completely meet the criteria for depression, patients with a personal or family history of alcoholism may benefit from antidepressants, especially if they remain moody, irritable, and dysphoric.

FAMILY ISSUES IN RELAPSE PREVENTION

Working with couples and families can be an essential element in preventing relapse, as this strengthens the support structure among intimates, particularly those in the same household as the primary patient. The term family is used broadly here, to include gay or lesbian partners, household members who may have no legal ties, and members of the extended family who are influential though they do not live in the patient's home. You may want to consider including any member of the patient's network who is involved in the addiction or who is likely to play a significant role in the patient's recovery (Galanter, 1994).

The terms "enabling" and "codependency" are frequently used in work with significant others, and it is important to avoid certain pitfalls with these concepts. Enabling refers to behaviors that perpetuate the addictive behavior. It can take the form of avoiding, shielding, minimizing, colluding, attempting to control the addicted person's behavior, taking over responsibilities, and otherwise protecting the addicted person from the consequences of behavior. Codependency refers to the unhealthy adjustments made by others in relation to the abuser. Attention shifts from their own needs and activities, and they become preoccupied with the behavior of the addicted person. Individuals gradually abandon their own interests, and family functioning becomes organized around the drinking and using of the identified patient. The therapeutic task is to restore a healthier equilibrium in which everyone's needs are taken into account.

Both "enabling" and "codependency" have come to be used by patients and therapists to express frustration, anger, and disapproval. It is important to keep in mind that the presence of significant others who care about your patient is an important positive prognostic sign. Your task is to shape their behavior, not to pathologize their attempts to help. Family members and others are often confused about what constitutes a desirable balance of engagement and detachment. They may label appropriate forms of support as negative. The therapeutic task is to help them get beyond epithets, examine specific situations in terms of what is or is not helpful, and adapt accordingly.

Domestic violence occurs in all social classes, and it is essential to include some questions on this subject in the assessment process. You can ask your patient and family members the following: Have you ever been hit, kicked, punched, or otherwise hurt by someone in the past year? If so, by whom? Do you feel safe in your current relationship? Is there a partner from a previous relationship who is making you feel unsafe now? Although substance use is typically involved in episodes of violence, it is important to remember that these patterns have a life of their own and may continue into periods of abstinence. Safety questions must always be addressed quickly in the treatment process, so it is important for you to clearly identify resources at your disposal. If continued drinking or using episodes put others at risk, you must formulate a plan that considers the needs of anyone at risk from the outset.

You will have to determine if doing the family work yourself is likely to interfere with your tasks with your primary patient, and include a family therapist in the treatment plan accordingly. It is very important that the family therapist understand the stages of recovery, so that he or she can synchronize treatment goals with recovery tasks. Focusing on conflict resolution prematurely is likely to precipitate relapse. It is important for the family therapist to be willing to help the family find solutions that protect the newly abstinent patient from excessive stress while giving others an appropriate outlet for their feelings.

On a more practical level, family members may feel that they previously lost the patient to the addiction and they are now losing him to self-help activities. A spouse and family members may feel jealous that the mate, who has created a huge wreckage, now acquires an extensive support system and they are asked not to undermine participation. They feel that they have formed the anchor, and each may ask, "What about me?" Helping them to be appropriately patient and weather the storms so that recovery rests on a solid foundation is a key task for the treatment team.

In the absence of problems such as domestic violence, it is useful to ask couples not to make major decisions about their relationship during the first year of recovery. Changes can be very dramatic, and it is difficult to know which problems will be enduring until a period of stability has been achieved. Many problems emerge from choosing a mate while actively addicted. One or both spouses may conclude they simply don't like each other and decide to terminate their relationship. In the early stages, encouragement to "focus on your recovery" can lead to a devaluation of the spouse, who is seen as remaining stagnant while the newly abstinent person is changing rapidly. Over time, the recovering partner may actually outgrow the mate as a result of the extended focus on self-examination. Partners may be involved in Al-Anon, psychotherapy, or another activity that promotes their own growth and increases their ability to exit an unhealthy relationship. For many, however, couple work allows them to renegotiate their relationship in a way that is satisfying.

As recovery progresses, many issues emerge that are not unique to addicted patients. The tendency to fuse and mesh with the partner requires a focus on clarifying personal boundaries so that neither partner swallows the other up. Some patients have an intense need for fusion in order to feel safe and must develop the capacity to be comfortable alone, even when not attached. Developing intimacy while retaining healthy autonomy is a challenge, especially if there is a long history of using alcohol and other drugs to feel connected.

Sexual problems may be evident in later-stage recovery, particularly in individuals who have used drugs to enhance their sexual experiences. Sex can be a trigger for renewed drug cravings and a relapse precipitant. Many patients are convinced that they cannot function sexually or genuinely enjoy sex without intoxicants. They cannot imagine getting through feelings of awkwardness and self-consciousness, particularly with a new partner. Therapy should address these issues when they arise. Past infidelities can pose a formidable challenge to the viability of the relationship (Schneider, 1988) and may be an insurmountable obstacle for some couples. Under the influence of alcohol and drugs, many individuals (particularly those who use stimulant drugs) engage in sexual behaviors and indiscretions that are uncharacteristic of them, but the partner's sense of betrayal is often profound and persists well into recovery. The partner's pent-up anger, disappointment, resentment, and pain can be overwhelming and create a formidable barrier to re-engaging in sex and intimacy.

As the formerly substance-dependent person builds clean and sober time, the power balance inevitably shifts in the couple's relationship. The actively addicted person does not want to call attention to herself, and the mate typically assumes major responsibilities and control, particularly if there are children. In early recovery, shame and guilt often preclude challenging the mate. With extended sobriety, however, other relationship problems emerge and the role of "identified patient" becomes unacceptable. The recovering partner becomes better able to stand up for her legitimate needs and tends to insist on more equality. This is particularly likely to play out over money and parenting issues. The anxieties and resistances of the mate must be handled sensitively, particularly if there has been a long period of irresponsibility during active use. It is important to remember that addicted spouses often seek to intimidate their mates, pathologize their behavior, and deny the validity of their concerns. The therapist must be attentive to the possibility that efforts to encourage mates to take their share of responsibility may elicit painful memories of past manipulation.

Will the relationship survive recovery? The complex challenge is described by Brown and Lewis (1999) in a developmental model that examines the critical tasks that couples face during the successive phases of active drinking, transition to abstinence, and then early and ongoing recovery. Certainly the couple's chances improve if the partner is willing to learn about addiction and recovery and use the opportunity to make the necessary changes. Couples may benefit from working with a skilled couples therapist who has in-depth knowledge of recovery issues. In our clinical experience, poor prognostic signs for the relationship surviving recovery include the following: (1) the relationship was formed while the addiction was active; (2) the partner has unrelenting hostility and resentment; (3) the partner refuses to take any responsibility for contributing to the relationship problems; (4) the partner is unable to see the need for personal change; (5) the partner is unwilling to engage in couple therapy, individual therapy, or self-help. However, it is important for you to avoid drawing premature conclusions, as some couples do manage to navigate through formidable obstacles and emerge eventually with a healthier and stronger relationship.

FINAL COMMENT

Relapse prevention strategies have become a standard feature of addiction treatment programs and group therapy approaches to treating addictions over the past two decades, and they can be integrated quite easily into individual treatment sessions in office-based practice. RP strategies emanate from the premise that the factors that help to initiate abstinence from addictive behaviors are different from those needed to maintain abstinence. These techniques are based primarily on a cognitive-behavioral and skills acquisition approach involving education, therapeutic confrontation, affect management, and coping skills development. Although slips and relapses should never be condoned or encouraged, clinicians should not only help patients face the reality that relapse is an ever-present danger, but also respond therapeutically if and when patients return to using alcohol and drugs again. Preventing slips from escalating into full-blown relapses is one of the primary goals of RP strategies. Helping patients to maintain abstinence and prevent relapse involves, among other things, teaching them how to recognize relapse warning signs and how to cope effectively with high-risk situations and other potential relapse precipitants. Therapists must be mindful of the potential for experiencing negative countertransference reactions to patients who relapse repeatedly. Although therapists must never downplay the potential dangers of relapses or ignore them, it is essential to show empathy, concern, and a positive problem-solving attitude that reframes relapses as avoidable mistakes, not tragic failures. A genuine belief that they can learn from these mistakes and move forward in their recovery should be conveyed to patients routinely. After abstinence has been firmly maintained for at least several months and the potential for relapse is markedly reduced, patients may benefit from more insight-oriented psychotherapy that focuses on a wider range of psychological issues in greater depth, as discussed in the next chapter.

CHAPTER 11

Psychotherapy in Ongoing and Later-Stage Recovery

The integrated approach addresses psychological issues that go beyond the patient's substance use behavior per se to explore other areas of the patient's psychological life, as in any psychotherapy. The ultimate goal here is not merely the acquisition of selfknowledge and insight, but fundamental change in an individual's habitually maladaptive ways of thinking, feeling, behaving, and interacting. Because people with long histories of substance abuse often lack the ability to identify, modulate, tolerate, and appropriately express feelings (especially negative ones), psychotherapy can play an important role in raising their awareness of these difficulties and in developing affect management skills to improve their functioning and to help prevent relapse over the long term. Ongoing therapy can also address, where indicated, couple issues and longstanding problems that may stem from parental alcoholism, physical and psychological abuse, and other developmental and life traumas. Each patient's treatment requires a focus on different sets of issues and themes as these arise in the course of the treatment. An important caution is that whenever such highly charged issues are being addressed, the therapist must be especially mindful of the patient's heightened potential for returning to alcohol and drug use. Even when exploration of these issues appears to be well tolerated, patients and therapists should always be alert to the possibility that focusing on these issues can and sometimes does reignite a person's desire to medicate emotional discomfort with alcohol and drugs. Thus, psychotherapy with these patients should never lose sight of the potential for relapse, no matter how motivated and stable they appear to be.

Many addiction specialists argue that psychological issues cannot be meaningfully addressed and psychotherapy is not likely to be beneficial while a patient continues to use intoxicants at any level (even if the patient is not intoxicated during therapy sessions) and not until a period of at least 3–6 months of uninterrupted abstinence has been achieved. This view is based on the assumption that use of intoxicants at any level poses an obstacle to making therapeutic progress. It is seen as preventing patients from developing a realistic perspective on their behavior, from getting in touch with internal feelings, and from acquiring nonchemical coping and affect management skills. There is also concern that while patients are focusing on the challenging task of changing their substance use behavior, they cannot channel sufficient energy into addressing and working through other issues. Regardless of these clinical concerns, many patients come to treatment with personal crises and other problems that beg for immediate attention. Some patients insist on addressing relationship problems or negative mood states (e.g., anxiety or depression) as their first priority rather than substance use. Although continued substance use can and often does hamper efforts to address other problems, the patient's immediate concerns and priorities must not be overridden or ignored by a therapist who insists on controlling the agenda of treatment. As discussed in Chapter 10, it is important to strike a balance between addressing SUDs and giving sufficient attention to problems that are of greater concern to the patient.

The need for ongoing psychotherapy as part of an overall recovery plan that extends beyond initial changes in substance use behavior, depends primarily on the patient's desire, readiness, and felt need for this type of treatment. Not all patients want or need ongoing individual therapy to maintain recovery. Some patients have little or no interest in engaging in ongoing psychotherapy, including those who are satisfied with having achieved their initial substance use treatment goals (whether reduction or abstinence), those who see their participation in 12-step programs rather than therapy as the mainstay of their recovery plan, those who are not actively distressed or emotionally unstable, and those who do not feel at high or imminent risk of returning to their former pattern of substance use.

Nonetheless, some individuals reach a point where they are disappointed to find that although remaining abstinent has brought substantial relief from problems caused by the substance use itself, it has not resolved other emotional difficulties that surface more clearly in the absence of alcohol and drug use. Others become receptive to engaging in ongoing psychotherapy only after relapsing repeatedly despite their intention to remain abstinent. They may develop a sense that perhaps there are unconscious conflicts and other forces operating beneath the surface that lead them back to using substances over and over again. Still others arrive at a point in recovery where they feel a need to find out *why* they developed a serious alcohol or drug problem in the first place, seeing identification and resolution of these issues as important to sustaining recovery over the long term.

Because psychotherapy is always highly individualized, it is counterproductive to try to proceed with the therapy according to a preconceived agenda. When the therapist imposes too much structure or tries to control the agenda too tightly, it may block the patient from raising meaningful issues spontaneously and thereby prevent the patient from acquiring a deeper, more meaningful understanding of the issues that are important to him. As with all patients, psychotherapy with patients attempting recovery must be highly individualized.

Kaufman (1994) defines several key psychological themes and issues that need to be addressed in ongoing psychotherapy with patients in recovery, particularly those in stable and later-stage recovery. These include (1) working through grief and loss centered on giving up alcohol and drugs and the lifestyle associated with using, as well as other losses resulting from death, divorce, and wasted time; (2) addressing childhood traumas, including abuse (both physical and psychological), neglect, and abandonment; (3) addressing transference and countertransference reactions; (4) relinquishing narcissistic vulnerabilities; (5) overcoming residual dysfunctional affects including chronic depression and anxiety; and (6) establishing healthy self-care.

FUNCTIONAL ROLE AND SIGNIFICANCE OF SUBSTANCE USE

A universal theme in ongoing psychotherapy for SUDs is examining the meaning and role of alcohol and drug use in the person's life. Typically, this involves focusing in detail on how substances may have been used to self-medicate intolerable affects and escape conflict. Exploration of these issues is valuable because it provides a basis for understanding that for individuals who develop chemical addictions, substance use is initially an attempt to cope and to resolve human problems (Dodes & Khantzian, 1991). Consistent with this view, it seems that individuals develop addictions only to those substances that work well for them in the early stages of use. They become victims of expecting that they can derive the beneficial self-medicating effects of alcohol and drugs without suffering the adverse consequences. In this context, it is not surprising that many patients experience intense grief reactions and considerable anxiety when they attempt to give up alcohol and drugs.

Some authors contend that without addressing and working through certain core issues, unique to each person, the prognosis for long-term recovery may be substantially diminished (Dodes & Khantzian, 1991; Kaufman, 1994). Contemporary psychodynamic theories of addiction have emphasized that in addition to the role of internal (unconscious) conflict and the object meaning of alcohol and drugs for an individual, deficits in ego and self-functioning are important contributors to reliance on psychoactive substances (Dodes & Khantzian, 1991). As mentioned previously in Chapter 4, Khantzian (1981) described certain types of self-regulatory impairments that require attention in ongoing psychotherapy with addicted patients: deficits in affect management, self-esteem maintenance, the capacity for self-care, and interpersonal relations. Problems in these areas may be evident during active addiction, but usually reveal themselves more clearly during periods of sustained abstinence. Similarly, therapy from a self-psychology perspective defines pathological narcissism as a core issue for people in recovery and defines the primary goals of psychotherapy in later-stage recovery as internalization of sobriety, remediation of structural deficits in the self, resolving intrapsychic conflicts, and building genuine self-esteem (e.g., Levin, 1995).

RELATIONSHIP AND INTIMACY ISSUES

Kaufman (1994) contends that achieving healthy intimate relationships is the single most important objective of recovery. He defines healthy intimate relationships as having certain defining features:

1. The partners are meaningfully connected, but not fused or enmeshed with one another. Each retains appropriate autonomy from the other, and boundaries are respected and kept clear.

2. The partners are able to freely express both positive and negative thoughts and feelings to one another without fearing reprisal, recrimination, or hostility from the other. Communication is respectful and well intentioned. The partners work hard on the difficult task of tolerating and processing anger appropriately with one another.

3. The partners are able to use their communication with one another to define and maintain boundaries of the relationship; to express caring, concern, and commitment; to negotiate rules and roles; and to resolve conflicts.

4. Sexual experience, which is not synonymous with intimacy but only one way of expressing it, is caring, nurturing, and affectionate and mutually satisfying for both partners. There is a balanced perspective about sex—it is neither made too important nor neglected. Sex between the partners is free of shame and guilt.

Married couples and others in intimate relationships are affected not only by a partner's active addiction, but also by profound changes that occur during recovery. Once active alcohol and drug use are no longer clouding the picture and serving as the primary focus or preoccupation of the relationship, other difficulties emerge more clearly, often revealing serious deficits in communication and intimacy. The partner in recovery may be at a disadvantage in not feeling that she has the right to voice dissatisfactions with certain aspects of the relationship, and it may become clearer that previous substance use was a way to avoid facing these problems. Sustained abstinence often brings destabilization in relationships as the power dynamics shift. Alcohol and other drug use may also have promoted an abusive dynamic, in which anger and irritability were used to intimidate the nonaddicted partner into submission. Once the substances are removed, communication and conflict resolution skills are needed as tools to renegotiate the interpersonal dynamics of the relationship (Brown & Lewis, 1999).

SEPARATION AND INDIVIDUATION ISSUES

Separation and individuation issues are common among substance-dependent patients, as evidenced most dramatically by severe enmeshement with their family of origin. This enmeshment often spills over into other relationships with spouses, friends, and co-workers in the form of boundary and unresolved dependency issues. In the presence of their parents, adults who have not yet achieved emotional or psychological autonomy often feel and act dependent, vulnerable, guilty, beholden, insecure, and even childlike. They also tend to feel manipulated, smothered, controlled, and unloved by parents and others with whom they are enmeshed. Because the intense anger, resentment, and self-loathing that this dynamic generates often contribute etiologically to development of addiction in many individuals and to an increased relapse potential, these feelings must be addressed and, it is hoped, resolved in order to sustain abstinence over the long term. Research shows that certain characteristics distinguish families of addicted individuals from families affected by other types of serious mental health problems (Stanton & Todd, 1982). These include: (1) a higher frequency of multigenerational addiction, particularly alcoholism, and a propensity for other addictive behaviors such as gambling; (2) more primitive and direct expression of conflict and hostility; (3) more overt alliances, as between an addicted son and an overinvolved mother; (4) retreat of the addicted person into a drug-oriented peer group following family conflict, thus fostering the illusion of independence or "pseudoindividuation"; (5) symbiotic, enmeshed child-rearing practices lasting longer into adulthood; and (6) frequent acculturation conflicts due to parent–child cultural disparity. If the parents separate or divorce, the unhealthy dynamics of the addicted person's family are likely to become even more exaggerated.

Helping adult patients separate appropriately from enmeshment with their parents and achieve genuine, lasting autonomy requires working through a number of critical issues. Patients who complain about their parents' being intrusive, controlling, and disapproving often do not recognize their own contribution to these troubling interactions. Thus, increasing patients' awareness of how they actively participate in these conflicts and helping them to take personal responsibility for this behavior is a critical first step. Other tasks include helping them to (1) become more aware of the degree to which their sense of self still depends on parental approval; (2) acknowledge their ambivalence about becoming more autonomous; (3) address their anxiety and fears about change and the negative reactions they anticipate from parents if they attempt to pull back; and (4) develop a vision of how they would act and how it actually might feel if they were more autonomous and less emotionally dependent on their parents. The ultimate goal for these individuals is to be able to make the choices in love, work, and personal values that are true to who they really are and allow them to be themselves rather than who their parents want them to be. An excellent self-help resource for patients embroiled in this autonomy and identity struggle is a book by Halpern (1976) that focuses on "breaking loose" from parental enmeshment and control.

A strategy to consider with adult patients attempting to untangle themselves emotionally from parents is based on the addiction recovery principle "act as if you were the person you aspire to be," which conveys that change often takes place from the outside in, as well as the inside out, and that resolving internal conflicts may not be necessary in order to change behavior. A conscious effort to handle situations in a new way despite discomfort can promote the development of new skills and internalization of new roles. For example:

Evelyn was strongly invested in making others comfortable and had difficulty setting boundaries in the service of self-protection. She was particularly vulnerable to family members' desires. She quickly learned she would have to face their disapproval once she refused to comply with their wishes, which she frequently detected without being openly asked. Although her initial efforts were focused on making it clear that she did not want to be offered alcohol or other drugs, she quickly noted that this was not the only issue on which she allowed her better judgment to be overtaken by family and other social pressures. She began to notice similar patterns in other areas of her life and made changes in how she handled her colleagues at work. She recognized that her desire to move into a managerial position required that she become less influenced by what others thought of her and more willing to be firm.

Thus, the need for rapid behavior changes produces many insights for the therapist and patient to explore.

SELF-ESTEEM ISSUES

Self-esteem problems are nearly universal among people who develop addictions. In some cases, this is evident in an individual's self-deprecating posture and passive reluctance to ask for what he needs. In others, problems of low self-esteem may be covered over by a hostile demanding attitude fueled by arrogance and grandiosity. These dynamics are likely to show up in the patient's transferential reactions to the therapist, providing an opportunity to address them therapeutically. Typically, self-esteem problems are rooted in developmental insults including the remnants of unattuned parenting as well as psychological abuse and neglect.

Also contributing to self-esteem problems are lingering feelings of shame, guilt, and self-recrimination stemming from the individual's behavior while actively addicted. These may include acts of dishonesty, irresponsibility, and infidelity. Many patients also lament wasted time, energy, and money associated with their alcohol and drug use. Although it is important to support your patients' willingness to accept personal responsibility for regretted behaviors, it is just as important to help them achieve self-forgiveness, realizing that many of things they did while addicted were part of the insanity of addiction and not characteristic of how they normally behave. It can be very difficult for individuals to achieve greater self-acceptance and make peace with the past while others adversely affected by the addiction (e.g., spouses) continue to express anger, hostility, distrust, and deep-seated resentment toward them. A helpful edict espoused in AA is that greater self-esteem results from performing estimable acts, such as being rigorously and unfailingly honest as well as humble and nondefensive about previous acts that have adversely affected others.

ISSUES RELATED TO CHILDHOOD TRAUMA AND POSTTRAUMATIC STRESS DISORDER

According to Young (1995), one of the greatest unacknowledged contributors to alcohol and drug relapse is the failure to identify and treat underlying childhood sexual abuse issues. She contends that the direct result of this trauma is an assault to the self and that various addictive behaviors are not only manifestations of the underlying self-impairment, but also mask the impairment and damaged sense of self. In many if not most cases, only after the addictive behavior has ceased for a while does recognition and repair of the original trauma become possible. Sustained abstinence from alcohol and drugs often leads to the emergence of repressed memories of sexual abuse that rekindle a person's desire to self-medicate. Sexual trauma survivors in addiction recovery are at risk for relapse in four major areas that need to be addressed as recovery proceeds (Young, 1995):

1. Memories of the abuse are unknown, but begin to surface
2. Affects associated with the abuse, as well as feelings in general, begin to emerge
3. Life experiences and problems are encountered without the aid of addictive behaviors
4. Addictive behaviors surface other than alcohol and drug addiction, such as sex and love addiction and compulsive eating.

Trauma issues related to early abuse or suffering other types of traumatic events (e.g., medical illness and disability, parental death, violent crime, financial ruination, acrimonious divorce and child custody disputes, etc.) can surface at any point in the recovery process, but the manner of handling them varies with the stage of recovery. In the early stages, the task is to help patients express or contain feelings and memories without drinking or using and to work on creating safety in their current life circumstances. As patients gain a more solid foothold in recovery, more intensive efforts toward trauma resolution can be undertaken and may be more effective. Discussion of specific techniques for treating coexisting SUDs, sexual abuse, and posttraumatic stress disorder (PTSD) is beyond the scope of this book but is available in the burgeoning literature on this topic (Evans & Sullivan, 1995; Ouimette & Brown, 2003).

THE IMPORTANCE OF IDENTIFYING POSITIVE BYPRODUCTS OF RECOVERY

As patients move through the later stages of recovery, they often become increasingly aware of how much their lives have improved along the way. It is not unusual to hear patients refer to their addiction and its consequences as a "wake-up call" that gave them the impetus not only to come to grips with the addiction, but also to make a variety of meaningful changes in their lives. Many believe that without this wake-up call these changes probably never would have occurred. This is exactly what people in recovery mean when they refer to themselves as "grateful addicts and alcoholics."

Research has shown that individuals who are able to find benefit from weathering various types of traumatic life events generally show better posttraumatic adjustment and clinical outcomes than individuals who remain stuck in feeling helpless and victimized (McMillen, 1999). These studies provide empirical support for the notions that "what doesn't kill you often makes you stronger" and "there is a silver lining in every cloud." Two recent studies (McMillen, Howard, Nower, & Chung, 2001; Washton & Washton, 2002) found that the types of positive byproducts reported by patients recovering from addiction were very similar to those commonly reported by people who have struggled with other kinds of adversities such as near fatal illnesses, catastrophic physical and psychological events (fires, tornadoes, rape), and various traumas (e.g., military combat, death of a loved one). The particular benefits reported most frequently by recovering patients included (1) greater appreciation for the simpler things in life; (2) positive reordering of life priorities; (3) greater acceptance of things that cannot be controlled or changed; (4) greater compassion, tolerance, and empathy for others; (5) greater honesty with oneself and others; and (6) enhanced self-knowledge. Moreover, the degree of perceived benefit was positively correlated with patients' length of time in recovery and level of involvement in AA. The most positive changes were reported by individuals who were further along in recovery and more meaningfully involved in AA (Washton & Washton, 2002).

Identifying positive benefits is important for patients in all stages of recovery because it can help to bolster their motivation to remain abstinent and continue to improve their lives. Thus, you should make a point of encouraging patients to compare their overall happiness, life satisfaction, and priorities during recovery versus prior periods of active addiction. You should also help them to periodically reassess positive benefits at various points along the way in recovery, as some benefits become apparent at later points in the process than others.

FINAL COMMENT

Ongoing individual psychotherapy is a valuable tool for addressing a variety of important problem areas, including intimacy, separation/individuation, self-esteem, childhood traumas, and relationships. It is crucial for the therapist to be continuously mindful of recovery issues and be prepared to shift the focus of therapy, as needed, to behaviors that support abstinence when the patient is tackling particularly painful issues or shows signs of letting up on practices that support recovery. It is also important to help patients identify and periodically reassess specific ways they have benefited from facing their addictions and channeling their energies into recovery. Patients in recovery can potentially benefit as much from ongoing psychotherapy as any other patients and often make rather striking and meaningful changes.

CHAPTER 12

Group Therapy

Although this book focuses on working with patients individually, it is important to recognize that group therapy offers unique benefits, especially for patients with SUDs, that individual therapy does not. Considering that group therapy continues to be the primary treatment modality and mainstay of addiction treatment programs, surprisingly few psychotherapists offer substance abuse groups in their office practices. Even clinicians who are experienced in treating SUDs typically refer patients for group therapy to local addiction treatment programs. Possible contributors are therapists' lack of familiarity with setting up and running these types of groups; lack of sufficient referral flow to start a group and maintain adequate group census; working in an office that is too small to accommodate groups; concern about the potential objection of landlords, office mates, and others to bringing "drug addicts" into the office; and refusal by many third party payers to reimburse for substance abuse group therapy not provided in a state-licensed addiction treatment program. Despite these obstacles, the potential clinical and financial benefits of providing substance abuse groups can be significant enough to warrant therapists investing the time, effort, and resources needed to make this type of treatment available in their private practices.

This chapter provides a general overview of how to set up and clinically manage substance abuse groups in office practice. Because group therapy techniques require much more extensive discussion than we can provide here, the reader is referred to other helpful resources for additional information (Brook & Spitz, 2002; Elder, 1990; Flores, 1988; Vannicelli, 1992; Velasquez et al., 2001; Washton, 2001, 2002; Yalom, 1995).

BENEFITS AND LIMITATIONS OF GROUP THERAPY

Perhaps the most striking benefit of substance abuse groups is an observation that most clinicians who have led these types of groups have witnessed time and again, namely, the remarkable ability of groups to support and encourage their members to make extraordinarily difficult changes that they had tried in vain to accomplish before joining the group. In substance abuse treatment groups, the patients' rate of change is often rapid and the nature of the change profound. When people in trouble join together in the pursuit of shared goals, a variety of potent forces are mobilized that motivate and inspire them to confront the problem and resolve it successfully. This same phenomenon is evident, for example, in how people respond to natural disasters and other extreme adversities.

The healing power of the group experience can be especially powerful for people with alcohol and drug problems, considering the pervasive social stigma and the intense feelings of shame, guilt, and self-recrimination often associated with these problems. The mutual identification, peer acceptance, social support, and role modeling that groups supply are powerful antidotes to these intense feelings. It is especially important to expose patients to positive role models who have "been there" to help to instill optimism and hope that successful recovery is attainable. Groups generate positive peer pressure, support, and accountability for making healthy changes that have no parallel in individual therapy. Under the guidance of a group leader, therapeutic (not aggressive) confrontation and realistic feedback can be provided, taking advantage of the astuteness and credibility of peers, while offering the benefits of a group process managed by a professional clinician. Significant benefits accrue from the exchange of factual information that takes place between group members both inside and outside of the group sessions. Patients also learn and have opportunities to practice in the group new behaviors and coping skills for managing the challenges at each stage of the treatment process.

Although many patients express trepidation about joining a substance abuse group, particularly if they are highly visible in their community, rapid acceptance into the group goes a long way toward overcoming these feelings. Forthright discussion gradually desensitizes newcomers who feel ashamed and exposed, particularly when other group members role model honest and open self-disclosure. Prospective newcomers should be reassured that many people with alcohol and drug problems, who consider themselves to be outsiders and loners, nonetheless derive great benefit from group participation. It is difficult for reluctant or quiet patients to "hide out" in small groups, because every member is regularly subjected to the scrutiny of the group. A healthy group culture places high value on self-disclosure, active participation, compliance with group norms (e.g., honesty, attendance, punctuality, behavior change, etc.), and facing rather than avoiding problems. The spirit of cooperation and positive support provided in groups can greatly enhance the work done in individual therapy. The bonding that occurs between group members can significantly enhance treatment adherence and retention.

Usually, groups are composed of 8–10 members and each group session lasts 1–2 hours. Group therapy has distinct economic advantages by allowing treatment intensity to be enhanced at lower cost than by adding more frequent individual sessions. Groups also allow practitioners to treat a larger number of patients as compared to individual therapy and thus make treatment more accessible to those with limited financial resources. Due to the lower per-session cost of group therapy and its reputation for being especially effective in treating substance abuse, many managed care organizations and other third party payers are more receptive to authorizing reimbursement for group rather than individual therapy for patients with SUDs.

Despite its many advantages, group therapy also has limitations. Concerns about loss of privacy and confidentiality can prevent some patients from joining a group. Patients must disclose their identities and many details about their private lives for the group to be helpful, and this can create problems for those who live in small communities where there is a good chance that they will encounter others in the group who may know them. Substance abuse often involves illegal or other antisocial behaviors which can intensify a patient's confidentiality concerns about divulging information to strangers. Although patient orientation to the group should stress the importance of maintaining strict confidentiality regarding group members' identities and the content of sessions, there is no guarantee that members will scrupulously adhere to this rule. Despite increasing public recognition that substance abuse is a health problem affecting a wide spectrum of people, unwanted disclosure can damage careers, reputations, and relationships. While it is important to be respectful of these concerns, it is also important to explore and help your patients work through them wherever possible. For many, their shame magnifies the dangers of disclosure. Once they have begun to make positive changes and have achieved some stability, they are often better able to face appropriate disclosure and later become more willing to take the risk of entering a group.

A second limitation of group therapy is that only a small portion of the session time is devoted to the needs of any one individual, and it may not be possible to give sufficient attention in a single session to every group member's issues. For this reason, the combination of individual and group therapy is often preferable particularly for patients in the early stages of treatment and those facing serious challenges in other areas of their lives. Although patients usually learn a great deal from discussions focused on other group members' issues, it is important recognize when a patient's needs are sufficiently pressing that adding concurrent individual therapy is indicated.

A third limitation of group therapy is that the content and pace of the group is determined by the members as a whole, and not by the needs of any one individual. Thus, the group's focus at times is unavoidably out of step with the needs of some members while simultaneously in sync with the needs of others.

A fourth limitation is that group therapy is not suitable for all patients. For example, patients suffering with psychiatric impairments that preclude meaningful involvement and communication with others may not be clinically appropriate for group therapy. Other patients may be clinically appropriate for group therapy, but flatly reject the idea of joining a group for a variety of reasons. Commonly stated objections to group therapy are "I'm a very private person. I don't see the point of talking about my personal problems with total strangers"; or "I'm here to help myself. I don't really want to spend time dealing with other people's problems." These and other objections can be taken as opportunities to educate patients about the unique therapeutic value of group therapy in general and how it may benefit them in particular. Nonetheless, it is important to respect the choice of patients who remain adamant about not joining a group, despite your recommendations to the contrary.

Lastly, there are certain practical obstacles to providing group therapy in an office-based practice. It takes time to gather enough patients to initiate a group, and in the interim some patients may change their minds, enter treatment elsewhere, or just fail to come back. It may be necessary to start with as few as three members in order to create a group for others to enter. Once the group is up and running, the therapist may still not have sufficient volume of newcomers to maintain an adequate group census, as some members inevitably leave upon completing treatment and others drop out prematurely. Another practical consideration is that the therapist's office and waiting room may not be large enough to comfortably accommodate a group of 8-10 patients. Generally speaking, a minimally furnished office that is at least 12' x 15' is required to accommodate a circle of 8–10 chairs (stackable chairs are recommended to minimize storage requirements when not in use). Even when the therapist's office is large enough, the waiting room may be too small to accommodate 8–10 people. One solution is to adjust your schedule so that group members can come directly into your office (the group room) when they arrive instead of assembling in the waiting room.

INTERFACE WITH INDIVIDUAL THERAPY

A combination of individual and group therapy, preferably with the same therapist, is optimal for many patients. When the patient's group leader also serves as his individual therapist, the usual problems of coordinating these two forms of treatment are eliminated. The dual role of the therapist provides an opportunity to directly observe a wider range of the patient's behavior first hand and to use the information obtained about the patient in one treatment context to maximize the effectiveness of interventions utilized in the other. For example, when patients display certain problems "live" in group sessions that have been previously discussed abstractly in individual sessions, the therapist has a unique opportunity to draw connections between the two. This type of interplay between individual and group therapy can have very potent synergistic effects, thereby accelerating treatment progress. Issues raised in group sessions often serve as catalysts for discussions in individual sessions and vice versa. Individual therapy also gives patients an opportunity to address certain sensitive or emotionally-charged issues that they may be reluctant to bring immediately if at all into group. The therapist should not rigidly insist that patients bring any and all personal matters discussed in individual sessions into the group. Similarly, the therapist must guard against violating the patient's confidentiality on certain issues. It is essential that the patient and therapist clarify with one another exactly which issues discussed in individual therapy sessions are not to be mentioned in group sessions. However, issues directly involving the patient's drug use must be categorically excluded from any such agreement: The therapist's hands cannot be tied when it comes to dealing with substance-related issues in the group and there can be no secrets among members regarding alcohol and drug use.

When patients are referred to you for group treatment by an outside practitioner who plans to continue seeing the patient for individual psychotherapy, you should obtain the patient's written permission to contact the individual therapist. When both clinicians communicate regularly and agree on a coordinated treatment plan, the two forms of treatment can work well together. Both therapists must guard against the splitting defense of some patients, particularly those with narcissistic and/or borderline personality features.

RELATIVE ROLES OF GROUP THERAPY AND SELF-HELP PROGRAMS

Many patients are unclear about the relative roles of group therapy and self-help meetings. It is important to clarify for prospective newcomers that group therapy and self-help meetings are not good substitutes for one another. Each can provide unique benefits and concurrent involvement in both often works synergistically to engender positive change. Those who regularly attend self-help meetings have ready access to an extensive peer support system that fosters healthy behaviors. Group meetings held by 12-step programs (e.g., AA, NA), by far the largest available self-help system worldwide, are led by peers (i.e., fellow members), not professionals, and feedback ("crosstalk") between members during a meeting is strictly prohibited. By contrast, in a professionally-led group, members are strongly encouraged to give feedback ("hold up the mirror") to one another adhering to certain basic guidelines that are role modeled by the group leader and by experienced group members (Washton, 2001, 2002). As compared to therapy groups, self-help meetings cannot provide the in-depth attention to psychological and personal issues that are addressed under the guidance of a professional group therapist. Also, the membership of therapy groups is relatively stable in comparison to self-help groups, and the size of the group is typically much smaller. This permits a different kind of self-exploration and intensive learning experience. Many individuals seek professional group therapy after realizing that their participation in 12-step programs alone cannot sufficiently address certain issues that continue to trouble them. The emphasis in 12-step programs on remaining "honest, open, and willing" can make these individuals excellent candidates for group therapy.

PATIENT SELECTION FACTORS

It is not possible to reliably ensure that the composition of patients placed together in a group will be optimal for accomplishing the therapeutic work. The best guideline for patient selection is to seek a balance between a reasonable degree of homogeneity and heterogeneity of group members. It is important that all group members find a modicum of common ground with at least some other members, because admitting a newcomer into the group who is different in very significant ways and shares few characteristics with other members may create problems that adversely affect the functioning of the group. At the same time, diversity enhances the richness of the group experience. Group members can differ in age, gender, race, socioeconomic status, educational level and other variables, as long as one member is not the lone "outlier" (Vannicelli, 1992). Patients need to be able to identify and bond with one another. Newcomers will fare better if there are at least one or two other group members with whom they can readily identify. Individuals who are different from all other group members in one or more important respects (e.g., one woman among a group of men, one gay person among heterosexuals, one seriously impaired person among highly functional people) are likely to feel out of place in the group (understandably so), not participate actively in group discussions, and/or drop out of the group prematurely.

Groups should not be restricted only to patients who have the same primary drug of choice, as the substance use disorder and the recovery process itself, not the drug, are the focus of the group's work. Heterogeneity in this regard can help group members realize that different substances usually lead to the same constellation of problems and that the types of changes required to deal effectively with these problems are similar, regardless of a person's substance(s) of choice. When a newcomer happens to be the only person in a group with a particular drug of choice, identification and bonding with other group members is often more difficult to accomplish. For example, a heroin user may feel out of place in a group where alcohol is the substance of choice of all other members. It is important to help such patients discover as soon as possible the similarities between different types of substance dependencies and encourage them to identify with the similarities rather than the differences in order to feel part of the group and derive maximum therapeutic benefit from being there. Despite the similarities, however, the group should not ignore some of the unique problems associated with using different types of substances such as residual cognitive impairments resulting from chronic alcohol use, lingering withdrawal symptoms of depression and insomnia following cessation of opioid use, and sexual acting-out behaviors associated with cocaine and methamphetamine use. Addressing substance-specific issues straightforwardly, proactively, and whenever they arise will help to promote group cohesiveness and more readily induct patients with different substances of choice into the group.

In addition to the above, other important patient selection factors such as the patient's desired treatment goals with regard to substance use, the patient's primary motivation or reasons for coming into the group and the patient's stage of readiness for change, should be taken into account when forming substance abuse groups.

Patients committed to the goal of total abstinence from all psychoactive substances usually do not mix well in groups with patients who choose non-abstinence goals such as harm reduction, moderation, or partial abstinence (i.e., abstinence from the most problematic substance, but not others). Those pursuing total abstinence often feel irritated, angered, and even demoralized by group members who are not committed to the same goal. Patients not committed to total abstinence are often labeled by others as "in denial," "resistant," or needing to "hit bottom," and may be treated with annoyance, pity, or even contempt by others who feel that the presence of group members with non-abstinence goals has a negative impact on their own motivation to refrain from all substance use and also distracts the group from its primary mission of supporting abstinence. Similarly, those not choosing total abstinence often view their counterparts as rigid and unreasonable. Obviously, these opposing camps are not likely to work well together in groups and their seemingly irreconcilable differences can consume the majority of the group's time and thwart the therapeutic work. Traditionally, substance abuse treatment groups have restricted membership to patients who are committed to to-

tal abstinence or at least willing to comply with an abstinence requirement during their tenure in the group. Recognizing that many patients
who seek help for SUDs are not ready or willing to accept total abstinence as their goal, harm reduction or moderation groups can be viable
alternatives for these patients, whether or not abstinence is their ultimate
goal (Little, 2002; Velasquez et al., 2001).

Potential group members may have different motivations and reasons
for coming into treatment. In this regard, mixing mandated and non-mandated patients can cause problems in the functioning of a group. Group
members who are mandated into treatment under threat of serious consequences (e.g., loss of personal freedom, job, driver's license, professional
licensure) are frequently mistrustful and reticent to open up and participate
actively in group discussions. Their presence in a group frequently disrupts
group cohesiveness and inhibits the participation of voluntary members
who may respond negatively toward those who are in the group only to
avoid severe consequences. This is not necessarily an insurmountable problem if properly addressed, but doing so consumes a substantial amount of
group time and requires a great deal of effort and patience from the group
leader who must help the group work through this difficult and often con-
tentious issue in a way that ideally benefits everyone in the group. We have
seen this happen in many of our own groups where grappling with this
issue has clearly enhanced the functioning of the group in several ways, not
the least of which was to afford group members the experience of successfully working through a thorny issue, particularly one that threatened the
group's integrity. Nonetheless, even with the group leader's best efforts,
there is no guarantee that this issue will be resolved to the satisfaction of all
group members and some of the non-mandated patients may end up leaving the group prematurely, feeling that it is simply not the best place for
them to get the help they need.

Recent work on the application of the stages of change model to
group therapy indicates that substance abuse treatment groups function
best when all members are in a similar stage of change (Velasquez et al.,
2001; Washton, 2001, 2002). Ideally, groups should be comprised of individuals either in the early stages of precontemplation and contemplation, or those in the latter stages of preparation, action and maintenance.
From a purely practical standpoint, however, offering separate groups for
patients in different stages of change may not be possible for many therapists because they do not have sufficient patient flow to establish and
maintain the census of several groups simultaneously. In these situations,
it is probably better to either form groups that are limited to patients in
the later stages and work individually with patients in the earlier stages,
or vice versa, depending on the types of patient referrals the therapist
receives.

GROUPS FOR DIFFERENT STAGES OF RECOVERY

Patients in the stages of precontemplation and contemplation are, by definition, not sure that their substance use is really a problem or they acknowledge it as a problem but are not yet ready to do anything about it. Groups designed specifically for patients in these early stages have been referred to variously in the literature as decision-making groups, transition groups, discovery groups, and self-evaluation groups (Matrix Center, 1997; Obert, Rawson, & Miotto, 1997; Washton, 2002), all of which rely heavily on motivation enhancement strategies to help participants more realistically examine their involvement with psychoactive substances and increase their readiness for change (Miller, 1999). These types of groups have been offered in mental health and primary care medical clinics, HIV treatment settings, and addiction treatment programs to give patients a chance to explore such issues without making an unwarranted assumption that they are in the action stage of change. As mentioned earlier, placing uncommitted patients into a group that is already operating under the premise that all members openly acknowledge that their substance use is a problem, and are actively working toward changing it, does not work very well. Group members committed to abstinence often attack the wavering newcomer's "denial," and everyone in the group can quickly become frustrated and demoralized. Thus, a major benefit of groups for patients in the earlier stages of change is to provide a safe environment in which they can explore their ambivalence, work on achieving greater clarity, and develop a clearer vision of their goals with regard to substance use. Such groups also allow the therapist to avoid the all too common trap of pressing prematurely for an abstinence commitment and immediate behavior change in patients who are likely to respond negatively to this approach.

Patients in the action stage who choose abstinence as their goal are best suited for groups commonly referred to as early abstinence or "beginners" groups that focus on achieving total abstinence from all psychoactive substances (Washton 2001, 2002). Length of an individual's participation in these groups often ranges from 3–6 months or more, depending on the individual's clinical needs and rate of progress. Newcomers entering an early abstinence group derive benefit from making connections with more experienced members who are often eager to take a beginner under their wing. This accelerates the newcomer's engagement and learning, and heightens the more experienced members' awareness of their own progress. The more experienced group members often appreciate having contact with beginners because it serves as a vivid reminder of their own mindset and of the problems they faced at earlier stages when they first entered the group. It helps to raise their level of awareness about their own relapse vulnerability, particularly if they have become complacent, overconfident, or are perhaps secretly harboring fantasies of returning to alcohol or drug use. An important task of early abstinence groups is to help all members begin to acquire the behavioral coping and affect-management skills needed to avoid using alcohol and drugs in response to stress and emotional discomfort. Group members learn to identify triggers that may elicit cravings and urges to use, and develop reliable strategies for avoiding or coping with these triggers without drinking or using. They also begin the process of identifying and changing some of the dysfunctional self-defeating cognitions, emotions, and behaviors that repeatedly lead them back to alcohol and drug use.

Patients in the maintenance stage are best suited for groups that focus on relapse prevention and other advanced recovery or later stage issues. These groups are typically open-ended and presume that members have achieved stable abstinence and made significant progress toward realizing other important goals, and are now able to work in greater depth on issues such as self-esteem, interpersonal relationships, sexuality, various self-defeating behaviors, and quality of life issues. At this point in recovery, the patient is better able to address and hopefully work through a wide range of issues that otherwise leave her prone to self-medication with alcohol and other drugs. In early recovery, mastering environmental triggers is a major challenge. In later recovery, relapses are more often triggered by patients' difficulties in managing stress, negative emotions, and other problems of daily living. With assistance from the group, patients continue to improve their ability to identify negative feelings, manage anger, be assertive without being aggressive, improve communication skills and learn to address interpersonal conflict, avoid impulsive decision-making, and give and take constructive feedback. Timing varies for each individual, but eventually the group can help members address long-standing problems such as those stemming from parental addictions, physical and sexual abuse, important losses, and other developmental and life traumas. It is crucial for you to remain aware that it is easy to underestimate relapse vulnerability, particularly in articulate and high functioning patients. Even when the patient appears to tolerate exploration of painful issues well, relapse is always a risk and both therapist and patient must remain attentive to warning signs. Good timing requires knowing when to press harder, back off, or provide more support.

GROUP MANAGEMENT ISSUES

Leadership Role and Style

Group leaders face many challenging tasks that influence the functioning and effectiveness of the group. Among the leaders' most important roles are: (1) to establish and enforce group rules in a caring, consistent, non-punitive manner so as to protect the group's integrity and progress; (2) to screen, prepare, and orient potential group members to insure suitability and proper placement in the group; (3) to keep group discussions focused on important issues and to do so in a way that maximizes the therapeutic benefit for all members; (4) to emphasize, promote, and maintain group cohesiveness; (5) to create and maintain a caring, nonjudgmental, supportive atmosphere in the group that not only counteracts self-defeating attitudes and behaviors, but also promotes self-awareness, expression of feelings, honest self-disclosure, alternatives to alcohol and drug use, and acquisition of adaptive coping skills; (6) to manage problem group members and problem group behaviors effectively to protect the other members and maintain the integrity of the group environment; and (7) to provide psychoeducation, where appropriate, to facilitate group members' ability to remain abstinent and develop non-drug coping skills.

Group leadership style is determined by many factors, not the least of which are the therapist's personality, theoretical orientation, and experience in facilitating groups. Substance abuse groups are usually conducted in a style that differs significantly from traditional psychotherapy groups, particularly in early abstinence groups. For example, the therapist in traditional group therapy gently guides and focuses the attention of group members on matters pertaining to group process, group dynamics, and the complex interpersonal interaction among members. Typically, the therapist remains fairly quiet and purposefully nondirective. By contrast, in early abstinence groups, the therapist must work actively to keep the group focused on specific issues that pertain directly to establishing and consolidating abstinence. The therapist is active and directive in questioning, confronting, advising, and educating group members, where indicated. It is important for these groups to remain task-oriented and reality-based, and maintain a focus on substance abuse issues as the primary (but not exclusive) priority of the group. The group leader facilitates a process in which members learn to interact with one another in an increasingly open, honest, empathic manner that promotes positive changes in behavior. Addressing issues related to honesty is of primary importance and the therapist must quickly address the many forms of denial, minimization, and fears of disapproval that lead patients to conceal their return to alcohol/drug use from other group members. When it becomes apparent that a patient has concealed a relapse, it is often appropriate to explore what obstacles within the patient or group prevented an honest disclosure.

When the group is working well, the leader stays largely in the background while the group takes most of the responsibility for the therapeutic work. When members become passive, the group leader should avoid doing a lot of talking and/or spending a lot of time exhorting members to join the discussion. Rather, the basic group therapy principles of addressing resistances and returning maximum responsibility should guide the group leader's behavior in these situations. The group should become reliably self-correcting when the discussion strays off track or becomes unproductive. Later stage recovery groups resemble traditional psychotherapy groups in their wide range of topics, with the caveat that it is always necessary to remain attentive to potential relapse warning signs, no matter what other issues are the focus of group discussion.

Preparing Newcomers for Group Entry

It is important to meet with new group members at least once or twice individually to orient and prepare them for attending their first group session. These preparatory sessions provide an opportunity for the therapist to educate newcomers about the basics of group therapy (especially for patients with no prior group therapy experience) and to give these patients an opportunity to ask questions and express their concerns. The group rules and guidelines should be discussed with newcomers and they should be asked to sign a form pledging to adhere to these stipulations (Washton, 1989, 2001). The purpose, goals, expectations, composition, content, and format of the group should be discussed with all newcomers and they should be given some idea of what usually happens during a group session. Newcomers also should be advised about how to give and receive constructive feedback in the group and how to differentiate between helpful and unhelpful group behaviors (Washton, 2001). Most newcomers simply do not yet know how to be good group members, thus one of the group leader's primary tasks is to teach them these skills through proper pregroup orientation followed by appropriate guidance and role modeling during group sessions (Vannicelli, 1992). When admitting a new member to the group, it is helpful to have an established introduction protocol to follow when the newcomer attends his first group session. For example, the leader asks all members to give the newcomer a brief (2–3 minute) synopsis of how and why they came into the group including an overview of their substance use and treatment history, what personal issues they are currently working on in the group, and something about their experience in the group thus far (both positive and negative). The newcomer is then asked to provide similar information and also explain how he expects to benefit from participating in the group and what issues he is hoping to work on in the group. Group members are then encouraged to ask the newcomer for clarification or additional information, offer feedback, and, where possible, describe how they identify with aspects of the newcomer's experiences. All of this is geared toward helping the newcomer feel welcome in the group and to initiate bonding between new and existing group members.

Outside Contact between Group Members

Group members should not be prohibited from maintaining contact with one another outside the group. In fact, especially in the early phases of treatment, this should be encouraged. (Again, this is very different from traditional psychotherapy, where outside contact among group members is viewed as undesirable "contamination" of group dynamics.) A list of telephone numbers of all group members should be routinely updated and distributed to all newcomers who enter the group. In order to promote rapid induction into the group and foster group cohesiveness, newcomers can be asked to call at least one other group member every day during their first two weeks in the group. Members should also be encouraged to go with one another to self-help meetings and to reach out to one another in times of need. One of the most important functions of the group, especially for newcomers, is to have an immediate support network to help prevent a return to substance use and serve as a buffer in dealing with various stressors.

Responding to Relapses

Addressing a group member's alcohol or other drug use since the last group session must be the topic of first priority in any group session, and the group leader's task is to help the group utilize the occasion as a learning opportunity for all concerned. It is important to maintain a leadership style that models clear, consistent, and non-punitive behavior. Group members usually have strong reactions in response to another member's use, and this must be placed into proper perspective. Many groups adopt a strategy for "debriefing" members who have used again (Washton, 2001, 2002; Washton, 1990b; Washton & Stone-Washton, 1990). Most groups respond supportively to a member's relapse; however, any member who repeatedly relapses eventually starts to lose the group's support as members start to disengage themselves from a member who is perceived as unmotivated or unable to make use of what the group can offer. If a group member is having trouble remaining abstinent and shows little evidence of utilizing previous suggestions offered by the group about how to prevent further use, other members may become intolerant and may feel that the person is undermining the group's purpose. The overall attitude of the relapsing member and the nature of his relationship with others in the group often determine how many relapses the group will tolerate. Group members have keen antennae for shifting commitment, and the leader should not allow the group to scapegoat or ostracize the member who is struggling with ambivalence. Sometimes it is best to remove a relapsing member from the group, at least temporarily, in order to protect both the individual and the group. Asking a relapsing member to leave the group can be humiliating for that patient and the group leader must handle this situation very carefully so as not to further exacerbate the patient's sense of shame and failure. Otherwise, removal from the group will likely be perceived as punishment rather than an appropriate change of treatment strategy intended solely to help, not hurt. While "on leave" from the group, the patient can be seen individually for more intensive work leaving open the possibility that he or she may return to the group once abstinence has been more firmly established and sufficient progress on contributing and related problems has also been achieved.

Confrontation and Feedback

The group feedback process is a powerful tool for helping members acquire a more realistic perspective on their maladaptive attitudes and behaviors. However, it is important to interrupt heavy-handed, excessive, and poorly timed feedback. Certain stereotypes about group therapy foster the belief that humiliation and aggressive confrontation are required to help resistant members face reality. Harsh confrontation is sometimes rationalized as an attempt to be "truly honest" with group members who are having difficulty in sustaining their motivation or otherwise violating group expectations and norms. The most frequent targets of attack are group members who relapse repeatedly, those who remain defiant, superficial or insincere, and those who minimize their problems and fail to bond with other members. A group leader must never allow members to be scapegoated or bludgeoned by their peers, even if the content of the communication is entirely accurate. Harsh or unrelenting confrontation can push unwanted members out of the group and promote premature dropout. Detailed guidelines for delivering effective, respectful confrontation in groups is described elsewhere (Washton, 1988, 2001).

Hostility

Some group members are routinely antagonistic, argumentative, volatile, and sarcastic. They may repeatedly devalue the group, complain about how poorly it is run, point out inconsistencies, and categorically reject advice or helpful suggestions from other group members and the group leader. Often the content of what is said in group is less important than the way it is said. The leader must attend vigilantly to group members' affect, body language, voice intonation, and overall communication style, and teach all group members how to do likewise. It is important to not allow sarcastic and aggressive statements to go unnoticed and unaddressed. An appropriate intervention by the group leader might be: "I wonder if others in the group are experiencing Howard's remarks as hostile and aggressive? Can some-one offer him feedback about how he is coming across and how it is affecting others in the group?" In these types of situations, you should carefully guide the ensuing discussion to make sure that group members do not use this as an opportunity to attack and berate the problem group member, but rather to help him see the self-defeating nature of his actions as well as the negative impact of his behavior on the rest of the group.

Failure to Participate

Some group members sit quietly on the sidelines as observers, content to have the focus of attention not be on them. Mandated patients, especially, may secretly harbor intense feelings of resentment and annoyance about being in the group and doubting whether the group is of any use to them. Other silent members may be harboring feelings of being bored, indifferent, insecure, out of place, or perhaps even superior. Some members are just shy and need gentle coaxing and encouragement from the group to open up. One possible intervention for addressing a silent member is to say: "I've noticed that Renee has not said a word during the last several group sessions. Maybe the group can try to find out what's holding her back and perhaps encourage or make it easier for her to participate in the group discussion?"

Similarly, circumspect or superficial presentations by group members that reveal little or nothing about their private thoughts and feelings is another form of resistance to participating in the group's therapeutic work. Without the group leader's intervention, the group may not see this behavior as resistance or "hiding out" since the presenter does in fact participate at some level even though she fails to bring up issues that are self-revealing or meaningful. In these situations, it might be helpful to say something like: "Nicole's statements about herself are usually brief and lacking in detail. I'm wondering whether other group members can ask Nicole what's going on for her and how we can encourage her to open up a bit more?"

Some group members present lengthy factual reports that recount external events and circumstances, devoid of feelings or emotional content. This is often indicative of a member who is just going through the motions of being in treatment. Consistent with the group's purpose to help members learn skills to deal with internals (emotions) rather than externals, this type of problem should be addressed whenever it arises and the group leader should role model how best to respond on these occasions. For example, the group leader might say: "Jeff, you've just given the group an extremely detailed account of what happened to you last week, but we've heard very little about how you felt about it or what all this means to you. Is everyone here getting the type of information from Jeff that they need in order to give him helpful feedback? I notice that some of you look distracted and bored. Can someone comment on what's happening here?"

Proselytizing and Hiding Behind the 12-Step Program

Patients who are meaningfully involved in 12-step programs such as AA and NA often add greatly to the richness of the group through the sharing of experiences related to their participation in these programs. However, some of these individuals are intolerant of those who do not embrace the 12-step programs unequivocally. They are quick to proselytize the benefits of 12-step participation, sometimes predicting failure and horrible consequences for others who do not follow the same path. Offering solutions to other members' problems, they may cite AA slogans or passages from the AA "Big Book" rather than engage more meaningfully in the group discussion. They may complain that there is not enough "recovery talk" in the group or that the group format does not conform sufficiently to that of 12-step meetings. Often these patients are deeply threatened by the idea that there may be pathways to recovery other than the one they have chosen. This is particularly problematic if the patient succeeds in polarizing the group along the lines of 12-step versus other approaches to recovery (Vannicelli, 1992; Washton, 2001). A patient's rigid attachment to the 12-step philosophy and refusal to consider anything short of strict adherence to that philosophy often reflects that person's deep-seated fears about the fragility of his own recovery. It appears of utmost importance for these patients to believe that the only way to avoid relapse is to do exactly what they are doing. The therapist can help these patients explore in the group what is so threatening about the idea that different people may choose different pathways to recovery. On a group level, it is important for the leader to support the unique therapeutic value of 12-step programs, but acknowledge that there is no one pathway for recovery that works best for everyone. The leader can then focus the group's attention on the process issue, such as feelings about the split in the group, why this issue stimulates such intense feelings on both sides, and how the conflict affects the safety of the group environment.

FINAL COMMENT

Group therapy can enhance the effectiveness of substance abuse treatment and provides unique therapeutic benefits that individual therapy alone cannot provide. Despite various obstacles that may prevent private practitioners from offering substance abuse groups in their offices, the potential clinical and financial benefits of doing so is potentially significant enough to warrant the investment of time, effort, and resources needed to overcome these obstacles. Setting up and running substance abuse groups is a highly challenging but rewarding task requiring skillful handling of various issues that emerge during different stages of the group process. The therapeutic power of groups is often quite remarkable.

CHAPTER 13

Facilitating Participation in Self-Help Programs

SELF-HELP PARTICIPATION IN EARLY RECOVERY

Self-help participation is widely viewed as a positive force in helping people overcome serious alcohol and drug problems, with or without formal treatment. It provides a subculture that supports recovery and a process for personal development that has no financial barriers. It is not a substitute for treatment and does not absolve therapists of the need to address issues related to alcohol and other drug use at all stages of recovery. However, it can immensely enhance the recovery process, augmenting therapeutic efforts and providing unique contributions beyond the scope of professional services.

Although a number of self-help groups have emerged (e.g., Moderation Management, SMART Recovery, LifeRing, etc.), the 12-step system is the largest in the world, with an immense variety of groups available in most urban environments and at least some activities in many rural communities. The more familiar you are with what goes on in self-help meetings, the more effective you will be in promoting the synergy that makes the combination of treatment and self-help effective.

"Twelve-step programs" is the generic name for the many descendants of Alcoholics Anonymous (AA), which was founded in 1935 and now has about 2 million people who call themselves members. The only requirement for membership is a sincere desire to stop drinking/using. Information about AA and a variety of other self-help programs within and outside the 12-step system can be found on their websites (see Appendix 4). The therapist's task when patients are in the stage of struggling to establish abstinence is to facilitate attendance and incorporate examination of resistance or issues generated by participation into the therapeutic process.

Those who go through an inpatient or residential addiction treatment program are almost always exposed to self-help meetings as part of an effort to help them get meaningfully connected to a recovery support network before discharge. Many of these programs are 12-step based—that is, they incorporate 12-step principles and activities into the programming, but have standard elements of professional treatment such as individual and group sessions and educational activities. Self-help groups by nature do not have a leadership hierarchy or any other objective means of holding the patient accountable. Twelve-step programs are fundamentally "programs of attraction," and you will know your patients are making use of them when they show familiarity with the language and concepts, gradually applying them to their own situations. Try to achieve the fine balance between getting someone over the initial obstacles to engagement and exerting a level of coercion that inspires rebellion. At the same time, reluctance to attending is often but not always a mirror of inner obstacles to addressing the addiction: minimization of the problem, shame about being an alcohol or drug user, and wanting to avoid exposure. Often the addiction problem is quite visible, but the patient is avoiding full recognition. Ask your patient to elaborate on his objections. These are therapeutic issues to explore, with the focused goal of promoting meaningful participation. You can convey to your patient your hope that he will at least give these groups a fair try at some point in the reasonably near future, but ongoing examination of negative feelings about getting involved in self-help programs is important for the treatment.

An example of an issue for examination is the patient's discomfort with the opening ritual in AA meetings in which participants state: "I am an alcoholic/addict." Patients voice many different objections: "I am much better off than those people"; "I don't miss work or other responsibilities; therefore, I am not alcoholic"; "I am not abusive like my father"; "My drinking is not at all like my mother's/father's"; "I only lose control sometimes and could eliminate that if I keep trying to improve my methods." Some of these are charged emotional issues, others require education as part of the therapist's intervention. For example, you can draw a patient out enough to recognize that she has intense and complicated feelings about her mother's drinking, without suggesting that now is the time to explore them in depth. You can then educate your patient to see that there are different kinds of destructive drinking patterns, and the fact that she does not drink to oblivion like her mother does not mean her drinking pattern is benign.

Other hesitations include basic challenges, such as discomfort at being the outsider in a self-help meeting. The palpable sense of group fellowship in self-help meetings can be a deterrent at the outset, where your patient may feel awkward at being the newcomer in a situation in which everyone else appears to know one another. This is a stressful event for most people, and many have bad childhood memories that compound their difficulties in getting to the first few meetings. Labeling the issue (e.g., stranger anxiety) can be helpful, as is providing support by discussing ways to make the situation more manageable. Merely knowing that the therapist will be interested in a report of the patient's initial experiences in meetings will often be encouraging for your patient. Other practical interventions include calling the AA central office to arrange for an escort to the meeting, or identifying "mentors," individuals currently or previously in treatment with you, who are willing to serve this function. It is common for those who balk at initial attendance to move quickly beyond this form of resistance once they find a group or groups they like.

Opposition to the idea of being engulfed by the group is another form of reluctance to attend meetings. It often takes the form of protesting, "I don't want to lose my identity," or some indication that the loss of uniqueness is a key issue. This may be based on the patient's insistence that he is different from those who participate: less addicted, less badly off, less crazy, less deteriorated. As someone in the later stages of recovery once described it, "When I first went to AA I was a star. Over time I learned to join the chorus." Gentle emphasis on the importance of focusing on what can be learned, not on the flaws, may be useful over time. Many patients take time to discover that their own methods are inadequate and they need to become willing to participate in activities that make them uncomfortable in order to make progress.

Another common objection to 12-step meetings is its focus on "that religious stuff." It is important to begin with how the patient understands the spiritual element of AA. The founders of AA are quite explicit that the program is nondenominational and participants need to identify their own "Higher Power," however they understand it. Meetings often reflect their communities and thus can acquire a specific religious tone, particularly if the meeting is held in a church. Many communities offer secular self-help groups (e.g., LifeRing), and religious tones may be diminished in meetings held in hospitals, mental health facilities, schools, and community centers. Patients can often direct one another to meetings in which the religious aspect is less visible.

Attitudes toward spirituality can reflect important clinical themes. Many patients who have had negative experiences with institutionalized religion in childhood find it difficult to distinguish between spirituality and religion. They need help in separating issues concerning harshness and control from a spiritual experience centering on wisdom, love, and compassion. Discomfort with spirituality may also be connected with negative experiences with abusive parental or other authority figures, and the therapist can help the patient distinguish between harsh powers and benevolent ones. For example, one patient's resistance to the spiritual dimension evaporated when she had an insight after months of rebellious feelings: "God is not my father. God is God and my father is my father." Connection to a positive inner force is considered important for healing, no matter how this force is labeled. It is understood that working out one's relationship with a Higher Power takes time, and you can emphasize the dictum "take what you need and leave the rest" while continuing to move the patient forward in an exploration of obstacles.

Social isolation is common in people with addiction problems, and it is also common for patients to announce, "I don't do groups." Patients may need time to discover that going it alone is not working and they must try another path. Dislike of groups in no way precludes benefits from self-help groups; many participants see themselves as misfits and isolates. In the initial engagement phase, you can explore whether the patient would be more comfortable in small meetings or large ones and proceed accordingly. Small meetings may seem less overwhelming, but they also tend to be more attentive to newcomers and may be intrusive in their efforts to welcome them. In larger meetings it is easier for your patient to regulate the distance from others and remain invisible if this seems necessary. Over time, it is important for patients to engage actively, but in early recovery the most important thing is to get them to attend regularly and develop a sense of comfort.

As part of your work, you can elicit a picture of what your patient thinks meetings are like and explore the charged issues. It is important to give permission to be ambivalent. Many meeting participants are enthusiastic and discuss their reservations only in the past tense. This can make it difficult for someone who currently has mixed feelings to feel comfortable. You can cultivate a productive stance by emphasizing "take what you need and leave the rest" and telling patients that if they get only one thing out of a meeting, the trip will be worth it. In the initial stage, your goal is to help them find meetings where they feel at home, where they hear "their story" and to begin to form the relationships that will keep them coming. It is important to provide a place for them to talk about their experiences on a regular basis. This will promote engagement and can raise broader therapeutic issues.

It is important to prepare patients on psychotropic medication for participation in meetings. Although AA is very clear that medication is compatible with recovery, meetings still need to be selected carefully. Hierarchy is minimized in the 12-step system and members may challenge those on medication, despite a clear statement that "no AA member is to play doctor" (Alcoholics Anonymous, 1984). "Double trouble" meetings exist in some communities for patients with co-occurring disorders, but such meetings are not numerous enough to constitute a sturdy support network by themselves. Alternative self-help groups such as LifeRing or SMART Recovery encourage appropriate use of medication. If you work with patients who are more disturbed, it is useful to develop a list of meetings that are more tolerant of eccentric behavior. Such patients should be coached on how to behave in meetings, and they may be too anxious or confused to grasp the social norms of the meeting quickly. The 12-step structure is often beneficial to such patients because it can provide stability without being intrusive.

Patients who use several drugs may wonder whether they should go to AA, NA, CA (Cocaine Anonymous), or some other variant. For those who are receptive to participating in a 12-step program, the first priority is to maximize engagement with the group. Stimulant users, for example, often prefer NA or CA because they feel they are much more likely to hear "their story." It is important to pick a place to start, and meetings of a group whose members are of a socioeconomic status similar to that of the patient, in the neighborhood of home or work, are often more comfortable for a beginner. For some, this may be more important than drug of choice. Others may prefer to start with meetings far from their usual territory to avoid recognition. Patient preferences may evolve quickly, as they "shop" for a "home meeting" they would like to attend regularly. They may come to dislike the "wired" feeling in some NA or CA meetings and settle into AA because of its calmer atmosphere. Although it is possible in a specific community to find NA meetings with many members who have long-term sobriety, AA meetings may have greater stability simply because they have a longer history.

You will be much more effective in connecting people to the self-help system if you have gone to local meetings yourself and have read the literature of the 12-step system or an alternative group. Contact information is included in the website list in Appendix 4. Open meetings are for anyone; closed meetings are for AA members. You can introduce yourself by name only, as a guest, or as a therapist. Notice the feelings you have in preparing to attend the meeting and multiply by 10 or more to gain a picture of what your patient might be feeling. Watch the ebb and flow of your feelings throughout the meeting. Observe the group process and reflect on the similarities and differences between this and a professionally led therapy group. What elements are strengths? What are the limits? When speakers share painful experiences, how are they comforted, given that there is no cross talk during the meeting? What is the purpose of the "no cross talk" rule? If possible, ask a recovering friend or colleague to take to you a favorite meeting. It is important for you to witness what makes this system generate such powerful enthusiasm and gratitude from so many thousands of people. The sense of vigor and fellowship is a powerful force that can augment the success of therapeutic intervention, and it is regrettable that some therapists adopt a competitive stance.

It is important to develop an understanding based on a variety of meetings, because they all have different "personalities." In this way, you will become better equipped to address the resistances patients will offer. Alternative self-help groups are growing and are certainly a fine resource. LifeRing is an example of an alternative self-help group that is expanding throughout the country. It is an abstinence-oriented group that stresses peer support with feedback in a secular setting. The program features an "open architecture," in which members structure their own individual recovery programs in a cooperative environment. There are no steps or sponsors, and groups include people whose addiction is to alcohol, drugs, or both. Unlike some other alternative groups, it does not adopt a competitive stance toward the 12-step system, and some patients are quite comfortable attending both.

Alternative groups are growing in number, but they usually do not offer a wide range of meetings, either in frequency or location. This may lessen their effectiveness for patients who need greater immersion. Those who are more stable may do well with a once-a-week LifeRing meeting, for example, but those trying to settle down their chaotic lives can benefit from more comprehensive support. You should encourage your patient to put together a firm structure from a variety of sources, especially during high-risk times.

SELF-HELP PARTICIPATION IN ONGOING AND LATER-STAGE RECOVERY

It is important to continue to monitor self-help participation, as it is a catalyst for the emergence of many issues important to the therapeutic process. "Telling your story" in a 12-step meeting can be viewed as a form of meditation that allows a person to view his life experiences from a position of greater awareness. The life story changes considerably as the person progresses in recovery and integrates new insights. Listening to many different stories will elicit a wide range of feelings in your patient, and exploring reactions can be quite productive:

Audrey had a tumultuous period of early recovery when she first stopped drinking, and finally settled down into a more stable state. After a while, she appeared to miss the excitement in her life and complained of being bored in her meetings. The therapist asked her to describe a recent meeting in which she felt bored, and it became apparent that "bored" was a blanket covering some difficult emotions. The speaker at the meeting had alluded to a history of childhood abuse and had stimulated Audrey's memories on taboo topics. Audrey had been accustomed to dissociating through her drinking and drug use, and she struggled to tune out during the meetings. The need to deal with her feelings in a new way became more pressing as she became invested in her sobriety. In the course of discussion with her therapist, she recognized that boredom represented an effort to turn off feeling states that made her anxious. In work with her therapist, she produced the image of a boat steadily riding the waves as a symbol of how she would like to be able to relate to her feelings.

In the relapse prevention stage, it is premature to explore child abuse issues in depth, but it is most appropriate to put the issue of learning to deal with feeling states in a new way near the top of the therapeutic agenda. Meetings, with their familiar and safe structure, can be occasions for patients to listen with openness and observe the ebb and flow of their feeling states. Meetings are a good vehicle for working on the concept of tolerating feelings without having to act. Patients will also bring you a variety of insights gleaned from listening to other speakers.

Finding a sponsor is a key element in successful engagement and fruitful participation in AA (Alcoholics Anonymous, 1983). A sponsor is an experienced recovering member who acts as an advisor, guide, or teacher on how to work a program of recovery. Research indicates that finding a sponsor is one indicator of engagement in AA that is associated with positive outcomes. A participant should be encouraged to find a sponsor quickly and chose someone with whom she can feel comfortable. Sponsors can be changed to meet evolving needs in recovery, so the commitment can be circumscribed and your patient can be encouraged to change sponsors if appropriate. Newcomers are encouraged to select someone with a year or more of sobriety, who appears to be enjoying sobriety. The sponsor should also be someone who is not an object of sexual or other interest that might distract from the primary purpose. Sponsors vary greatly in how they interpret this role; their involvement may range from making suggestions to attempting to control your patient's decisions.

Research on AA participation has shown that working with a sponsor is one of the signs of successful affiliation that is associated with improvement (Brown, Seraganian, Tremblay, & Annis, 2002; Humphreys, 2003; Kaskutas, Bond, & Humphreys, 2002; Kelly, McKellar, & Moos, 2003; Kelly & Moos, 2003; Longabaugh, 2003; Longabaugh, Wirtz, Zweben, & Stout, 1998; McKellar, Stewart, & Humphreys, 2003; Morganstern et al., 2003; Morgenstern, Labouvie, McCrady, Kahler, & Frey, 1997; Owen et al., 2003; Staines et al., 2003; Tucker, Vuchinich, & Rippens, 2004). The sponsor relationship can present a difficult clinical challenge to therapists. Triads are inherently difficult, and the relationship to the 12-step system and the sponsor can be intense. It is crucial that the therapist have a good understanding of stages of recovery and the range of healthy sponsor relationships in order to determine what constitutes an appropriate intervention. Patients certainly can chose sponsors who bring out some of the worst of their authority conflicts, and it is important address these situations without getting drawn into an unresolved family drama.

The therapist must distinguish between a relationship that is pathological by any standards, and one based on assumptions that differ from the therapist's orientation. Stephanie Brown (1985) notes that it is important for therapists to appreciate the patient's need to maintain a behavioral focus on early recovery. Resistance to insight-oriented work that stirs up anxiety may be adaptive for the patient who has not consolidated an abstinent lifestyle. Statements and attitudes that appear to run counter to the therapy may be manifested as a division between the sponsor and the therapist. Timing traps may be unrecognized, because a patient who has been abstinent for 3–6 months can look a great deal better and appear less vulnerable than he is. The therapist may wish to resume "real therapy" and explore charged issues, and the patient may be unable to articulate concerns or may feel caught in the middle. Thus, it is important for the therapist to frame therapeutic tasks but give the patient latitude to control the pace.

Both patients and therapists have concerns about how long and how frequently patients need to attend meetings. The answer is, as long as it takes. Part of the power of the self-help system is that patients replace their relationships with alcohol and other drug users with new friendships formed within the groups. This gives an ongoing social structure in which they do not have to drink and use in order to belong. The social factors that keep many engaged for years after giving up drinking or using is an actual risk and may progress to include activities only tangentially related to recovery. Members may form important new friendships and expand their interests in a variety of directions once they become involved in this community.

Some question whether the meetings themselves can become an "addiction," and the answer lies in the presence or absence of adverse consequences. The therapist needs to help the patient explore the balance of benefits and detrimental factors, keeping in mind that premature disengagement is more common and more hazardous. Patients in their first year of recovery, who have not resolved their shame and guilt issues, may wish to regard their addiction as "the problem I used to have" and discontinue without much self-examination. Reduction or elimination of meeting attendance is often a reliable indicator of relapse risk. You should ask the patient how she made the decision to disengage. Was the decision planned, impulsive, or not even conscious? Ask how your patient expects to replace the recovery resources available within the self-help system. Once their time is no longer consumed with focusing on their addiction, many patients become involved in recreational, social, or religious activities that are incompatible with drug use and may not need meetings as a form of social support. However, there are still recovery tasks related to the psychological processing of issues related to the addiction.

Total disengagement usually eliminates an arena where these issues remain on the table and can be continuously explored. It is not necessary for all patients to maintain regular and frequent attendance in order to secure their recovery, but it is useful to remain in sufficient contact to maintain the sense of affiliation. This will ensure that issues around the addiction do not become totally submerged and that patients can feel they are returning to a comfortable base when a life crisis occurs.

FINAL COMMENT

Self-help programs are powerful forces for change that can enormously augment the therapeutic work. They supply a rich subculture that supports the recovery process in a variety of ways. For patients in early recovery, these programs offer an essential time structure and specific strategies for achieving abstinence. They offer a place where patients can feel less dreadfully unique and shameful, and more understood. Many are drawn by the earthy honesty that has been missing from their lives. As recovery progresses and participation in self-help continues, patients have ongoing access to a program for personal development that does not have financial barriers and is complementary to the therapeutic process. They learn, not only from telling their own stories and seeing them evolve, but by hearing the life stories of others who have struggled with many of the same issues. Patients who are working the steps in earnest often make good psychotherapy patients, as the process is quite similar despite the differences in the way it is described. Therapists who become familiar with the philosophy and practices of self-help programs are in the best position to enhance their work with addicted patients.

Appendices

Self-Administered Patient Questionnaire

HISTORY OF SUBSTANCE USE

Substance	Age at first use	Time since last use	Currently a "problem"?	Ever a "problem"?	Longest time able to remain abstinent from this drug when you were deliberately trying to stop using it
Cocaine powder					
Crack cocaine					
Methamphetamine "crystal"					
Alcohol					
Heroin					
Methadone					
Prescription narcotics/painkillers (Vicodin, Percoset, codeine, OxyContin, etc.)					

Marijuana/hashish					
Benzodiazepines (Valium, Xanax, Ativan, Klonopin, etc.)					
Barbiturates					
Hallucinogens (LSD, mescaline, psilosybin, etc.)					
"Ecstasy" (MDMA)					
Amyl nitrate ("snappers")					
"Special K" (ketamine)					
PCP ("angel dust")					
GHB ("G")					
Rohypnol ("roofies")					
Nitrous oxide					
Other (specify):					

Alcohol and Drug Use during the *Past Week*

	Substances used	Amounts used
Today		
Yesterday		
2 days ago		
3 days ago		
4 days ago		
5 days ago		
6 days ago		

SUBSTANCE USE PROFILE

1. Have you ever found yourself thinking a great deal about alcohol/drugs or being preoccupied with using?
   [ ] Yes [ ] No

2. Have you ever experienced cravings or a strong compulsion to use alcohol/drugs?
   [ ] Yes [ ] No

3. Have you ever had difficulty in reducing or totally stopping your alcohol/drug use?
   [ ] Yes [ ] No [ ] Never tried to stop

4. Have you ever used more frequently and/or in larger amounts than you intended to?
   [ ] Yes [ ] No

5. Have you ever been under the influence of alcohol/drugs while driving a car or operating other dangerous machinery?
   [ ] Yes [ ] No

6. Has alcohol/drug use ever caused you to miss days of work and/or impaired your productivity, effectiveness, or judgment at work?
   [ ] Yes [ ] No

7. Have you ever become less sociable, socially withdrawn, or isolated as a result of using alcohol/drugs?
   [ ] Yes [ ] No

8. Have you ever given up recreational activities, exercise, or other healthy pursuits because of alcohol/drug use?
   [ ] Yes [ ] No

9. Has your self-esteem or self-image ever been negatively affected by your alcohol/drug use?
   [ ] Yes [ ] No

10. Have you ever engaged in "STD-risky" sexual behavior, such as having sexual encounters with unknown partners or having unprotected sex with someone other than your primary mate while under the influence of alcohol/drugs?
    [ ] Yes [ ] No

11. Have relationships with a mate, family members, or significant others been damaged by your alcohol/drug use?
    [ ] Yes [ ] No

12. Have you ever used alcohol/drugs to "medicate" yourself for depression, anxiety, or other negative moods?
    [ ] Yes [ ] No

13. Do you feel a need for professional help to deal with your alcohol/drug problem?

[ ] Yes [ ] No [ ] Not sure

Total number of "Yes" responses _____

CONSEQUENCES OF ALCOHOL AND DRUG USE

Psychological: [ ] irritability, short temper [ ] self-hate [ ] depression [ ] suicidal thoughts or actions [ ] homicidal thoughts or actions [ ] paranoia, suspiciousness [ ] memory problems [ ] anxiety or panic attacks [ ] other (describe):

Sexual: [ ] loss of sexual desire [ ] sexual obsession [ ] sex with strangers [ ] AIDS-risky sex [ ] inability to achieve orgasm [ ] inability to achieve or sustain erection [ ] other (describe):

Relationships: [ ] arguments with mate [ ] violence with mate [ ] breakup of marriage or relationship [ ] loss of friends [ ] arguments with parents or siblings [ ] other (describe):

Job or financial: [ ] job loss or threatened job loss [ ] lateness or absenteeism [ ] less productive at work [ ] in debt [ ] falling behind in paying bills [ ] other (describe):

Legal: [ ] arrested for possession of illegal drugs [ ] arrested for sale of illicit drugs [ ] arrested for DWI [ ] other (describe):

TREATMENT HISTORY

Inpatient Addiction Treatment (in a Hospital, Detox, Rehab, or Residential Program)

Facility name	Reason for admission	Admission date (mo/yr)	Length of stay	Results (completed/ dropped out)

Outpatient Addiction Treatment (in a Clinic or Program)

Facility name	Reason for admission	Admission date (mo/yr)	Length of stay	Results (completed/ dropped out)

POSITIVE EFFECTS OF SUBSTANCE USE

Please check all positive effects you have experienced from using alcohol/drugs, even if presently you no longer get these positive effects when you use.

[ ] more relaxed [ ] less anxious [ ] less depressed [ ] better able to have fun [ ] increased sexual desire [ ] better able to perform sexually [ ] easier to meet sexual partners [ ] more talkative [ ] less anxious or awkward in social situations [ ] less critical of myself [ ] more energy [ ] less angry [ ] more productive at home or work [ ] other positive effects (specify):

PHYSICAL PROBLEMS RELATED TO SUBSTANCE USE

[ ] sleep problems [ ] poor nutrition [ ] abnormal blood test results [ ] heart or circulation problems [ ] liver problems [ ] stomach or digestion problems [ ] vomiting [ ] bleeding [ ] seizures [ ] shaking [ ] panic anxiety attacks [ ] paranoia [ ] HIV [ ] hepatitis C [ ] other infections or diseases (specify) [ ] withdrawal symptoms when you have tried to stop using (specify) [ ] other medical or physical problems (specify):

SEXUAL BEHAVIOR AND SUBSTANCE USE

Has your alcohol or drug use *ever* been associated with sex? [ ] Yes (answer all questions below) [ ] No (stop here)

When using substances do you get involved in (check all that apply): [ ] compulsive masturbation [ ] sex with prostitutes/escorts [ ] strip clubs [ ] porno movies [ ] telephone sex [ ] Internet pornography [ ]sadomasochistic sex [ ] asphyxiation [ ] sex with transvestites [ ] other (specify):

Approximately how often does your substance use involve sexual thoughts, feelings, fantasies, or behaviors? [ ] always [ ] almost always [ ] most of the time [ ] sometimes [ ] almost never [ ] never

1. Does your substance use stimulate your sex drive and fantasies?

2. Does your substance use impair your sexual performance (e.g., prevent orgasm and/or erection) ?

3. Are you more likely to have sex (e.g., intercourse, oral sex, masturbation, etc.) when using substances?

274

4. Are you more likely to have sex with a prostitute, pickup, other unknown partner, or someone besides your spouse or primary mate when using substances?

5. Has your use of substances increased your preoccupation and obsession with sex or made your sex drive abnormally high?

6. Do you think your substance use is so strongly associated with sex that the two are difficult for you to separate from one another?

7. In prior attempts to stop using substances, have sexual thoughts, feelings, and/ or fantasies perpetuated your drug use and contributed to relapse?

8. Are you concerned that if you stop using this substance, sex will not be as interesting or pleasurable for you?

9. Have sexual fantasies or desires ever increased your chances of using substances?

10. If you try to stop using substances, are you concerned that your sexual fantasies or desires will make it harder for you to stop ?

11. If you are heterosexual, have you experienced homosexual fantasies or engaged in sex with a same-sex partner while under the influence of substances?

12. Are you less likely to practice safe sex under the influence of substances (e.g., not use condoms, be less careful about whom you choose as a sex partner, etc.)?

13. Has your sexual behavior under the influence of substances caused you to feel that you are sexually perverted or have a sex problem?

14. Prior to getting involved with substances, were you ever concerned that your sex drive was abnormally high or that you were preoccupied or obsessed with sex?

15. Prior to getting involved with substances, were you ever concerned that your sex drive was abnormally low or that your sexual performance was inadequate?

16. Do you feel that your treatment should address substance-related sexual issues?

10 Tips for Cutting Down on Your Drinking

1. **Write down your specific reasons for changing your drinking habits.** Is it to improve your health and avoid illness, to sleep better, to feel better about yourself, or to get along better with family or friends? Whatever your reasons, write them down.

2. **Set a realistic goal and time frame.** Make sure that you choose a target level and frequency of alcohol consumption that all but guarantees that you will experience no negative consequences from your drinking. For example: "I will have no more than one drink with dinner, no more often than three times a week, and not go above that drinking level for at least 3 months." Similarly, if you choose to not drink at all for a while, set a firm quitting date and then try to maintain abstinence for at least several weeks or months.

3. **Keep a drinking diary.** Keep a daily log of every drink you have for a period of 3–4 weeks to monitor how well you stick to your goal.

4. **Drink slowly.** Sip your drinks and space them at least 1 hour apart. Drink soda, water, or juice after an alcoholic beverage. Don't drink on an empty stomach. Eat before you drink and between drinks.

5. **Designate certain nondrinking days.** Choose a day or two or three each week when you will not drink at all. Or try not drinking at all for an entire week. Observe how you feel physically and emotionally on your nondrinking days.

6. **Practice drink refusal skills.** You do not have to drink when other people drink. You do not have to accept a drink when it is given to you. Practice ways

to say no politely. For example, you can tell people that you just feel much better when you drink less or not at all.

7. **Avoid temptations and pressures to drink.** Stay away from people who drink a lot and from bars or parties where there is strong pressure to drink. Avoid places where you previously drank a lot ,because they can stimulate your desire to drink excessively again.

8. **Don't drink when you are emotionally upset.** Do not drink when you are angry, sad, lonely, frustrated, hurt, anxious, or generally having a bad day. Try talking things out with a trusted friend or relative rather than numbing your upset with alcohol.

9. **Get support and stay active.** Ask family members and close friends for support to help you change your drinking habits. Keep busy to avoid boredom.

10. **Don't give up!** Drinking habits are not always easy to change. Don't get discouraged. Persistence is the key to success.

Inventory of "Triggers" for Alcohol and Drug Use

SITUATIONAL TRIGGERS
(PEOPLE, PLACES, THINGS)

- Bars
- Clubs
- Parties
- Dealers
- Drug paraphernalia
- Hidden "stashes" of drugs/paraphernalia in your home, car, office, clothing
- Other people who abuse alcohol/drugs—family members, friends, coworkers, sex partners
- Certain anniversaries, holidays, celebrations, etc.
- Having a lot of cash on hand (e.g., payday)
- ATM card
- Sex partners (e.g., escorts, prostitutes, pickups)
- Pornography

INTERNAL (EMOTIONAL) TRIGGERS

- Anger
- Frustration
- Boredom

- Depression
- Hopelessness
- Helplessness
- Anxiety
- Stress
- Uncertainty
- Loneliness
- Sadness
- Exhaustion
- Excitement
- Joy
- Sexual arousal

CHEMICAL TRIGGERS

- Alcohol
- Any other mood-altering drugs of abuse
- Sedating antihistamines, cough medicines, sleep remedies
- Sleeping pills, tranquilizers
- Prescription painkillers (narcotics)
- Large doses of caffeine
- Nicotine

Substance Abuse Websites

Addiction Technology Transfer Center
www.nattc.org

Addiction Training Center–University of California, San Diego
www.atc.ucsd.edu

Addiction Treatment Forum
www.atforum.com

Alcoholics Anonymous
www.alcoholics-anonymous.org

Alcohol Medical Scholars Program
www.alcoholmedicalscholars.org

American Academy of Addiction Psychiatry
www.aaap.org

American Association for the Treatment of Opioid Dependence (AATOD)
www.aatod.org

American Bar Association
Standing Committee on Substance Abuse
www.abanet.org/subabuse

American Psychological Association
The Addictions Newsletter
www.kumc.edu/addictions_newsletter/

American Psychological Association College of Professional Psychology
Certificate of Proficiency in the Treatment of Alcohol
and Other Substance Use Disorders
www.apa.org/college

American Society of Addiction Medicine
www.asam.org

Brown University Center for Alcohol and Addiction Studies–Brown University
www.caas.brown.edu

Buprenorphine
www.buprenorphine.samhsa.gov

College on Problems of Drug Dependence
www.cpdd.vcu.edu/

DanceSafe
www.dancesafe.org

Debtors Anonymous
www.debtorsanonymous.org

Drug Evaluation Network System (DENS)
www.densonline.org

Drug Policy Alliance
www.drugpolicy.org

Dual Disorders
www.treatment.org/Topics.dual.html

Dual Recovery Anonymous
www.draonline.org/

East Bay Community Recovery Project
www.ebcrp.org

Faces & Voices of Recovery
www.facesandvoicesofrecovery.org

Gamblers Anonymous
www.gamblersanonymous.org

Hazelden
www.hazelden.org

Institute for Research on Pathological Gambling
and Related Disorders–Harvard
www.hms.harvard.edu/doa/institute/

Institute of Behavioral Research at Texas Christian University
www.ibr.tcu.edu

Integrated Substance Abuse Programs–UCLA
www.uclaisap.org

Join Together
www.jointogether.org

LifeRing
www.unhooked.com

Marijuana Anonymous
www.marijuana-anonymous.org

Matrix Institute on Addictions
www.matrixinstitute.org

Mothers Against Drunk Driving (MADD)
www.madd.org

Motivational Interviewing Network of Trainers
www.motivationalinterview.org

Narcotics Anonymous
www.na.org

National Advocates for Pregnant Women
www.advocatesforpregnantwomen.org

National Association of Alcohol and Drug Abuse Counselors
(NAADAC)
www.naadac.org

National Association of State Alcohol/Drug Abuse Directors (NASADAD)
www.nasadad.org

National Center on Addiction and Substance Abuse at Columbia University
(CASA)
www.casacolumbia.org

National Clearinghouse for Alcohol and Drug Information
www.health.org

National Council on Alcoholism and Drug Dependence
www.ncadd.org

National Institute on Alcohol Abuse and Alcoholism (NIAAA)
www.niaaa.nih.gov

National Institute on Drug Abuse
www.nida.nih.gov

Office of National Drug Control Policy (ONDCP)
www.whitehousedrugpolicy.gov

Partnership for a Drug-Free America
www.drugfreeamerica.org

Recovery Network
www.recoverynetwork.com

Recovery Options
www.recoveryoptions.us

Sober.com
www.sober.com

Substance Abuse and Mental Health Services Administration (SAMHSA)
www.samhsa.gov

SMART Recovery
www.smartrecovery.org

Sober Housing
www.soberhouses.com

The Other Bar
www.otherbar.org

Therapeutic Communities of America
www.therapeuticcommunitiesofamerica.org

Treatment Improvement Exchange
Co-Occurring Dialogues Electronic Discussion List
treatment.org/Topics/DualDialogues.html

Treatment Research Institute (TRI)
www.tresearch.org

Women for Sobriety, Inc.
www.womenforsobriety.org

References

Alcoholics Anonymous World Services, Inc. (1976). *Alcoholics Anonymous: The story of how many thousands of men and women have recovered from alcoholism* (3rd ed.) New York: Author.

Alcoholics Anonymous World Services, Inc. (1983). *Questions and answers on sponsorship.* New York: Author.

Alcoholics Anonymous World Services, Inc. (1984). *The AA member—medications and other drugs. Report from a group of physicians in AA.* New York: Author.

Allen J. P., & Columbus M. (1995). *Assessing alcohol problems: A guide for clinicians and researchers* (Treatment Handbook Series 4, NIH Publication No. 95-3745). Bethesda, MD: National Institute on Alcoholism and Alcohol Abuse.

American Psychiatric Association. (1994). *Diagnostic and statistical manual of mental disorders* (4th ed.). Washington, DC: Author.

Berg, I. K., & Miller, S. D. (1992). *Working with the problem drinker: A solution-focused approach.* New York: Norton.

Biernacki, P. (1986). *Pathways from heroin addiction: Recovery without treatment.* Philadelphia: Temple University Press.

Bierut, L. J., Dinwiddie, S. H., Begleiter, H., Crowe, R. R., Hesselbrock, V., Nurnberger, J. I., et al. (1998). Familial transmission of substance dependence: Alcohol, marijuana, cocaine, and habitual smoking. *Archives of General Psychiatry, 55,* 982–988.

Blume, S. B., & Lesieur, H. R. (1987). Pathological gambling in cocaine abusers. In A. Washton (Ed.), *Cocaine: A clinician's handbook* (pp. 208–213). New York: Guilford Press.

Bouza, C., Magro, A., Munoz, A., & Amate, J. M. (2004). Efficacy and safety of naltrexone and acamprosate in the treatment of alcohol dependence: A systematic review. *Addiction, 99,* 811–828.

Bovasso, G. (2001). Cannabis abuse as a risk factor for depressive symptoms. *American Journal of Psychiatry, 158,* 2033–2037.

Brook, D. W., & Spitz, H. I. (Eds.). (2002). *The group therapy of substance abuse.* Binghamton, NY: Haworth Medical Press.

Brown, S. (1985). *Treating the alcoholic: A developmental model of recovery.* New York: Wiley Inter-Science.

Brown, S., & Lewis, V. (1999). *The alcoholic family in recovery: A developmental model.* New York: Guilford Press.

Brown, T. G., Seraganian, P., Tremblay, J., & Annis, H. (2002). Matching substance abuse aftercare treatments to client characteristics. *Addictive Behavior, 27,* 585–604.

Carnes, P. (1991). *Don't call it love: Recovering from sexual addiction.* New York: Bantam.

Carroll, K. M. (1998). *A cognitive-behavioral approach: Treating cocaine addiction* (Vol. 1). Rockville, MD: U.S. Department of Health and Human Services.

Carroll, K. M. (1999). Behavioral and cognitive-behavioral treatments. In B. S. McCrady & E. E. Epstein (Eds.), *Addictions: A comprehensive guidebook* (pp. 250–267). New York: Oxford University Press.

Carroll, K. M., Libby, B., Sheehan, J., & Hyland, N. (2001). Motivational interviewing to enhance treatment initiation in substance abusers: An effectiveness study. *American Journal on Addictions, 10,* 335–339.

Connors, G. J., Donovan, D. M., & DiClemente, C. C. (2001). *Substance abuse treatment and the stages of change: Selecting and planning interventions.* New York: Guilford Press.

Daley, D. C. (2000). *Relapse prevention workbook: For recovering alcoholics and drug-dependent persons.* Holmes Beach, FL: Learning Publications.

Daley, D. C., & Lis, J. A. (1995). Relapse prevention: Intervention strategies for mental health clients with comorbid addictive disorders. In A. M. Washton (Ed.), *Psychotherapy and substance abuse: A practitioner's handbook* (pp. 243–263). New York: Guilford Press.

Denning, P. (2000). *Practicing harm reduction psychotherapy: An alternative approach to addictions.* New York: Guilford Press.

Denning, P., Little, J., & Glickman, A. (2004). *Over the influence: The harm reduction guide for managing drugs and alcohol.* New York: Guilford Press.

DiClemente, C. C. (2003). *Addiction and change: How addictions develop and addicted people recover.* New York: Guilford Press.

Dodes, L. M., & E. J. K. (1991). Individual psychodynamic psychotherapy. In S. I. Miller (Ed.), *Clinical textbook of addictive disorders* (pp. 391–405). New York: Guilford Press.

Dole, V. (1988). Implication of methadone maintenance for theories of narcotic addiction. *Journal of the American Medical Association, 260,* 3025–3029.

Dole, V., & Nyswander, M. (1967). Heroin addiction: A metabolic disease. *Archives of Internal Medicine, 20,* 19–24.

Dole, V. P., & Nyswander, M. M. (1965). A medical treatment for diacetylmorphine (heroin) addiction. *Journal of the American Medical Association, 193,* 646–650.

Drake, R. E., Essock, S. M., Shaner, A., Carey, K. B., Minkoff, K., Kola, L., et al. (2001). Implementing dual diagnosis services for clients with severe mental illness. *Psychiatric Services, 52,* 469–476.

Earle, R., & Crow, G. (1989). *Lonely all the time: Recognizing, understanding, and overcoming sex addiction, for addicts and codependents.* New York: Simon & Schuster.

Eisenhandler, J., & Drucker, E. (1993). Opioid dependency among the subscribers of a New York area private insurance plan. *Journal of the American Medical Association, 269,* 2890–2891.

Elder, I. R. (1990). *Conducting group therapy with addicts.* Brandenton, FL: Human Services Institute.

Evans, K., & Sullivan, J. M. (1995). *Treating addicted survivors of trauma.* New York: Guilford Press.

Fairburn, C., & Brownell, K. D. (Eds.). (2001). *Eating disorders and obesity: A comprehensive handbook.* New York: Guilford Press.

Fertig, J. B., & Allen, J. P. (1995). *Alcohol and tobacco: From basic science to clinical practice.* Washington, DC: U.S. Government Printing Office.

Fiore, M. C., Bailey, W. C., Cohen, S., Dorfman, S. F., Goldstein, M., Gritz, E. R., et al. (2000). *Treating tobacco use and dependence: Clinical practice guidelines.* Rockville, MD: U.S. Public Health Service.

Flores, P. (1988). *Group psychotherapy with addicted populations.* New York: Haworth.

Flowers, L. K., & Zweben, J. E. (1996). The dream interview method in recovery-oriented psychotherapy. *Journal of Substance Abuse Treatment, 13,* 99–105.

Flowers, L. K., & Zweben, J. E. (1998). The changing role of "using dreams" in addiction recovery. *Journal of Substance Abuse Treatment, 15,* 193–200.

Galanter, M. (1994). Network therapy for the office practitioner. In M. Galanter & H. D. Kleber (Eds.), *Textbook of substance abuse treatment.* Washington, DC: American Psychiatric Press.

Gawin, F. H., & Kleber, H. D. (1986). Abstinence symptomatology and psychiatric diagnosis in cocaine abusers. *Archives of General Psychiatry, 43,* 107–113.

Gerstley, L., McLellan, A. T., Alterman, A. I., Woody, G. E., Luborsky, L., & Prout, M. (1989). Ability to form an alliance with the therapist: A possible marker of prognosis for patients with antisocial personality disorder. *American Journal of Psychiatry, 146,* 508–512.

Giannini, A. J., & Slaby, A. E. (Eds.). (1989). *Drugs of abuse.* Oradell, NJ: Medical Economics.

Gold, M. S. (1998). The pharmacology of marijuana. In A. W. Graham, T. K. Schultz, & B. B. Wilford (Eds.), *Principles of addiction medicine* (2nd ed., pp. 147–152). Chevy Chase, MD: American Society of Addiction Medicine.

Gorski, T. (1988). *The staying sober workbook: Exercise manual.* Independence, MO: Independence Press.

Gorski, T., & Miller, M. (1986). *Staying sober: A guide for relapse prevention.* Independence, MO: Independence Press.

Graham, A. W., & Schultz, T. K. (Eds.). (1998). *Principles of addiction medicine* (2nd ed.). Chevy Chase, MD: American Society of Addiction Medicine.

Graham, A. W., Schultz, T. K., Mayo-Smith, M., & Ries, R. K. (2003). *Principles of addiction medicine* (3rd ed.). Chevy Chase, MD: American Society of Addiction Medicine.

Green, B. E., & Ritter, C. (2000). Marijuana use and depression. *Journal of Health and Social Behavior, 41,* 40–49.

Greenstein, R. A., Arendt, I. C., McLellan, A. T., O'Brien, C. P., & Evans, B. (1984). Naltrexone: A clinical perspective. *Journal of Clinical Psychiatry, 45,* 25–28.

Halpern, H. M. (1976). *Cutting loose: An adult's guide to coming to terms with your parents.* New York: Fireside.

Hser, Y.-I., Hoffman, V., Grella, C., & Anglin, M. D. (2001). A 33-year follow-up of narcotics addicts. *Archives of General Psychiatry, 58,* 503–508.

Humphreys, K. (2003). Alcoholics Anonymous and 12-step alcoholism treatment programs. *Recent Developments in Alcoholism, 16,* 149–164.

Humphreys, K., Noke, J. M., & Moos, R. H. (1996). Recovering substance abuse staff members' beliefs about addiction. *Journal of Substance Abuse Treatment, 13*(1), 75–78.

Hunt, W. A., Barnett, L. W., & Branch, L. G. (1971). Relapse rates in addiction programs. *Journal of Clinical Psychology, 27,* 455–456.

Imhof, J., Hirsch, R., & Terenzi, R. E. (1983). Countertansferential and attitudinal considerations in the treatment of drug abuse and addiction. *International Journal of Addictions, 18,* 491–510.

Imhof, J. E. (1995). Overcoming countertransference and other attitudinal barriers in the treatment of substance abuse. In A. M. Washton (Ed.), *Psychotherapy and substance abuse: A practitioner's handbook* (pp. 3–22). New York: Guilford Press.

Institute of Medicine. (1990). *Broadening the base of treatment for alcohol problems.* Washington, DC: National Academy Press.

Jellinek, E. M. (1960). *The disease concept of alcoholism.* New Brunswick, NJ: Hillhouse Press.

Kadden, R., Carroll, K., Donovan, D., Cooney, N., Monti, P., Abrams, D., Litt, M., & Hester, R. (Eds.). (1995). *Cognitive-behavioral coping skills therapy manual.* Rockville, MD: U.S. Department of Health and Human Services.

Kaskutas, L. A., Bond, J., & Humphreys, K. (2002). Social networks as mediators of the effect of Alcoholics Anonymous. *Addiction, 97,* 891–900.

Kaufman, E. (1994). *Psychotherapy of addicted persons.* New York: Guilford Press.

Kelly, J. F., McKellar, J. D., & Moos, R. (2003). Major depression in patients with substance use disorders: Relationship to 12-step self-help involvement and substance use outcomes. *Addiction, 98,* 499–508.

Kelly, J. F., & Moos, R. (2003). Dropout from 12-step self-help groups: Prevalence, predictors, and counteracting treatment influences. *Journal of Substance Abuse Treatment, 24,* 241–250.

Kendler, K. S., & Prescott, C. A. (1998). Cannabis use, abuse and dependence in a population-based sample of female twins. *American Journal of Psychiatry, 155,* 1016–1022.

Kessler, R. C., Crum, R. M., Warner, L. A., Nelson, C. B., Schulenberg, J., & Anthony, J. C. (1997). Lifetime co-occurrence of DSM-III-R alcohol abuse and dependence with other psychiatric disorders in the National Comorbidity Survey. *Archives of General Psychiatry, 54,* 313–321.

Kessler, R. C., McGonagle, K. A., Zhao, S., Nelson, C. B., Hughes, M., Eshleman, S., et al. (1994). Lifetime and 12-month prevalence of DSM-III-R psychiatric disorders in the United States. *Archives of General Psychiatry, 51,* 8–19.

Kessler, R. C., Nelson, C. B., & McGonagle, K. A. (1996). The epidemiology of co-occurring addictive and mental disorders: Implications for prevention and service utilization. *American Journal of Orthopsychiatry, 66,* 17–31.

Kessler, R. C., Sonnega, A., Bromet, E., Hughes, M., & Nelson, C. B. (1995). Posttraumatic stress disorder in the National Comorbidity Survey. *Archives of General Psychiatry, 52*(12), 1048–1060.

Khantzian, E. J. (1981). Some treatment implications of the ego and self disturbances in alcoholism. In M. H. Bean & N. E. Zinberg (Eds.), *Dynamic approaches to the understanding and treatment of alcoholism* (pp. 163–193). New York: Macmillan.

Khantzian, E. J. (1997). The self-medication hypothesis of substance use disorders: A reconsideration and recent applications. *Harvard Review of Psychiatry, 4,* 231–244.

Khantzian, E. J., Halliday, K. S., & McAuliffe, W. E. (1990). *Addiction and the vulnerable self: Modified dynamic group therapy for substance abusers.* New York: Guilford Press.

Kiefer, F., Jahn, H., Tarnaske, T., Helwig, H., Briken, P., Holzbach, R., et al. (2003). Comparing and combining naltrexone and acamprosate in relapse prevention of alcoholism. *Archives of General Psychiatry, 60,* 92–99.

Koob, G. F. (2000). Neurobiology of addiction: Toward the development of new therapies. *Annals of the New York Academy of Sciences, 909,* 170–185.

Koob, G. F., & Le Moal, M. (2001). Drug addiction, dysregulation of reward, and allostasis. *Neuropsychopharmacology, 24,* 97–129.

Kosten, T. R., Fontana, A., Sernyak, M. J., & Rosenheck, R. (2000). Benzodiazepine use in posttraumatic stress disorder among veterans with substance abuse. *Journal of Nervous and Mental Disease, 188,* 454–459.

Krystal, H. (1988). *Integration and self healing: Affect, trauma, alexithymia.* Hillsdale, NJ: Analytic Press.

Leshner, A. L. (1997). Addiction is a brain disease, and it matters. *Science, 278,* 45–47.

Levin, J. D. (1995). Psychotherapy in later stage recovery. In A. M. Washton (Ed.), *Psychotherapy and substance abuse: A practitioner's handbook* (pp. 264–284). New York: Guilford Press.

Little, J. (2002). Harm reduction group therapy. In A. Tatarsky (Ed.), *Harm reduction psychotherapy: A new treatment for alcohol and drug problems* (pp. 310–346). Northvale, NJ: Aronson.

Longabaugh, R. (2003). Involvement of support networks in treatment. *Recent Developments in Alcoholism, 16,* 133–147.

Longabaugh, R., Wirtz, P., Zweben, A., & Stout, R. L. (1998). Network support for drinking, Alcoholics Anonymous and long-term matching effects. *Addiction, 93*(9), 1313–1333.

Lowinson, J. H., Ruiz, P., Millman, R. B., & Langrod, J. G. (Eds.). (2005). *Substance abuse: A comprehensive textbook* (2nd ed.). Baltimore: Williams & Wilkins.

Margolis, R. B., & Zweben, J. E. (1998). *Treating patients with alcohol and other drug problems: An integrated approach.* Washington, DC: American Psychological Association.

Marlatt, G. A. (1985). Relapse prevention: A general overview. In G. A. Marlatt & J. R. Gordon (Eds.), *Relapse prevention: Maintenance strategies in the treatment of addictive behaviors* (pp. 3–16). New York: Guilford Press.

Marlatt, G. A., & Gordon, J. R. (Eds.). (1985). *Relapse prevention: Maintenance strategies in the treatment of addictive behaviors.* New York: Guilford Press.

Matrix Center. (1995). *The Matrix intensive outpatient program: Therapist manual.* Los Angeles: Author.

Matrix Center. (1997). *Matrix model of early intervention.* Los Angeles: Author.

Matrix Center. (1999a). *The Matrix introduction to recovery program.* Los Angeles: Author.

Matrix Center. (1999b). *The Matrix model of outpatient chemical dependency treatment: Family education guidelines and handouts.* Los Angeles: Author.

McKellar, J., Stewart, E., & Humphreys, K. (2003). Alcoholics Anonymous involvement and positive alcohol-related outcomes: Cause, consequence, or just a correlate? A prospective 2-year study of 2,319 alcohol-dependent men. *Journal of Consulting and Clinical Psychology, 71,* 302–308.

McLellan, A. T., Arndt, I. O., Metzger, D. S., Woody, G. E., & O'Brien, C. P. (1993). The effects of psychosocial services in substance abuse treatment. *Journal of the American Medical Association, 269,* 1953–1959.

McLellan, A. T., Grissom, G. R., Brill, P., Durell, J., Metzger, D. S., & O'Brien, C. P. (1993). Private substance abuse treatments: Are some programs more effective than others? *Journal of Substance Abuse Treatment, 10,* 243–254.

McLellan, A. T., Lewis, D. C., O'Brien, C. P., & Kleber, H. D. (2000). Drug dependence, a chronic medical illness: Implications for treatment, insurance, and outcomes evaluation. *Journal of the American Medical Association, 284*(13), 1689–1695.

McLellan, A. T., Woody, G. E., Luborsky, L., & Goehl, L. (1988). Is the counselor an "active ingredient" in substance abuse rehabilitation?: An examination of treatment success among four counselors. *Journal of Nervous and Mental Disease, 176,* 423–430.

McMillen, J. C. (1999). Better for it: How people benefit from adversity. *Social Work, 44,* 455–468.

McMillen, J. C., Howard, M. O., Nower, L., & Chung, S. (2001). Positive byproducts of the struggle with chemical dependency. *Journal of Substance Abuse Treatment, 20,* 69–79.

Mercer, E., & Woody, G. E. (1999). *An individual drug counseling approach to treat cocaine addiction: The collaborative cocaine treatment study manual* (NIH Publication No. 99-4380). Washington, DC: U.S. Government Printing Office.

Milkman, H., & Sunderwirth, S. (1987). *Craving for ecstacy: The consciousness and chemistry of escape.* Lexington, MA: Lexington Books.

Miller, N. S. (1991). *The pharmacology of alcohol and drugs of abuse and addiction.* New York: Springer-Verlag.

Miller, W. R. (1983). Motivational interviewing with problem drinkers. *Behavioral Psychotherapy, 11,* 147–172.

Miller, W. R. (1999). *Enhancing motivation for change in substance abuse treatment* (Vol. 35). Rockville, MD: U.S. Department of Health and Human Services.

Miller, W. R., & Brown, S. A. (1997). Why psychologists should treat alcohol and drug problems. *American Psychologist, 52,* 1267–1279.

Miller, W. R., & Muñoz, R. F. (2005). *Controlling your drinking: Tools to make moderation work for you.* New York: Guilford Press.

Miller, W. R., & Page, A. C. (1991). Warm turkey: Other routes to abstinence. *Journal of Substance Abuse Treatment, 8,* 227–232.

Miller, W. R., & Rollnick, S. (1991). *Motivational interviewing: Preparing people to change addictive behavior.* New York: Guilford Press.

Miller, W. R., & Rollnick, S. (2002). *Motivational interviewing (2nd ed.): Preparing people for change.* New York: Guilford Press.

Miller, W. R., Zweben, A., & Rychtarik, R. G. (1994). *Motivational enhancement therapy manual.* Rockville, MD: U.S. Department of Health and Human Services.

Minkoff, K., & Drake, R. E. (Eds.). (1991). *Dual diagnosis of major mental illness and substance disorder.* San Francisco: Jossey-Bass.

Minkoff, K., Zweben, J. E., Rosenthal, R., & Ries, R. K. (2003). Development of service intensity criteria and program categories for individuals with co-occurring disorders. In D. Gastfriend (Ed.), *Addiction treatment matching: Research foundations of the American Society of Addiction Medicine (ASAM) criteria.* New York: Haworth.

Mirin, S. A., & Weiss, R. D. (1991). Substance abuse and mental illness. In R. J. Frances & S. I. Miller (Eds.), *Clinical textbook of addictive disorders* (pp. 271–298). New York: Guilford Press.

Monti, P. M., Kadden, R. M., Rohsenow, D. J., Cooney, N. L., & Abrams, D. B. (2002). *Treating alcohol dependence: A coping skills training guide.* New York: Guilford Press.

Morgan, T. J. (2001). Behavioral treatment techniques. In F. Rotgers, D. S. Keller, & J. Morgenstern (Eds.), *Treating substance abuse: Theory and technique.* New York: Guilford Press.

Morganstern, J., Bux, D. A., Labouvie, E., Morgan, T., Blanchard, K. A., & Muench, F. (2003). Examining mechanisms of action in 12-step community outpatient treatment. *Drug and Alcohol Dependence, 72,* 237–247.

Morgenstern, J., Labouvie, E., McCrady, B. S., Kahler, C. W., & Frey, R. M. (1997). Affiliation with Alcoholics Anonymous after treatment: A study of its therapeutic effects and mechanisms of action. *Journal of Consulting and Clinical Psychology, 65,* 768–777.

Mueser, K. T., Noordsy, D. L., Drake, R. C., & Fox, L. (2003). *Integrated treatment for dual disorders: A guide to effecive practice.* New York: Guilford Press.

Murphy, S. L., & Khantzian, E. J. (1995). Addiction as a "self-medication" disorder: Application of ego psychology to the treatment of substance abuse. In A. M. Washton (Ed.), *Psychotherapy and substance abuse: A practitioner's handbook* (pp. 161–175). New York: Guilford Press.

Najavits, L. M. (2002). *Seeking safety: A treatment manual for PTSD and substance abuse.* New York: Guilford Press.

National Consensus Development Panel on Effective Medical Treatment of Opioid Addiction. (1998). Effective medical treatment of opioid addiction. *Journal of the American Medical Association, 280*(22), 1936–1943.

National Institute on Alcohol Abuse and Alcoholism. (2000). *10th special report to the U.S. Congress on alcohol and health*. Rockville, MD: U.S. Department of Health and Human Services.

National Institute on Drug Abuse. (1999). *Principles of addiction treatment: A research-based guide*. Rockville, MD: National Institutes of Health.

Obert, J. L., Rawson, R. A., & Miotto, K. (1997). Substance abuse treatment for "hazardous users": An early intervention. *Journal of Psychoactive Drugs, 29*(3), 291–298.

O'Malley, S., Jaffe, A. J., Chang, G., Shottenfeld, R., Meyer, R., & Rounsaville, B. (1992). Naltrexone and coping skills therapy for alcohol dependence. *Archives of General Psychiatry, 49,* 881–887.

Ouimette, P., & Brown, P. J. (2003). *Trauma and substance abuse: Causes, consequences, and treatment of comorbid disorders*. Washington, DC: American Psychological Association.

Ouimette, P. C., Moos, R., & Finney, J. W. (1998). Influence of outpatient treatment and 12-step group involvement on one-year substance use substance abuse treatment outcome. *Journal of Studies on Alcohol, 59,* 513–522.

Owen, P. L., Slaymaker, V., Tonigan, J. S., McCrady, B. S., Epstein, E. E., Kaskutas, L. A., et al. (2003). Participation in Alcoholics Anonymous: Intended and unintended change mechanisms. *Alcoholism, 27,* 524–532.

Payte, J. T., Zweben, J. E., & Martin, J. (2003). Opioid maintenance therapies. In A. W. Graham, T. K. Schultz, M. M. Smith, R. K. Ries, & B. W. Wilford (Eds.), *Principles of addiction medicine* (3rd ed.). Bethesda, MD: American Society of Addiction Medicine.

Peele, S., & Brodsky, A. (1991). *The truth about addiction and recovery*. New York: Simon & Schuster.

Pickens, R. W. (1997, November 17). *Genetic and other risk factors in opiate addiction*. Paper presented at the effective medical treatment of heroin addiction, William H. Natcher Conference Center, National Institutes of Health, Bethesda, MD.

Pickens, R. W., Preston, K. L., Miles, D. R., Gupman, A. E., Johnson, E. O., Newlin, D. B., et al. (2001). Family influence on drug abuse severity and treatment outcome. *Drug and Alcohol Dependence, 61,* 261–270.

Polcin, D. L., Prindle, S. D., & Bostrom, A. (2002). Integrating social model principles into broad-based treatment: Results of a program evaluation. *American Journal of Drug and Alcohol Abuse, 28*(4), 585–599.

Prochaska, J. O., & DiClemente, C. C. (1986). Toward a comprehensive model of change. In W. R. Miller & N. Heather (Eds.), *Treating addictive behaviors: Processes of change* (pp. 3–27). New York: Plenum Press.

Prochaska, J. O., DiClemente, C. C., & Norcross, J. C. (1992). In search of how people change: Applications to addictive behaviors. *American Psychologist, 47,* 1102–1114.

Project MATCH Research Group. (1997). Matching alcoholism treatments to client heterogeneity: Project MATCH post-treatment drinking outcomes. *Journal of Studies on Alcohol, 58,* 7–29.

Rawson, R. A. (1999). *Treatment for stimulant use disorders* (Vol. 33). Rockville, MD: U.S. Department of Health and Human Services.

Rawson, R. A., Obert, J. L., McCann, M., & Marinelli-Casey, P. (1993). Relapse prevention strategies in outpatient substance abuse treatment. *Psychology of Addictive Behaviors, 7,* 85–95.

Rawson, R. A., Obert, J. L., McCann, M. J., Smith, D. P., & Ling, W. (1990). Neurobehavioral treatment of cocaine dependency. *Journal of Psychoactive Drugs, 22,* 159–172.

Rawson, R. A., Obert, J. L., McCann, M. J., Smith, D. P., & Scheffy, E. H. (1989). *The neurobehavioral treatment manual: A therapist manual for outpatient cocaine addiction treatment.* Beverly Hills, CA: Matrix Center.

Rawson, R. A., Washton, A., Domier, C. P., & Reiber, C. (2002). Drugs and sexual effects: Role of drug type and gender. *Journal of Substance Abuse Treatment, 22,* 103–108.

Rawson, R. A., & Washton, A. M. (1998, April 18). *Stimulant abuse and compulsive sex.* Paper presented at the American Society of Addiction Medicine, New Orleans, LA.

Reilly, P. M., & Shropshire, M. S. (2002). *Anger management for substance abuse and mental health clients: A cognitive behavioral therapy manual.* Rockville, MD: U.S. Department of Health and Human Services.

Resnick, R. B., Schuyten-Resnick, E., & Washton, A. M. (1979). Narcotic antagonists in the treatment of opioid dependence: Review and commentary. *Comprehensive Psychiatry, 20,* 116–125.

Resnick, R. B., Schuyten-Resnick, E., & Washton, A. M. (1980). Assessment of narcotic antagonists in the treatment of opioid dependence. *Annual Review of Pharmacology and Toxicology, 20,* 463–474.

Resnick, R. B., & Washton, A. M. (1978). Clinical outcome with naltrexone. *Annals of the New York Academy of Sciences, 311,* 241–247.

Resnick, R. B., Washton, A. M., Thomas, M. A., & Kestenbaum, R. S. (1978). Naltrexone in the treatment of opiate dependence. *NIDA Research Monograph, 19,* 321–332.

Rettig, R. A., & Yarmolinsky, A. (1995). *Federal regulation of methadone treatment.* Washington, DC: National Academy Press.

Rogers, R. L., & McMillan, C. S. (1989). *Don't help: A positive guide to working with the alcoholic.* New York: Bantam.

Rotgers, F., Kern, M. F., & Hoeltzel, R. (2002). *Responsible drinking: A moderation management approach for problem drinkers.* Oakland, CA: New Harbinger.

Sanchez-Craig, M. (1993). *Drink wise: How to quit drinking or cut down.* Toronto: Addiction Research Foundation.

Schneider, J. P. (1988). *Back from betrayal: Recovering from his affairs.* Center City, MN: Hazelden.

Schuckit, M. A. (1989). Biomedical and genetic markers of alcoholism. In H. W. Goedde & D. P. Agarwal (Eds.), *Alcoholism: Biomedical and genetic aspects* (pp. 290–302). New York: Pergamon Press.

Schuckit, M. A. (1996). Recent developments in the pharmacotherapy of alcohol dependence. *Journal of Clinical and Consulting Psychology, 64,* 669–676.

Schuckit, M. A. (2000). *Drug and alcohol abuse: A clinical guide to diagnosis and treatment.* New York: Kluwer Academic/Plenum.

Schuckit, M. A., & Smith, T. L. (1996). An 8-year follow-up of 450 sons of alcoholic and control subjects. *Archives of General Psychiatry, 53*, 202–210.

Sees, K. L., Delucci, K. L., Masson, C., Rosen, A., Clark, H. W., Robillard, H., et al. (2000). Methadone maintenance vs. 180-day psychosocially enriched detoxification for treatment of opioid dependence. *Journal of the American Medical Association, 283*(10), 1303–1310.

Shaffer, H. J., & Gambino, B. (1990). Epilogue: Integrating treatment choices. In H. B. Milkman & L. Sederer (Eds.), *Treatment choices for alcoholism and substance abuse* (pp. 351–375). Lexington, MA: Lexington Books.

Siegel, R. K. (1989). *Intoxication: Life in pursuit of artificial paradise*. New York: Dutton.

Sobell, L. C., Ellingstad, T. P., & Sobell, M. B. (2000). Natural recovery from alcohol and drug problems: Methodological review of the research with suggestions for future directions. *Addiction, 95*, 749–764.

Sobell, M. B., & Sobell, L. C. (1993). *Problem drinkers: Guided self-change treatment*. New York: Guilford Press.

Staines, G., Magura, S., Rosenblum, A., Fong, C., Kosanke, N., Foote, J., et al. (2003). Predictors of drinking outcomes among alcoholics. *American Journal of Drug and Alcohol Abuse, 29*, 203–218.

Stanton, M. D., & Todd, T. C. (1982). *The family therapy of drug abuse and addiction*. New York: Guilford Press.

Stoffelmayr, B. E., Mavis, B. E., Sherry, L. A., & Chiu, C. W. (1999). The influence of recovery status and education on addiction counselors' approach to treatment. *Journal of Psychoactive Drugs, 31*, 121–127.

Substance Abuse and Mental Health Services Administration. (2003). *The DAWN Report: Narcotic analgesics*. Rockville, MD: Office of Applied Studies, Substance Abuse and Mental Health Services Administration.

Sullivan, J. M., & Evans, K. (1994). Integrated treatment for the survivor of childhood trauma who is chemically dependent. *Journal of Psychoactive Drugs, 26*, 369–378.

Tatarsky, A. (Ed.). (2002). *Harm reduction psychotherapy: A new treatment for alcohol and drug problems*. Northvale, NJ: Aronson.

Taylor, E. (Ed.). (1988). *Dorland's medical dictionary*. Philadelphia: Sanders.

Tonigan, J. S., Toscove, R., & Miller, W. R. (1996). Meta-analysis of the literature on Alcoholics Anonymous: Sample and study characteristics moderate findings. *Journal of Studies on Alcohol, 57*, 65–72.

Tsuang, M. T., Lyons, M. J., Meyer, J. M., Doyle, T., Eisen, S. A., Goldberg, J., et al. (1998). Co-occurrence of abuse of different drugs in men. *Archives of General Psychiatry, 55*, 967–972.

Tucker, J. A., Vuchinich, R. E., & Rippens, P. D. (2004). Different variables are associated with help-seeking patterns and long-term outcomes among problem drinkers. *Addictive Behavior, 29*, 433–439.

Vaillant, G. E. (1995). *The natural history of alcoholism revisited*. Cambridge, MA: Harvard University Press.

Vannicelli, M. (1992). *Removing the roadblocks: Group psychotherapy with substance abusers and family members*. New York: Guilford Press.

Vanyukov, M. M., & Tarter, R. E. (2000). Genetic studies of substance abuse. *Drug and Alcohol Dependence, 59*, 101–123.

Velasquez, M. M., Maurer, G. G., Crouch, C., DiClemente, C. C. (2001). *Group treatment for substance abuse: A stages-of-change therapy manual*. New York: Guilford Press.

Verebey, K. (Ed.). (1982). *Opioids in mental illness: Theories, clinical observations, and treatment possibilities* (Vol. 398). New York: New York Academy of Sciences.

Volkow, N. D., Chang, L., Wang, G. J., Fowler, J. S., Franceschi, D., Sedler, M., et al. (2001). Loss of dopamine transporters in methamphetamine abusers recovers with protracted abstinence. *Journal of Neuroscience, 21*, 9414–9418.

Volpicelli, J. R., Altterman, A. I., Hayashida, M., & O'Brien, C. P. (1992). Naltrexone in the treatment of alcohol dependence. *Archives of General Psychiatry, 49*, 876–880.

Washton, A. (2001). Group therapy: A clinician's guide to doing what works. In R. H. Coombs (Ed.), *Addiction recovery tools* (pp. 239–256). Thousand Oaks, CA: Sage.

Washton, A. (2002). Outpatient groups at different stages of substance abuse treatment: Preparation, initial abstinence, and relapse prevention. In D. W. Brook & H. I. Spitz (Eds.), *The group psychotherapy of substance abuse* (pp. 99–119). Binghamton, NY: Haworth Medical Press.

Washton, A. M. (1988). Preventing relapse to cocaine. *Journal of Clinical Psychiatry, 49*, 34–38.

Washton, A. M. (1989). *Cocaine addiction: Treatment, recovery, and relapse prevention*. New York: Norton.

Washton, A. M. (1990a). *Quitting cocaine*. Center City, MN: Hazelden.

Washton, A. M. (1990b). *Staying off cocaine*. Center City, MN: Hazelden.

Washton, A. M. (1990c). *Maintaining recovery*. Center City, MN: Hazelden.

Washton, A. M. (Ed.). (1995). *Psychotherapy and substance abuse: A practitioner's handbook*. New York: Guilford Press.

Washton, A. M., & Boundy, D. (1989). *Willpower's not enough: Recovering from addictions of every kind*. New York: HarperCollins.

Washton, A. M., Gold, M. S., & Pottash, A. C. (1984a). Naltrexone in addicted physicians and business executives. *NIDA Research Monograph, 55*, 185–190.

Washton, A. M., Gold, M. S., & Pottash, A. C. (1984b). Successful use of naltrexone in addicted physicians and business executives. *Advances in Alcohol and Substance Abuse, 4*(2), 89–96.

Washton, A. M., Gold, M. S., & Pottash, A. C. (1985). Opiate and cocaine dependencies: Techniques to help counter the rising tide. *Postgraduate Medicine, 77*, 293–297, 300.

Washton, A. M., & Stone-Washton, N. (1990). Abstinence and relapse in outpatient cocaine addicts. *Journal of Psychoactive Drugs, 22*, 135–147.

Washton, A. M., & Washton, L. J. (2002). *Finding silver linings in the clouds: Addiction as a catalyst for positive life changes*. Paper presented at the Annual Medical–Scientific Conference of the American Society of Addiction Medicine, Atlanta, GA.

Yalisove, D. (2004). *Introduction to alcohol research: Implications for treatment, prevention, and policy*. Boston: Pearson/Allyn & Bacon.

Yalom, I. D. (1995). *The theory and practice of group psychotherapy* (4th ed.). New York: Basic Books.

Young, E. B. (1995). The role of incest issues in relapse and recovery. In A. M. Washton (Ed.), *Psychotherapy and substance abuse: A practitioner's handbook* (pp. 451–469). New York: Guilford Press.

Zackon, F., McAuliffe, W. E., & Ch'ien, J. M. N. (1993). *Recovery training and self-help: Relapse prevention and aftercare for drug addicts* (NIH Publication No. 93-3521). Rockville, MD: National Institute on Drug Abuse.

Zweben, J. E. (1989). Recovery oriented psychotherapy: Patient resistances and therapist dilemmas. *Journal of Substance Abuse Treatment, 6,* 123–132.

Zweben, J. E. (2002). Special issues in treatment: Women. In A. W. Graham, T. K. Scultz, M. May-Smith, R. K. Ries, & B. B. Wilford (Eds.), *Principles of addiction medicine* (3rd ed., pp. 171–182). Chevy Chase, MD: American Society of Addiction Medicine.

Zweben, J. E., & Clark, H. W. (1991). Unrecognized substance misuse: Clinical hazards and legal vulnerabilities. *International Journal of the Addictions, 25,* 1431–1451.

Index

t indicates table

Abstinence
  cessation techniques, 186–187
  concurrent disorders and, 92–93, 94,
    95–97, 102
  cravings and, 199
  developing a support system, 194–
    195
  disease model and, 34–35, 84
  drug dreams and, 203–204
  establishing structure and external
    controls, 193–194
  goals and, 73, 163–170, 187–188
  later-stage recovery and, 232–234
  maintenance stage of change and, 78,
    79
  polysubstance use and, 200–201,
    218–219
  slips and, 211–212
  treatment and, 35–36, 106, 113,
    188, 247–248
  trial period of, 185
Abstinence violation effect, 216–217.
    See also Relapse; Slips
Abuse, substance, 26, 36–39, 48, 148–
    149
Acamprosate, 106. *See also*
    Pharmacotherapy

Action stage of change. *See also*
    Stages-of-change model
  group therapy and, 249
  in the integrated approach, 75
  overview, 77–78
  presenting and explaining the
    diagnosis to the patient and, 153
  treatment planning and, 172*t*, 178–
    179
Action strategies. *See also* Interventions
  cessation techniques, 186–187
  concurrent disorders and, 204–205
  dealing with triggers, cravings and
    urges, 195–198, 198–200
  developing a support system, 194–
    195
  drug dreams and, 203–204
  establishing structure and external
    controls, 193–194
  frequency of sessions and, 188
  managing withdrawal, 192–193
  moderation and harm reduction
    techniques, 185–186
  overview, 184, 205
  polysubstance use, 200–201
  post-acute withdrawal syndrome
    and, 202